Rae L. Schnuth, PhD
MSU Dept. OB-GYN
1200 E Michigan Avenue, Suite 730
Lansing, MI 48912
PH   517.364.5940

INDICATORS OF
CHRONIC HEALTH CONDITIONS

INDICATORS OF CHRONIC HEALTH CONDITIONS

Monitoring Community-Level Delivery Systems

Edited by

Robert J. Newcomer
A. E. Benjamin

THE JOHNS HOPKINS UNIVERSITY PRESS
Baltimore & London

© 1997 The Johns Hopkins University Press
All rights reserved. Published 1997
Printed in the United States of America on acid-free paper
06 05 04 03 02 01 00 99 98 97   5 4 3 2 1

The Johns Hopkins University Press
2715 North Charles Street
Baltimore, Maryland 21218–4319
The Johns Hopkins Press Ltd., London

A catalog record for this book is available from the British Library.

Library of Congress Cataloging-in-Publication Data

Indicators of chronic health conditions : monitoring community-level
delivery systems / edited by Robert J. Newcomer and A. E. Benjamin.
      p.   cm.
   Includes index.
   ISBN 0-8018-5491-1 (alk. paper). — ISBN 0-8018-5494-6 (pbk. :
alk. paper)
   1. Chronic diseases—United States—Epidemiology—Statistical
methods. 2. Health status indicators—United States. 3. Community
health services—United States—Evaluation. 4. Chronically ill—
Medical care—United States. 5. Medical care—Needs assessment—
United States. 6. Public health surveillance—United States.
I. Newcomer, Robert J.   II. Benjamin, A. E.
RA644.6.I53   1997
362.1'2'0973—dc20   96-42207
                                                        CIP

CONTENTS

v

PREFACE

Several attempts have been made over the past twenty years to develop data systems that generalize to the city, county, or substate level. For simplicity, these are often grouped under the term "community." The most ambitious of these include the Cooperative Health Statistics System (CHSS), the National Health Planning and Resources Development Act, and the establishment of hospital discharge databases. These efforts have left a legacy of experience and an infrastructure upon which any current efforts can build. The CHSS, for example, was initiated in 1969 by the National Center for Health Statistics (NCHS) with the idea of producing uniform definitions and standards so that data related to health status, health work force, and services could be compared among states and local areas. Federal funding for this program was phased out during the early 1980s, but all states have continued to support their State Centers for Health Statistics, which were first implemented under this initiative. At a minimum, these centers collect and analyze vital statistics within the state. Some centers have broader information and policy development roles. The NCHS, as it did from the outset, provides newsletters and technical assistance to these centers.

The National Health Planning and Resources Development Act of 1975 authorized a national network of health systems agencies (HSAs) and required states to designate a state health planning and development agency. The HSAs were responsible for community-level health service planning, regulation of medical facility development, and the use of new technology within these catchment areas. When federal support for HSAs ended in 1986, many information-collection and planning roles were transferred to state health planning agencies. These agencies continue to compile data on hospital, nursing home, and related health care service supply and utilization patterns.

Twenty-eight states currently maintain hospital discharge databases, which collect patient-level data across all payers, and which have been used since 1970 to produce state and national estimates of diagnoses and treatment patterns. The National Association of Health Data Organizations (NAHDO) was established in 1986, in part, to help standardize hospital discharge data collection methods. These efforts continue, but they have not yet been expanded to outpatient care.

While the preceding suggests some optimism about community-level experience and data systems, it is also about abandoned or scaled-back data infrastructure. In formulating our indicator recommendations, we have tried to be sensitive to factors that affect the use and perpetuation of data systems. Key among these are cost, an identifiable client for the information, and a focus on information that is actionable. Where appropriate, we have tried to parallel the indicator models developed by such organizations as the Institute of Medicine, the U.S. Public Health Service, and the National Committee on Quality Assurance (NCQA). In many circumstances, our proposed phased or staged indicator model for chronic conditions could perhaps readily supplement these other systems—particularly that of NCQA. Unlike these other efforts, our proposals have not gone through extensive consensus development. This remains to be done, as does the empirical testing of the political and programmatic utility of the proposed indicators.

In addition to other community-level data systems, a number of books have been important to us because of their insights into the problems of, and approaches to, the measurement and monitoring of social policy and program effects using indicators and other data systems. Among these books are M. Millman, ed., *Access to Health Care in America* (Washington, D.C.: National Academy Press, 1993); S. M. Teutsch & R. E. Churchill, eds., *Principles and Practice of Public Health Surveillance* (New York: Oxford University Press, 1994); Institute of Medicine, *The Future of Public Health* (Washington, D.C.: National Academy Press, 1988); D. Patrick & P. Erickson, *Health Status and Health Policy—Allocating Resources to Health Care* (New York: Oxford University Press, 1993); and J. Innes de Neufville, *Social Indicators and Public Policy* (New York:, Elsevier Scientific Publishing Company, 1975).

How does our book differ from these others? None of the recent publications addresses the central issues of our book: the conceptualization and development of community-oriented indicators that link and monitor health and other delivery systems for persons with chronic conditions. Most of these other materials discuss either refinements within national indicator systems or the need to reorganize and strengthen the responsibilities of state- and local-level public health and other delivery systems.

In short, this literature suggests a renewed interest in indicator systems and begins staging and operationalizing issues.

Our book explores the practicality of community-level health and delivery system indicators for persons with chronic illness by focusing on seven subpopulations: children, persons with developmental disabilities, individuals with severe mental illness, adults with physical disability, adults with chronic degenerative illness, chronic alcohol and drug abusers, and the aged. These provide an in-depth illustration of the complexity of chronic health conditions, the likely service needs over time of those with these conditions, and the health and social service delivery systems that potentially respond to these "service careers." Data systems and measures that are in place, or that could be modified, to track and monitor need and delivery responsiveness are also discussed. The conclusions emerging from these background chapters are placed into a historical context by an extensive review of indicator systems and the major governmental programs and initiatives in place. This is done to highlight the factors that have been necessary in the past to effect and maintain indicator systems. The concluding chapter integrates the common themes and dimensions from the subpopulation chapters and proposes a framework for conceptually organizing indicators into domains and for staging the compilation of measures.

This book bridges the professional fields of public health, city planning, and social welfare, as well as a number of categorical populations and the professions that serve them. Graduate programs in these respective areas form one primary target audience. Most such programs offer coursework on service need estimation, program planning, and program evaluation. Additionally, public health, nursing, and health administration courses concerned with quality assurance and continuous quality improvement would likely find this material of use. Professionals and policymakers involved in health and social service planning and delivery are another major target audience. This includes individuals working within government (including congressional and state legislative staff), health plans, health insurance companies, and advocacy organizations.

ACKNOWLEDGMENTS

The preparation of this book was funded by the Robert Wood Johnson Foundation under grant number PC-292/UCSF. This funding enabled us to assemble a distinguished group of experts who authored the eight major chapters of this book and a second group who served as an advisory committee to the project. We are extremely grateful to the background paper authors for the thoroughness with which they approached their papers and the thoughtfulness of their writing.

The advisory committee complemented the perspective of the authors with their own extensive expertise. The committee met with the authors during the formulation of the chapter outlines and after reviewing the initial drafts. The eight members of the national advisory committee are Susan Allen, Ph.D., Associate Professor of Medical Science, Department of Community Medicine, Brown University; Andrew Bindman, M.D., Assistant Professor, Departments of Medicine and Epidemiology and Biostatistics, University of California, San Francisco; Mary Anne Freedman, Ph.D., Special Assistant to the Director, National Center for Health Statistics; Ira Kaufman, Ph.D., Associate Clinical Professor of Medicine, University of Medicine and Dentistry, Robert Wood Johnson Medical School; David McQueen, Sc.D., Chief, Behavioral Surveillance Branch, Centers for Disease Control & Prevention; Dorothy Rice, Sc.D. (Hon), Professor Emeritus (in Residence), Institute for Health & Aging and Department of Social and Behavioral Sciences, University of California, San Francisco; Thomas Rundall, Dr.P.H., Professor, Social and Administrative Health Sciences, School of Public Health, University of California, Berkeley; and Zili Sloboda, Sc.D., Director, Division of Epidemiology and Prevention Research, National Institute of Drug Abuse.

We are also grateful to Dianne Barker, M.P.H., Project Officer, and James Knickman, Ph.D., Vice President for Research of the RWJ Foundation, for their assistance in recruiting individuals to this project and their general support throughout its implementation.

Finally, we would like to acknowledge the contributions of our University of California colleagues Dorothy Rice, Sc.D., and Catherine Hoffman, Sc.D., whose preparation of a *Chronic Care Chartbook* for this project enriched our thinking and provided useful analyses on current trends; Shay Starkey, M.S.W., who was a tireless research librarian both for us and for Dr. Hoffman; and Barbara Paschke, M.Ed., whose editorial competence and easy-going professional manner greatly enriched the clarity of this manuscript.

CONTRIBUTORS

A. E. Benjamin, Ph.D., Professor, Department of Social Welfare, School of Public Policy and Social Research, University of California, Los Angeles, California

Lindsey A. Criswell, M.D., M.P.H., Assistant Professor, Department of Medicine, University of California, San Francisco, California

Catherine Hoffman, Sc.D., Senior Policy Analyst, Henry J. Kaiser Family Foundation, Menlo Park, California

Judith Kasper, Ph.D., Associate Professor, Department of Health Policy and Management, School of Hygiene and Public Health, The Johns Hopkins University, Baltimore, Maryland

Bryan J. Kemp, Ph.D., Associate Clinical Professor, Departments of Family Practice and Psychiatry and Behavioral Science, and Associate Research Professor of Gerontology, University of Southern California, Los Angeles, California

K. Charlie Lakin, Ph.D., Director, Research and Training Center on Community Living, Institute on Community Integration, University of Minnesota, Minneapolis, Minnesota

Anthony Lehman, M.D., Professor, Department of Psychiatry, School of Medicine, University of Maryland, Baltimore, Maryland

Jay S. Luxenberg, M.D., Associate Clinical Professor of Medicine, Institute on Aging, University of California, San Francisco, California

Robert J. Newcomer, Ph.D., Professor and Chair, Department of Social and Behavioral Sciences, University of California, San Francisco, California

James Perrin, M.D., Associate Professor, Department of Pediatrics, Harvard Medical School, Boston, Massachusetts

Donald M. Steinwachs, Ph.D., Professor and Chair, Department of Health Policy and Management, School of Hygiene and Public Health, The Johns Hopkins University, Baltimore, Maryland

Carol L. Such, Ph.D., Senior Public Administration Analyst, Arthritis Research Group, University of California, San Francisco, California

Constance Weisner, Ph.D., Associate Adjunct Professor, School of Public Health, University of California, Berkeley, California

Edward H. Yelin, Ph.D., Adjunct Professor of Medicine and Health Policy, Arthritis Research Group, University of California, San Francisco, California

1/ COMMUNITY-LEVEL INDICATORS OF CHRONIC HEALTH CONDITIONS

A. E. Benjamin and Robert J. Newcomer

Together, chronic health conditions and disabilities are the largest public health problem affecting the U.S. population. About 45 percent of those not living in institutions—88.5 million people—have one or more chronic conditions (Hoffman & Rice, 1995). In addition, another 1.5 million adults residing in nursing homes or personal care homes are disabled as a result of chronic conditions (Lair & Lefkowitz, 1990). According to recent prevalence estimates, the number of persons with functional limitations and disabilities measured by activity limitation due to chronic conditions is 39.3 million, or 15.5 percent of the noninstitutionalized civilian population (Benson & Marano, 1994). Of these, 8.1 million working-age adults were unable to work because of their disability.

The economic costs attributable to chronic conditions are equally staggering. In 1990, total health care costs resulting from chronic conditions—including both direct and indirect costs—were estimated at $650 billion (Hoffman & Rice, 1995). The direct costs of care were $425 billion. Hospitals ($167 billion) and nursing homes (just over $50 billion) account for the largest share of these costs. All told, more than 75 percent of personal health care expenditures are incurred by those with chronic conditions. These direct service cost estimates are conservative, because they do not include social, educational, and other community services commonly used by persons with disabilities.

When human resources are lost because a person with a chronic condition is temporarily or permanently unable to work or dies prematurely, society's potential productivity is decreased: these are indirect costs. In 1990, indirect costs added approximately $234 billion to the direct medical care costs incurred by those with chronic conditions: $161 billion

1

from premature death and $73 billion from people's inability to work or perform their usual activities (Hoffman, Rice, & Sung, 1996).

Although older persons constitute the majority of the population with serious chronic-care needs and the risk of disability increases with age and reaches its apex among the very old, chronic conditions are not the exclusive province of older persons. Roughly 40 percent of people requiring chronic-care services are under age sixty-five (LaPlante, 1992), and the disproportionately high use of services for those with chronic conditions holds for all age groups. For example, nearly 25 percent of children have a chronic condition, and this subgroup uses almost half of all children's medical care dollars. Among the elderly, where chronic conditions affect 88 percent of the population, those with chronic conditions account for 96 percent of total direct medical care dollars.

The importance of chronic conditions to the health of society and to health care cost has been recognized as a national concern since at least the mid-1940s (Commission on Chronic Illness, 1957). For example, the first National Health Survey (and all subsequent ones) was conducted in part to determine the extent of chronic health problems. Moreover, as early as 1977, the Centers for Disease Control began to redefine its role to include an emphasis on primary prevention of chronic disease and personal injury. Paralleling these concerns has been a continuing refinement in the measurement of health through surveys and administrative records, and several efforts at service-appropriateness monitoring.

In addition to current expenditures, a number of developments have focused attention on those with chronic conditions. First of all, the number of younger persons living with disabilities has continued to grow as medical science has increased the prospects for survival of persons disabled by birth defects, disease, or injury. Second, the deinstitutionalization movement has had an impact well beyond its effects on the elderly in nursing homes, shifting many nonelderly persons with disabilities into the community and increasing the visibility of the care needs of various people who were once confined to institutional settings. The effective politicization of disability and chronic disease by advocacy groups and lobbies is a third factor. One example of their success is passage of the Americans with Disabilities Act. Following that success, these coalitions have turned to other issues, such as expanded services to people with disabilities in the home and community, which has helped redefine the cast and content of the chronic-care debate. A fourth factor heightening the political visibility of chronic conditions is the experience of more than a decade of budget crises at the federal and state levels. Many advocates as well as professionals have been sobered by the competition among groups with similar needs, each struggling for a share of a shrinking budget pie. Reducing service fragmentation and inefficiency within delivery systems, as well as ensuring equity in service access, has become important to all.

A variety of approaches to financing and organizing care for the chronically ill and the general population has been formulated over the years. These approaches, arrayed along a continuum of complexity, include tightened benefit eligibility, case management review and authorization of benefits to ensure more appropriate service targeting, consolidation of programs, enrollment of beneficiaries into "managed care" systems, establishment and enforcement of treatment and rehabilitation protocols for selected health conditions, and efforts to identify and moderate behaviors and conditions that increase the risk of disability or chronic disease. These approaches are being used with varying focus and intensity and in varying combinations by insurance companies, health plans, and state and local governments across the country.

MONITORING PREVALENCE AND SYSTEM PERFORMANCE

The recent and rapid changes in health care financing (including those involving managed care systems) and the recognized need to expand the monitoring of prevalence and service delivery performance for chronic conditions are taxing the capability of the "public health" system to conduct such needed functions as ongoing health condition assessment, policy development, and assurance of adequate care.[1] For purposes of this discussion, we broadly define the public health system to include the official governmental apparatus of public health (e.g., state and local health departments), governmental agencies responsible for the financing of care (e.g., Medicare and Medicaid), and those responsible for ensuring quality of care from private insurance and health plans. Included under the concept of assessment are such activities as disease surveillance, identifying service needs, analyzing the causes of problems, monitoring and forecasting trends, and evaluating delivery outcomes.

The assurance of adequate care implies that necessary services are provided and that avoidable causes of problems are minimized. The role of assurance does not inherently require that all services be provided by the public sector or through governmental financing, although government is often the provider of last resort in the U.S. health and human service system. We are concerned with those functions of assurance that help society reach agreed-upon goals and that encourage responsiveness to these goals. Encouragement can take many forms, including regulatory requirements of particular private sector providers, reimbursement for care, and facilitation of communication between providers, financing entities, and beneficiaries. Strategies for the appropriate distribution of responsibility and authority between federal, state, and local government or for delineation of the role of government versus that of the private sector have yet to coalesce into a clear or unitary direction. There does seem to be consensus about the importance of understanding whether given systems and policies are meeting the intended needs. Disagreements remain, however, over which conditions to measure, the viability of state- and community-level monitoring systems, the form of public oversight into the "private" health sector's performance, and the allocation of responsibility for data monitoring.

Established data systems exist to provide the basis for prevalence estimates and general trends in health care use. These include births, deaths, causes of death, disease registries, surveillance surveys, and various periodic surveys (such as those undertaken by the National Center for Health Statistics); also included would be such measures as crime and employer roles in social services. Most commonly, survey data provide national or regional estimates. Other data systems often provide state- or community-level measures, but they do not necessarily aggregate into national estimates.

Special studies and demonstration evaluations are also common and are usually targeted to specific interventions. Their fundamental purpose is to expand basic knowledge, rather than to provide systematic and ongoing systems performance measurement. A third type of data source is administrative records, such as those created by hospital discharge abstracts and Medicare service claims. Administrative data are employed to track utilization rates, practice patterns, and health outcomes at both national and community levels. Further refinement in the use of administrative records has come from efforts to monitor the appropriateness of care by individual providers or health plans. While most of these data systems and studies are limited to public expenditures, there are exceptions, such as the hospital discharge database and the recent private sector initiative to develop health plan "report cards" and to implement total quality management (TQM).

Momentum is building for more systematic collection and use of community-level health and social service information. Among the factors influencing this are community variations in practice, the potential cost shifting between levels of care and the payers of this care, the desire to reduce public and private expenditures, and a recognition that state governments, under their constitutional role and the decentralization of federal programs (begun in the 1970s and likely to continue), have accumulated many responsibilities for the design and management of the "local" delivery system. Examples of emerging systems are the community-level indicators being formulated in response to the U.S. Public Health Service Healthy People 2000 program, Health Plan Employer Data and Information Set (HEDIS) health plan "report cards" from the National Committee on Quality Assurance (NCQA), and the quality assurance tracking systems within Medicare. The constituency for such data include accreditation bodies and regulators (e.g., the Joint Commission on Accreditation of Health Care Organizations, state health departments, and peer review organizations [PROs]), payers (such as health plans, insurance companies, Medicare, and Medicaid), and professional organizations.

The objective of this book is to explore the practicality of community-level indicators of chronic conditions and the community systems that serve this population. We are trying to determine whether a meaningful framework that is common to multiple conditions and populations can be formulated and to identify the data available or needed for its implementation. The starting point for our emphasis on chronic conditions has already been outlined. The emphasis on the community level is equally basic: since services are delivered locally, it may be appropriate to have mechanisms to monitor the performance of local- or community-level delivery systems and the conditions that affect the encounters between clients and the delivery system.

The adoption of indicators and the refinement of data systems require enormous resources (including time) to establish consensus about the measures and to come to agreement on their operational and policy meaning. Quite reasonably, the indicators proposed by recent efforts (such as those noted above) and by the Institute of Medicine (IOM) (Millman, 1993) are constrained by existing data sources and the assumptions that connect indicators of treatment access with outcomes. We endorse this practicality in areas where there is agreement on basic principles, such as the relevant delivery system elements, and where there is a reasonable research basis for the assumed connection of service elements to outcomes. However, as shown by the service-use histories discussed in the following chapters, quality of care and service responsiveness for those with chronic conditions are more appropriately measured by considering multiple delivery systems (e.g., social, educational, and other service systems), rather than just those of the health sector. In other words, obtaining agreement on the delivery system components is a first step in community and chronic condition indicator development. The conceptualization of the care system has ramifications as to data sources, geographic and other aggregations for the indicators, and even the organizations that may be responsible for data management and decision making.

Another major problem affecting indicator development is the conceptual and clinical complexity of defining salient conditions and of tracing these conditions to disability or other risks and health outcomes. This complexity is heightened with chronic conditions, because multiple dimensions of health status are often statistically associated with one another. For example, depressive symptom levels, number of chronic illnesses, number of physician office visits, absence of an exercise program, higher alcohol consumption, and more physical dependencies are often found to be associated. Such intercorrelation compounds the task of assessing causal pathways or creating analytical models that can disaggregate these multiple associations. Another implication is that measurement—whether from diagnoses, standardized assessment, procedure coding, death certificates, or other sources—will likely have a high degree of error. It will not always be possible to distinguish "program" effects from changes in rates that are caused by "improved" reporting. The fact that multiple conditions often use similar services adds to these complications.

Most existing indicators, including those in national surveys, have little direct connection between cause and effect. The IOM, in its landmark report *Access to Health Care in America* (Millman, 1993), and HEDIS illustrate similar perspectives on how to respond to this information problem. Both organizations have selected broad, but nevertheless informative, measures to reflect various aspects of delivery system accessibility and outcome. For example, the percentage of pregnant women obtaining adequate care is represented by physician utilization rates, which in turn are considered jointly with such outcomes as infant birthweight and mortality. Preventable childhood diseases are reflected in immunization rates and the incidence of communicable diseases. Early detection and diagnosis of treatable diseases are measured by such procedures as breast and cervical cancer screening and the incidence of late-stage cancers. The IOM indicators are largely based on existing national data systems and yield national performance estimates. The HEDIS system at this point is experimental and built on information generated by health plans. It is generally intended to provide a "report card," by which one health plan can be compared with another. Both the IOM and HEDIS approaches reflect a substantial effort at consensus on the measures and what they reflect.

DEFINING THE SUBPOPULATIONS OF INTEREST

Because consideration of the populations living with chronic conditions is generally organized by categorical sources of funding or with a focus on specific subpopulations, there is no consensual framework in the literature for connecting these diverse groups. For purposes of diversity in our case examples, we have defined the following seven subsets of elderly and nonelderly populations, each with varying forms of chronic conditions and the ensuing prevalence of disability.

- *Children with chronic illness.* About 2 percent of children have severe functional limitations that require sustained, supportive care. Known as "children with special health needs," this population has grown as medical technology has made it possible to save children who only a decade or two ago would have died at or soon after birth.
- *Adults with developmental disabilities.* From 2 to 3 percent of the U.S. population are identified as having mental retardation or developmental disability during their preadult years, and a much smaller number (perhaps 0.5 percent) are considered moderately to profoundly retarded into adulthood and in need of supportive care.
- *Adults with physical disabilities.* Medical science has greatly improved the likelihood that adults with physical disabilities caused by disease and injury will survive and, with required support, lead productive lives into old age. Visual impairment and mobility impairment are among the chronic conditions included under the rubric of "adults with physical disabilities."
- *Adults with chronic illness.* This classification includes persons with illnesses such as rheumatoid arthritis, diabetes, hypertension, or HIV, with the focus being the subset of conditions for which there is a prominent role of medical care. Because the epidemiology

of disability and ancillary resource use is quite different for children than for adults, we limit this category to persons aged eighteen and older. Also, as patterns of disability and resource use vary between physical and mental conditions, we have confined adults with chronic illness to those affected by physical health conditions.

- *Adults with chronic mental illness.* Included in this classification is an estimated 1 percent of the adult population who suffer recurrent episodes of mental illness, most notably schizophrenia. This population requires a blend of clinical, rehabilitative, and supportive services to address what can be severe limitations in functioning.

- *Chronic substance abusers.* We are now aware of a (still inadequately defined) number of long-term abusers of alcohol and drugs whose needs for supportive services overlap substantially with those of more traditional recipients of chronic-care services. While relatively little is known about these "chronic alcohol and drug abusers," a small percentage of alcohol and drug users apparently is not amenable to current treatment interventions and requires tailored version(s) of chronic care.

- *Aged.* Finally, we consider the elderly population, looking primarily at highly prevalent conditions that have either a risk for secondary complications or avoidable acute care use, or that produce severe functional limitations.

DEFINING COMMUNITY AND COMMUNITY SYSTEMS

Need, delivery system responsiveness, and operational effectiveness vary among the many "market areas" comprising the U.S. health and human service systems. This variation was documented in the work of the health systems agencies of the 1970s and by the more recent small area analyses of medical and surgical service use (e.g., Chassin et al., 1986), hospital admission rates and mortality (e.g., Wennberg, Freeman, & Clup, 1987), length of stay; and such specific problems as admissions for respiratory distress (e.g., Richardson et al., 1991). Similarly, within social services there are wide variations between states and communities in such areas as per capita spending on education and community-based care (DuNah et al., 1993; Harrington, DuNah, & Bedney, 1993; Miller, 1992; Swan & Benjamin, 1990, 1993).

Service supply and delivery variation are thought to be caused (at least in part) by the mix of public and private providers and benefit structures, the diversity of populations and their differential service needs, and the competition for resources inherent in the financing and delivery of care. Large discrepancies in the rates at which various activities have been performed, without apparent adverse consequences, have been acknowledged by an audience of policymakers eager to identify inappropriate or ineffective care. The policy concern has mainly involved cost reduction, but it has also been an important stimulus to a refinement of quality assurance efforts by organized medicine, insurance companies, regulators, PROs, and the U.S. Congress (e.g., Leape, 1990).

To understand community service systems as we discuss them throughout the book, it may be useful to clarify a few basic terms. We have broadly defined "community" to include both the public and private (including the voluntary) sectors, since both are significant sources of financing and service provision for persons with chronic conditions. Similarly, we have broadly defined "service systems" to include acute health care, rehabilitation, prevention, institutional long-term care, and community-based social services or supportive care.

Regardless of the type of chronic condition, many service needs are common. Among these are primary care, assistance with activities of daily living (e.g., bathing, dressing, eating, toileting, transferring), and assistance with instrumental activities of daily living (e.g., housekeeping, meal preparation, medication use, shopping, transportation).

This use of the same or similar service providers suggests, at least at some level of abstraction, that there is a single service system affecting and affected by a community's population. Within such a closed system, the populations in need of care compete in their demand for access, financing, and even labor. The more communities are constrained by limited resources, the more obvious is the "single system-ness."

There are, of course, risks in oversimplification. If the conceptualization of the service system is too general, it may be inadequately sensitive to specific conditions, illnesses, and populations. On the other hand, if it too specifically reflects the experience of familiar populations, such as the elderly and people with physical disabilities, it will again fall short of addressing the full range of needs of other groups with chronic health conditions. We have tried for balance in these concerns and have approached the commonality of service system definitions and performance as a question rather than as an assumption in this work.

Leaving open the issue of whether there is a single service system or subsystems for each constituent group, it is nevertheless helpful to have a framework that helps conceptualize and identify potential elements in a delivery system. We have chosen a market framework for this purpose (e.g., Paringer, 1985). A market framework distinguishes factors that determine the "demand" for a particular service and the "supply" of services provided within the price structure of this demand. This perspective, considered in the context of a balance between demand and supply or conditions where demand exceeds supply (or supply exceeds demand), helps to explicate the market (or community-level) factors that may affect who receives services, what needs are addressed, and what levels of care are provided. For example, when excess demand is present and providers are financially motivated to prefer private patients to public beneficiaries, state or federal policies that alter the demand for a service by public program eligibles (e.g., by increasing accessibility through broadened eligibility standards) are likely to have little or no impact on use. Increasing the number of people eligible for a particular program (or the types of services for which they might be eligible) without also increasing the supply of providers results in either lengthened queues for service or other forms of rationing or service targeting. Overall use will not change. In contrast, when use falls short of demand, policies that expand supply—such as increased reimbursement rates or a lowering of licensing standards—may increase use.

In short, we define the performance of community service systems in terms of "responsiveness" and "effectiveness" and recognize that these comparisons are most effectively made in the context of local balances between service supply and demand. Without this additional control, an indicator system may produce misleading results in describing the responsiveness of a community in the realms of system access, coordination, and integration. Similarly, without appropriate contextual controls, responsiveness may be mistakenly attributed to other market or structural conditions.

Responsiveness

Responsiveness is concerned with the extent to which communities adopt policies and practices that are consistent with the needs and preferences of various groups—in this case, those with particular chronic health conditions. To understand the responsiveness of community service systems over time, several data elements are necessary, including an assessment of

1. needs and preferences of relevant groups;
2. structure of benefits, or the availability of insurance coverage for services;
3. supply of providers and facilities, or the availability of needed services; and
4. presence and absence of barriers to access to services.

Effectiveness

Effectiveness is concerned with the extent to which community service systems function to improve the lives of people with chronic health conditions. To understand effectiveness, one needs to measure

- service utilization;
- system coordination and integration; and
- outcomes.

Although probably not exhaustive, these dimensions suggest the range of conceptualization that is needed to measure the performance of community service systems.

THE ORGANIZATION OF THE BOOK

This volume examines seven populations with chronic conditions in terms of their service needs, the responsiveness and effectiveness of service systems in meeting these needs, and sources of data for monitoring chronic care service use and impact. Chapter 2 reviews the history of efforts to develop and maintain community-level indicators and data systems in health care. This review provides a practical and pragmatic perspective on the types of data systems that have been developed in the past, the time frame for their effective implementation, and the factors associated with continued vitality or declining support for these systems. Chapter 2 also analyzes the limited attention that has so far been given to multiple delivery systems and describes the emerging data sources that have the potential for effective system monitoring.

Different subpopulations with chronic conditions or illness are considered in chapters 3 through 9, each authored by recognized experts in those areas. These chapters are structured around four core themes, the first of which is epidemiology, particularly data on prevalence, to provide an estimate of the size and composition of the group within the larger context of persons with chronic illness. Second, one or more highly prevalent conditions is used to illustrate the condition trajectory and the service history or career likely to be associated with those conditions. We have done this to emphasize the mixture of health, social, and related services that are likely to be needed (and delivered in a more or less coordinated manner) over time. The focused examples also illustrate the implications of effective and ineffective service delivery for patients and their families and the potential points of interaction with other delivery systems. The third core theme looks at service system issues by examining the fit between prominent service needs and availability and access to services that are assumed to address these needs. Key funders and programs are identified, factors limiting access are considered, and more broadly, the fit between actual and ideal service experiences is assessed. Finally, each author identifies existing data sources and considers potential indicators of service system performance. While the primary focus is existing data sets and their potential utility and limitations, the authors also suggest new approaches to data collection and new data indicators that merit attention.

The final chapter synthesizes the primary themes and conclusions of the population group chapters and suggests the next steps to be taken in building a conceptual framework for organizing community-level indicators and data sources that might be useful in monitoring the experience of persons with chronic illness. There is also consideration of the types of measures or dimensions that might be common across a range of subpopulations. We place the material in this volume in the context of emerging efforts to strengthen chronic care monitoring and available data systems. Our conclusions about the development of local data systems are presented as a staged progression from minimum indicators into a more complex data system.

One perspective that has influenced the content and organization of this book and its conclusion is our assumption that the politics of indicators and system maintenance are much too complex for any single work to dictate a universally accepted approach. We want to stimulate positive thinking and discussion about ways to approach these issues in those who already have responsibility for indicator systems, and we want to illustrate the benefits of broadening the delivery systems and stakeholders who are included in indicator design and interpretation. We are trying to suggest a process and framework for constructively moving ahead with a variety of indicators. Much work remains, such as testing the proposed measures for reliability and measurement error across time and communities. Similarly, the predictive value of trigger or sentinel events (including the rates that define an issue as problematic) needs further testing and refinement.

With the roles of federal and state governments in transition relative to each other, and with the likelihood that managed care systems will become even more predominant, it seems prudent to develop an indicator system that can simultaneously serve the information needs of multiple decision makers. This we have tried to do.

Note

1. It is the sense of some observers, including the Institute of Medicine (1988), that this combination of health and social services financing and planning programs was not adequately addressing the public health functions even before the rapid escalation of changes in the health care system and its reorientation to market competition. A number of factors are thought to contribute to this. Among these are that a substantial portion of public funding for health departments is allocated to the provision of direct care for those without private health insurance or without entitlement eligibility. Another major contributing factor is the fragmented delivery system itself. Both public and private payers and public and private providers are involved in the planning, provision, and financing of care. The range or level of care is, moreover, often affected by multiple regulators. This process is further complicated by the evolving roles of government relative to managed health care systems and by a reevaluation of the relationships between federal, state, and local government.

References

Benson, V., & Marano, M. A. 1994. Current estimates from the NHIS: United States, 1993. *Vital and Health Statistics*. Series 10, no. 190. Washington, D.C.: DHHS Publication no. (PHS) 95–1518, 106–9.

Chassin, M., Brook, R., Park, R., et al. 1986. Variations in the use of medical and surgical services by the Medicare population. *New England Journal of Medicine 314*: 285–90.

Commission on Chronic Illness. 1957. *Chronic Illness in the United States, Prevention of Chronic Illness*. Cambridge, Mass.: Harvard University Press.

DuNah, R., de Wit, S., Harrington, C., Swan, J., Bedney, B., & Clark, C. M. 1993. *State Date Book on Longterm Care Program and Market Characteristics*. San Francisco: Institute for Health & Aging, University of California.

Harrington, C., DuNah, R., & Bedney, B. 1993. *The Supply of Community-Based Long Term Care Services in the States in 1992*. San Francisco: Institute for Health & Aging, University of California.

Hoffman, C., Rice, D., & Sung, H.-Y. 1996. Persons with chronic conditions—their prevalence and costs. *Journal of the American Medical Association 276*: 1473–79.

Institute of Medicine. 1988. *The Future of Public Health.* Washington, D.C.: National Academy Press.

Lair, T., & Lefkowitz, D. 1990. Mental health and functional status of residents of nursing and personal care homes. *NMES Research Findings 7:* AHCPR Publication no. 90–8470. Rockville, Md.: Agency for Health Care Policy Research.

LaPlante, M. 1992. How many Americans have a disability? *Disability Statistics Abstract, no. 5.* Washington, D.C.: National Institute on Disability and Rehabilitation Research.

Leape, I. 1990. Practice guidelines and standards: An overview. *Quality Review Bulletin 16:* 42–49.

Miller, N. A. 1992. Medicaid 2176 home and community-based care waivers: The first ten years. *Health Affairs 11:* 162–71.

Millman, M. (ed.). 1993. *Access to Health Care in America.* Washington, D.C.: National Academy Press.

Paringer, L. 1985. Medicaid policy changes in long term care: A framework for impact assessment. In C. Harrington, R. Newcomer, C. L. Estes & Asociates, *Long Term Care of the Elderly* (pp. 233–50). Beverly Hills, Calif.: Sage Publications.

Richardson, S. L., Renz, K. K., Vogel, T. T., Graham, J. E., & Kaufman, J. 1991. Small area analysis shows differences in utilization. *Quality Assurance and Utilization Review 6:* 91–94.

Swan, J. H., & Benjamin, A. E. 1990. Medicare home health utilization as a function of nursing home market factors. *Health Services Research 25:* 479–500.

Swan, J. H., & Benjamin, A. E. 1993. Nursing home queues and home health users. *Home Health Care Services Quarterly 14:* 157–73.

U.S. Public Health Service. 1992. *Healthy People 2000: National Health Promotion and Disease Prevention Objectives.* Washington, D.C.: Government Printing Office.

Wennberg, J. E., Freeman, J. L., & Clup, W. J. 1987. Are hospital services rationed in New Haven or over-utilized in Boston? *Lancet 1:* 1185–89.

2/ A History of Health Indicators

From Vital Registration to Report Cards

Catherine Hoffman

Measuring the health status of Americans has steadily grown in importance over the last century. In the past, health care policies and priorities have been shaped by the kinds of health information available at the time; in many ways, any system's future depends in large part on how and how accurately it measures its own performance. The need for useful health indicators is even more pronounced today, as society deals with an economic crisis in the health care system and pushes toward some form of health care reform.

While this book focuses on the complex task of understanding the dimensions of chronic conditions and proposing relevant health indicators, this chapter aims to provide a broad historical context. It is not a comprehensive history of health indicators, but rather a rendering of notable U.S. milestones (with a modicum of interpretation) that have contributed to the current state of the art. The chapter begins with the early history of three major sources of health information and then recounts the modern history of health measurement, beginning with the social indicator movement of the 1960s and including efforts to revitalize the public health system in the 1980s. The chapter concludes with a discussion of developments in the field, framed by the contemporary issues shaping the health care system and its information infrastructure: access to health care, escalating costs, and concerns about quality of health care. These problems have generated an even greater need for better health indicators to gain control of a system in crisis.

THE BEGINNINGS OF HEALTH MEASUREMENT IN THE UNITED STATES

The systematic collection of health information in the United States has gradually evolved since the mid-1800s, leading to three fundamental means of measuring the nation's health status: vital registration, disease reporting, and health survey.

Vital Statistics

Vital statistics are the roots of U.S. health information. Their precursors, vital records, began in colonial times as accounts of births, marriages, and deaths, which were used to settle inheritance and property right disputes. They were seldom used for health purposes until local health boards in eastern port cities began to use death records to monitor epidemics and institute quarantines.

While clearly useful to the community, official systems of vital statistics failed to catch on in the United States until the mid–nineteenth century. Several medical and scientific organizations in the United States, including the newly formed American Statistical Association (1847), were impressed by the outstanding quality of annual health reports compiled from centralized registry data by Dr. William Farr in England; these organizations worked toward the enactment of birth and death registration laws—one state at a time. Consequently, the collection of vital statistics became a state versus a federal function, while the complete registration of births and deaths for the entire nation, as was done in England, was a distant goal. To fill the gap, the Office of the Census added vital statistics questions to its forms between 1850 and 1900; however, a decennial count was inadequate to monitor trends in epidemics.

In 1902, the Office of the Census was formally established as a bureau and was authorized to create registration areas. Only ten states had sufficiently complete systems to qualify as such by the bureau's standards. The Bureau of the Census standardized local efforts by providing model certificates, detailed handbooks on the registration process, and personnel training. In addition, the federal government paid the costs of sending copies of records to Washington. By 1933, all states qualified, and the United States finally had a system of birth and death registration for the entire country, nearly a century later than England (Duncan & Shelton, 1978). Vital statistics were increasingly used for public health purposes:

Table 2.1. Milestones in Health Measurement in the United States

1799	U.S. Marine Service, forerunner of the Public Health Service, congressionally authorized within the Act for the Relief of Sick and Disabled Seamen
1840s	Medical and scientific organizations begin push for state registration of vital statistics
1850	Vital statistic questions added to U.S. census forms, and mortality statistics published
1874	Massachusetts State Board of Health establishes voluntary plan for physician reporting of diseases by postcard
1878	National quarantine system begins to collect data to supervise epidemic disease control
1883	Michigan becomes first state to require reporting of specific communicable diseases
1887	*Public Health Reports* first published
1893	Quarantine Act authorizes weekly morbidity data collection from states and cities (voluntary)
1901	All state and municipal laws require notification to local authorities of selected communicable diseases
1902	Office of the Census officially established and vital registration standardized
1912	Public Health and Marine Hospital Service reorganized; name changed to Public Health Service (PHS), and field studies authorized
1914	PHS personnel appointed to state health departments to telegraph incidence reports weekly to the PHS
1916	PHS conducts cotton mill community surveys to study causes of pellegra (Goldberger & Sydenstricker)
1920	PHS community surveys continue—first general population survey conducted in Hagerstown, Md., by Sydenstricker
1925	All states now participating in morbidity reporting following serious epidemics
1930	National Institutes of Health (NIH) established
1932	Committee on the Cost of Medical Care releases study of health care economics, finding health care not affordable for the middle class
1933	Uniform birth and death registration accomplished in all states
1933	*Recent Social Trends in the United States* published—chapter by Sydenstricker focuses on disabling chronic illnesses
1935	Federal Social Security Act—dealt primarily with economic security, but also created Social Security Board to conduct health care research
1936	First National Health Survey conducted by PHS
1946	Administration of vital statistics shifted to the PHS
1946	Communicable Disease Center established as a unit within the PHS
1948	World Health Organization defines health broadly, including physical, mental, and social well-being
1948	National Committee on Vital and Health Statistics established, linking public and private interests in health statistics
1949	Commission on Chronic Illness established; a private and public sector effort, also conducts community surveys
1951	Conference of State and Territorial Epidemiologists Standard develops reporting procedures for notifiable diseases
1952	*Public Health Reports* adds morbidity data; later matures into *Morbidity and Mortality Weekly Report (MMWR)*

(continued)

Table 2.1.   *(continued)*

1953	Department of Health, Education, and Welfare (HEW) established to coordinate programs and enrich federal research
1957	First U.S. National Health Interview Survey (NHIS) conducted
1960	National Center for Health Statistics (NCHS) instituted within the PHS, administratively joining the National Office of Vital Statistics and the NHIS
1960	*HEW Indicators* and *HEW Trends* first published; continued until 1967
1961	CDC authorized to maintain the National Notifiable Diseases Surveillance System
1962	Social Security Administration reports national expenditures for health
1965	Medicare and Medicaid programs enacted
1966	PHS report *Estimating the Cost of Illness* released
1969	*Toward a Social Report* published; covers a variety of social topics and calls for a system of social reporting
1969	Cooperative Health Statistics System (CHSS) proposed by NCHS; later affirmed in several federal laws
1971	First Health and Nutrition Examination Survey (NHANES) conducted
1971	Surveillance, Epidemiology, and End Results Program (SEER) mandated under the National Cancer Act
1973	First of three triennial compendiums of *Social Indicators* published
1975	National Health Planning and Resources Development Act authorizes local planning agencies
1976	First of annual *Health, United States* published
1979	*Healthy People*—Surgeon General's report on health promotion and disease prevention
1980	First National Medical Expenditures Survey conducted; repeated in 1987
1980	Strategic plan set by the PHS: *Promoting Health/Preventing Disease: Objectives for the Nation*
1981	Behavioral Risk Factor Surveillance System initiated by CDC
1990	*Healthy People 2000* objectives published

assessing maternal and child health needs, communicable disease patterns, and the growth in chronic conditions. Because of these broader applications, the Public Health Service (PHS) took over the vital registration system from the Bureau of the Census in 1946. Today's vital registration system produces health indicators that are of routine usefulness to policymakers. Indicators such as infant mortality and life expectancy are acknowledged as reliable gauges of the success of the health care delivery system of a nation, a state, and even a county.

Early Public Health Surveillance: Disease Reporting

Recognizing that a system of regular monitoring or surveillance was needed to assess and prevent epidemics of infectious disease, Congress authorized the PHS as early as 1878 to collect reports on quarantined disease in port cities. In 1893, Congress enacted the Quarantine Act, authorizing collection of weekly morbidity data from states and cities; thus began the current system of national notifiable disease reporting (Lawrence, 1976).[1] Surveillance activities at the time focused solely on infectious disease reporting. This information was published promptly in *Public Health Reports;* many cities and states, however, did not contribute to this effort initially, because unlike vital statistics registration, it was a voluntary system.[2]

Gradually, all states came to require reporting of specific infectious diseases to local authorities. By 1914, personnel in state health departments were designated as collaborating epidemiologists with the responsibility to telegraph weekly reports to the PHS. Full participation in national morbidity reporting by all states did not occur until 1925, following serious epidemics of poliomyelitis and influenza (Thacker & Berkelman, 1988).

Several significant infectious disease threats established support for federally organized public health surveillance efforts. Malaria had ravaged the southern states throughout the 1930s to such an extent that by the time the United States entered World War II, the disease was considered a threat to troops and wartime industries located there. The Malaria Control in War Areas (MCWA) unit was set up within the PHS and centered in Atlanta for lack of room in Washington, D.C. The threat of an epidemic was crushed by the MCWA's aggressive program of mosquito control.[3]

Through its malaria surveillance program, the MCWA established its expertise to meet the practical public health needs of the states. Following the war in 1946 (with no resistance from the National Institutes of Health [NIH]) with its focus on basic research and chronic illnesses), the MCWA evolved into the Communicable Disease Center, the first agency to use the acronym CDC and the forerunner of today's Centers for Disease Control and Prevention (Etheridge, 1992).[4] The future of the CDC, however, with its emphasis on infectious disease, was uncertain, because by this time, chronic diseases were recognized as the nation's biggest health concern.[5]

Given the CDC's experience, it was the natural home for notifiable disease reporting within the PHS. Efforts to standardize disease reporting, which had been highly variable from the start, were first initiated in 1951 by the Conference (now Council) of State and Territorial Epidemiologists (CSTE), a unit of the Association of State and Territorial

Health Officials. They began by determining which diseases should be reported to the PHS and developing standard reporting procedures. Since 1961, the CDC has had the responsibility for maintaining the National Notifiable Diseases Surveillance System (NNDSS). Today, the CSTE meets annually and, in collaboration with the CDC, issues recommendations for state standards in morbidity surveillance, determining which diseases should be reported nationally. Recently, the CSTE began approving standardized case definitions for nationally notifiable diseases, which is expected to greatly improve comparison of surveillance data.

Today, forty-nine infectious diseases and related conditions are reported routinely. National numbers for most of these are published weekly in the *Morbidity and Mortality Weekly Report (MMWR)*; however, states collect information on a much larger set of health concerns. In a recent survey of state statutes and regulations, over three hundred diseases or conditions (including occupational diseases, environmental diseases, and congenital conditions) were identified (Chorba et al., 1989).[6]

Over the next several decades, the CDC continued to refine its surveillance expertise when challenged by new infectious diseases, the most daunting being the AIDS epidemic. Eventually, all these skills, combined with working relationships established over time with state health departments, would be applied to other public health problems, but only gradually and in limited ways to chronic health conditions.

Health Surveys

By the early 1900s, vital registration and surveillance of infectious conditions were not enough to portray the full range of health problems in the United States. Health could no longer be defined sufficiently by the ability to escape fatal diseases. Richer information was needed to understand nonfatal diseases—their costs, the disabilities they caused, and the behavioral and social conditions associated with them—information that could be obtained only by asking people directly. In the tradition of infectious disease monitoring, the entire community was examined. Berkman and Breslow (1983) summarized the early history of health surveys in the United States, beginning around 1916 with the work of Goldberger and Sydenstricker, who were sent by the PHS to South Carolina to study pellagra (the number-two killer in the state at the time). They conducted household surveys in seven cotton-mill villages, and by studying the relationship between disabling illnesses, pellagra, and various dietary and social factors, they eventually identified a dietary deficiency as the causative agent for pellagra.

Sydenstricker, the first appointed statistician in the PHS, was encouraged by the surveys and continued to conduct them, primarily in communities of industrial workers. In Hagerstown, Maryland, in the early 1920s, this work was extended to the first general population survey of "illnesses, as ordinarily understood" by persons of all ages and sexes. The PHS collected morbidity information over seven months from nearly two thousand households. Among the findings were that the causes of death were quite different from the major causes of illness in the population and that self-reported health data showed fair agreement with Sydenstricker's earlier estimates of the prevalence of illness.

Measuring Social Consequences of the Great Depression

The PHS continued to conduct community morbidity surveys throughout the 1920s and early 1930s, publicizing the growing morbidity from chronic conditions and laying the groundwork for the first National Health Survey. During this time, several organizations, including the Metropolitan Life Insurance Company, the Rockefeller Institute, the Massachusetts Department of Public Health, and the Montefiore Hospital for Chronic Invalids in New York, began to respond to the challenge raised by chronic conditions; however, policymakers and the press devoted most of their attention to infection and the cure of illness (Fox, 1989).

The idea that a country needed a societal profile from which to judge change caught on in the late 1920s. In the face of the Great Depression, a presidential committee was formed, enlisting scholars to review a variety of contemporary social issues, such as education, occupations, health care, and the changing role of women. Their efforts produced a massive report titled *Recent Social Trends in the United States*. Published in 1933, it is considered the first significant review of "social indicators," a term coined much later, in the 1960s. The project revealed interrelationships among different sectors of society and stimulated new thinking on social concerns (Ferriss, 1979).

"The Vitality of the American People" was addressed in the committee's report by Edgar Sydenstricker (1933). Besides describing general trends in mortality (based on mortality data from the ten states that had

had active registries since 1900), he reported morbidity data from several large-scale surveys, which corroborated much of what he had found in his PHS surveys of industrial workers.[7] Because of the growing numbers of disabled adults, Sydenstricker stressed the significance of chronic conditions: "In spite of the reduction in the death rate among younger persons and the prevention of many infectious diseases, the American people are not enjoying the full extent of their vitality before they die. . . .The available evidence on the prevalence of chronic diseases and organic as well as functional impairments, although incomplete, also reveals that a large proportion of the population is thus rendered more or less inefficient" (659). Furthermore, he concluded that the most important area for further "conservation of vitality" was among those over age forty. Unfortunately, what was known about chronic disease came entirely from unrepresentative surveys. While these surveys were the best available, Sydenstricker's report raised awareness that the extent of America's major health problems was actually unknown, which in turn advanced the notion of a nationwide survey.

The harsh social and economic times of the Depression helped expose the costly nature of chronic conditions, as those on public relief roles were frequently burdened by chronic health problems as well. Subsidized by federal funds under the New Deal, state relief agencies began to pay for physicians' services. Once government took on the function of health insurance payer, a significant stimulus for improved health information was created. The federal government now needed the ability to assess the extent of the nation's health problems to predict the magnitude of health care costs and in turn, the potential costs to be paid by tax dollars.

The President's Research Committee on Social Trends called for improvements in the U.S. statistical system and suggested the need for a national advisory council to consider the basic social problems of the nation, goals that are often echoed today. Despite the opportune timing of these recommendations, the National Resources Planning Board and the Central Statistical Board (the two national boards established in response to the recommendations) were not in a position to be proactive; as a result, the impact of the report was small (Innes de Neufville, 1975).

The Committee on Economic Security, appointed by President Roosevelt in 1934, examined a wide spectrum of economic problems confronting the country, including health care issues. The committee noted that research on the issue of national health insurance (NHI) should continue, but in the face of strong opposition from the American Medical Association (AMA), the report on NHI was never published (Dobson & Bialek, 1985). Even though political support for NHI could not be mustered, the year 1935 marked the beginning of a deliberate national policy to address the consequences of chronic conditions, part of which was the decision by the PHS to conduct the first National Health Survey (Fox, 1989).[8]

The National Health Survey involved over 700,000 households—almost three million people—and provided many significant insights about chronic conditions. Nearly one-quarter of Americans had a chronic disease. These diseases were costly, and the poor received less medical care than the nonpoor, even though they were sicker. Increasingly, general hospitals, not just public hospitals, were caring for persons with chronic illness, and there were not enough hospitals to meet the growing needs (Pihlbland, 1937). Further supplements to the National Health Survey were conducted in the 1940s under contract by the Bureau of the Census, but the national survey did not gain a permanent status until the next decade.

Social statistical activities slowed during World War II, but as the war wound down and the economy began to prosper, attention turned to problems at home. The relationship between chronic conditions and economic dependence in the United States became evident when characteristics of persons still on relief rolls were examined. Chronic conditions were now being viewed as a social, not just a medical, concern. By the early 1940s, many local and state voluntary health agencies began to address the problems of persons with disabilities. For example, a major change in vocational rehabilitation programs occurred in 1943, when funds were made available for a broad range of medical and social services to enable people with disabilities to be gainfully employed.

Postwar America

After the war, the United Nations began its efforts to define "quality of life," so that a range of conditions in addition to economic indices could be measured to evaluate a country's growth. To this end, the World Health Organization (WHO) broadly characterized health in their 1948 U.N. charter as "a state of complete physical, mental, and social well-being and not merely the absence of disease or infirmity" (Culyer, 1983). While this definition has been criticized as idealistic and difficult to quantify, it represents a positive nondisease perspective and a framework that does not limit the goals of health care to only those that can be achieved by the medical profession.

Interest in data gathering and health care research resumed after the war. Successful new treatments for war injuries fueled societal support for medical research, and confidence in science and technology was high, because of their significant contributions to the outcome of the war. Since the 1930s, the NIH had expanded into several disease-specific centers of research.

Recognizing that an organized attack on the problems of chronic conditions was needed, four professional associations banded together: the American Hospital Association, the AMA, the American Public Health Association (APHA), and the American Public Welfare Association. These organizations agreed that "something more was needed and by the late forties the time was most auspicious for a broader approach. . . . Although effective in other activities such as clinical research, the one-disease-at-a-time approach did not fill the need for pooling resources and combining efforts to meet the many problems common to most chronic illness" (Commission on Chronic Illness, 1957, 287).

They also agreed that local efforts were often poorly planned (sometimes unsound administratively and professionally) and that lack of coordination would result in further social and economic losses. In 1949, a formal Commission on Chronic Illness was established.[9] In its bylaws, the commission agreed to direct their efforts

- To modify the attitude of society that chronic illness is hopeless; to substitute for the prevailing overconcentration on the provision of institutional care, a dynamic program designed as far as possible to prevent chronic illness, to minimize its disabling effects, and to restore its victims to a socially useful and economically productive place in the community.
- To define the problems arising from chronic illness among all age groups, with full realization of its social as well as its medical aspects.
- To coordinate separate programs for specific diseases with a general program designed to meet more effectively the needs which are common to all the chronically ill
- To stimulate in every state and locality a well-rounded plan for the prevention and control of chronic disease and for the care and rehabilitation of the chronically ill (Commission on Chronic Illness, 1957, 294).

In its seven-year life, the commission made progress toward many of these sizable goals. It gathered information about the size and nature of the problem, developed recommendations, and, through publications and conferences, stimulated other groups to take up the charge.

To gather descriptive information about chronic illness, the commission undertook two significant community surveys. Targeting rural America, they first studied chronic illness in Hunterdon County, New Jersey, a demonstration of "local initiative and interest in survey planning."[10] Interviews with over four thousand families and clinical evaluations of a subsample were conducted, which enabled comparison of physician and respondent responses. In addition to interviews and clinical evaluations, the urban survey in Baltimore conducted a medical screening and a demonstration of vocational rehabilitation (Commission on Chronic Illness, 1957).

A Continuous National Health Survey

The surveys conducted for the Commission on Chronic Illness, like the community surveys conducted before the National Health Survey of 1935, helped raise awareness of the value of an ongoing national survey effort (Berkman & Breslow, 1983). To enrich federal research and coordinate programs, the Department of Health, Education, and Welfare (HEW) was formed in 1953. Meanwhile, researchers in public health and biostatistics were rapidly developing probability sampling methods, and the subcommittee of the National Committee on Vital and Health Statistics (an advisory committee to the secretary of health, established in 1948 to link public and private sector interests) recommended a permanent National Health Survey be started, using scientific sampling techniques. Legislation authorizing such a survey passed in 1956, and the first Health Interview Survey was launched the following year. The National Center for Health Statistics (NCHS) was instituted in 1960 within the PHS, administratively joining the National Office of Vital Statistics and the National Health Interview Survey (NHIS).[11]

The United States was not the first to recognize the need for better information to profile the health status of a nation. Two other countries had already begun large-scale national surveys to capture morbidity and disability and their attending costs. Great Britain was the first to collect morbidity data, beginning in 1943 with a nine-year Survey of Sickness. A decade later, Japan began its continuing health survey, which included examinations and clinical tests (Armitage, 1976).[12]

The creation of the NHIS is a significant landmark in the history of health measurement in the United States. Since 1957, face-to-face household interviews of the civilian noninstitutionalized population have been conducted, using multistage probability sampling. The survey collects information about all illnesses, impairments, and injuries (providing prevalence estimates of roughly one hundred chronic conditions), health care use, and the extent of disability associated with health problems. Besides marking the beginning of a federal commitment to monitor health status on a regular basis, findings from the NHIS have made policymakers aware of the demands that chronic conditions create upon the health care system. It continues to be the primary source of information on the extent of chronic conditions and disability.

THE SOCIAL INDICATORS MOVEMENT

Health measurement benefited in the 1960s from a force outside the health field. Theory-based economic indicators were beginning to influence federal policy significantly, and the practicality of other social indicators was newly appreciated (Culyer, 1983).[13] Measuring social issues had grown more important as national goals were focused by President Lyndon Johnson's Great Society domestic agenda. The National Commission on Technology, Automation, and Economic Progress, appointed by Johnson in 1964, studied evidence of changes in socioeconomic conditions and recommended that the Council of Economic Advisers begin to develop a system of social accounts. About the same time, the National Aeronautics and Space Administration (NASA) commissioned a study of potential unforeseen social, political, and economic effects, the "second-order consequences" of the space program. The resulting book, *Social Indicators,* coined the broad catchword under which many interests were to gather, and the social indicators movement was launched (Bauer, 1966).

As early as 1960, HEW had begun publishing key measures of social issues through two periodicals: *HEW Indicators* and *HEW Trends* (Department of Health, Education, and Welfare [DHEW], 1960–66; 1960–63). Both series depicted trends in national conditions and social programs related to the work of the department (Ferriss, 1979). *HEW Indicators* was a monthly publication containing tables and graphs describing regularly featured topics. *HEW Trends* summarized this information, presenting it in time series in an annual supplement. Regularly featured health indicators, primarily from NHIS data, included rates of acute conditions and accidents, disability days, and employee sick days. Besides the regular data tables, different topics were featured each month. These focused on current health policy concerns, for example, racial differences in infant mortality and PHS cancer programs. Both HEW publications continued until 1967, when they presumably were to be replaced by a more comprehensive monitoring effort.

In 1967, Senator Walter Mondale introduced legislation providing for a council of social advisors to produce an annual social report with recommendations to the president and Congress (Land & Spilerman, 1975). Although reintroduced in sessions over the next decade, the bill never passed.

The administration also tried to institutionalize social indicators. A deputy secretary for social indicators was appointed within HEW. Working under HEW's direction, the Panel on Social Indicators prepared working papers, which were published in a now classic document titled *Toward a Social Report* (1969). The topics covered were health and illness, social mobility, the physical environment, income and poverty, public order and safety, learning, science and art, and participation and alienation. Data used in the chapter on health and illness were limited to mortality rates, life expectancy, and bed-disability rates.[14] The chapter identified health status differences and the costs of medical care within the United States and made international comparisons. Like others before it, the full report outlined the need for future reports of social indicators. In the introduction, HEW Secretary Cohen referred to the document as a "preliminary step toward the evolution of a system of social reporting" (Land & Spilerman, 1975).

The discontinuance in 1967 of *HEW Indicators* and *Trends* left a void in serial reporting of social indicators that was never filled (Ferriss, 1979). While the Mondale bill and the publication of *Toward a Social Report* failed to generate sufficient support for a continuous system of social monitoring, some objectives were nevertheless advanced. The federal government's main efforts produced a series of three triennial compendiums of social indicators *(Social Indicators 1973, Social Indicators 1976,* and *Social Indicators III),* presenting a variety of statistics "on important aspects of our current social situation and their underlying historical trends" (Bureau of the Census, 1980, xix). Tables and figures were compiled from data from a variety of federal agencies and national organizations, much of which had been published in other formats. Although this federal series held potential for policy application, there is little evidence to suggest that it was used in this way. One survey of 115 upper level government officials found that no more than 4 percent made use of the 1973 volume at all (primarily for speech writing and background references), only 22 percent expressed any awareness of the report, and no one reported that its data played an important role in any policy decision (Caplan & Barton, 1978). The triennial series was discontinued after the third volume.

Encouraged by the federal government's interest, the private sector was equally active in the social indicator movement. The efforts of the Russell Sage Foundation toward improved social measurement are particularly noteworthy. The foundation supported a program dedicated to exploring all facets of social indicator research, including conceptualization work, methodology, and compilation of statistics (Ferriss, 1979). Social science journals committed volumes to social indicator work (*The Annals of the American Academy of Political and Social Science,* in particular), and a new journal emerged, *Social Indicators Research,* fully dedicated to the field.

The social indicator movement slowed after the 1970s, but progress in health measurement did not seem to falter. Federal health survey activity grew rapidly following the early years of the NHIS. For example, between 1971 and 1975, the first Health and Nutrition Examination Survey (NHANES) was conducted. The purpose of NHANES I and the six national examination surveys that followed has been to gather health data by physical examination and laboratory tests; these data are uniformly collected by a traveling staff of health professionals using mobile examination centers. This survey continues to provide normative distributions for the U.S. population, estimates of disease prevalence, risk factors, reference values (e.g., blood pressure, serum cholesterol levels, and visual acuity), and to estimate unmet needs for health care. Because of the representativeness that can be achieved through sampling, many national health surveys have been added to the U.S. health information base since the 1970s (an inventory of which is beyond the scope of this historical chapter).[15]

At roughly the same time that the *Social Indicators* reports were being produced, Congress enacted legislation mandating the secretary of HEW to assemble and submit an annual report to the president and the Congress focusing specifically on health indicators. The NCHS and the National Center for Health Services Research were assigned the responsibility, and they published the first in the series of *Health, United States* (for

1975) in 1976. Starting as a descriptive account of four major areas—health costs and finances, resources, use of services, and health status—the annual report grew to include a more analytical interpretation of health data; in more recent years, it has expanded to track measures of health prevention. While considerable effort is necessary to sustain the report, the series is considered to be useful to a wide audience as a summary of the health and health care system of the nation. For this reason, the congressional requirement of periodic data has never been waived, even in lean budget years (DHEW, 1977; D. Rice, personal communication, January 1994).

REVITALIZING THE PUBLIC HEALTH SYSTEM IN THE INFORMATION AGE

While the major advancements in the health status of the U.S. population in this century have occurred through public health efforts, such as control of infectious disease and safer food and water, the stature of public health had diminished by the 1970s. Health measurement benefited tremendously from a serious evaluation of the public health system and its information base, begun in the late 1970s.

Healthy People

Recognizing that the mission of public health needed direction, enormous efforts were initiated to focus the work of public health by setting objectives and to organize states and communities as the foundation of a more effective system. The leadership for this renewal came from the WHO. Beginning in the early 1980s, the WHO laid out a blueprint for prioritizing national health goals. Health indicators were organized under a framework of goals referred to as *Health for All* goals. Member countries received assistance in setting up systematic monitoring and evaluation, and an international database became a realizable goal. The WHO identified four broad categories of indicators:

1. health policy indicators (e.g., resource allocation, distribution of health resources, political commitment);
2. health status indicators (e.g., infant mortality, nutritional status of children, life expectancy);
3. indicators of the provision of health care (e.g., primary health care coverage);

4. social and economic indicators related to health (e.g., adult literacy rate, housing and food availability).

This broad and inclusive framework was put forward with the idea that countries would select those indicators most appropriate to the health needs of their population and that the framework would trickle down to guide even community-level public health efforts (WHO, 1981, 1985).

The United States launched its public health assessment initiative in 1979 with the publication of *Healthy People: The Surgeon General's Report on Health Promotion and Disease Prevention.*[16] This report originated in the CDC under the direction of William Foege, who recognized that the agency's mission needed to be reformulated to include chronic conditions. To do this, he sought advice from people outside the CDC. In 1977, the "Red Book Committee" (composed of sixteen health professionals and laymen, some of whom were former CDC staff) was formed to study the nation's leading causes of morbidity and mortality and to define the CDC's role in controlling them. They agreed that primary prevention was the best way to improve the nation's health and that the CDC was in a unique position to lead the charge. Building on its strong relationship with the states, the CDC could apply surveillance and epidemiology—the successful tools of infectious disease control—to the widespread problems of chronic conditions and personal injury. CDC staff then drafted a document outlining prevention strategies for the nation. When the surgeon general reviewed their work, he proposed that it be adopted by the entire PHS (Etheridge, 1992).

The impact of *Healthy People* was further extended the following year, when a strategic plan was outlined in *Promoting Health/Preventing Disease: Objectives for the Nation* (USPHS, 1980).[17] Specific Department of Health and Human Services agencies were assigned responsibility for developing implementation plans (published in 1983) and for preparing regular progress reports on the priority areas. Good data were needed to monitor progress. While most objectives could be measured, no data source was available to evaluate more than one-quarter of the 1990 objectives (Office of Disease Prevention and Health Promotion, 1986). As the objectives were applied over the next decade, the need for more health indicators became increasingly apparent.

By the time the *Healthy People 2000* objectives were written (Table 2.2), it was clear that weaknesses in surveillance and data systems needed

Table 2.2.   Healthy People 2000: National Health Promotion and Disease Prevention Objectives

Priority areas:

Health promotion

1. Physical activity and fitness	5. Family planning
2. Nutrition	6. Mental health and mental disorders
3. Tobacco	7. Violent and abusive behavior
4. Alcohol and other drugs	8. Educational and community-based programs

Health protection

9. Unintentional injuries	12. Food and drug safety
10. Occupational safety and health	13. Oral health
11. Environmental health	

Preventive services

14. Maternal and infant health	18. HIV infection
15. Heart disease and stroke	19. Sexually transmitted diseases
16. Cancer	20. Immunization and infectious diseases
17. Diabetes and chronic conditions	21. Clinical preventive services

Surveillance and data systems

22. Surveillance and data systems

Source: Data from U.S. Public Health Service, 1990.

Note: Each priority area has specific objectives categorized as (1) health status objectives, (2) risk reduction objectives, and (3) services and protection objectives. Many of the objectives have subobjectives targeting special populations. An example of each kind of objective, using the priority of "Tobacco," follows.

3.	*Tobacco*
3.3	Slow the rise in deaths from chronic obstructive pulmonary disease to achieve a rate of no more than 25 per 100,000 people. (Age-adjusted baseline: 18.7 per 100,000 in 1987.)
3.5	Reduce the initiation of cigarette smoking by children and youth so that no more than 15% have become regular cigarette smokers by age 20. (Baseline: 30% of youth had become regular cigarette smokers by ages 20 through 25 in 1987.)
3.10	Establish tobacco-free environments and include tobacco use prevention in the curricula of all elementary, middle, and secondary schools, preferably as part of quality school health education. (Baseline: 17% of school districts totally banned smoking on school premises or at school functions in 1988; antismoking education was provided by 78% of school districts at the high school level, 81% at the middle school level, and 75% at the elementary school level in 1988.)

to be addressed.[18] A separate priority area (number 22) was established, with seven objectives that targeted expanded state-based assessment activity, improved data on minorities, improved information transfer among levels of government, enhanced data processing for quicker application, and creation of new data sources (Table 2.3). The first objective (22.1) called for the adoption of a common set of health status indicators that could be used by federal, state, and local health agencies. A consensus set of eighteen indicators was developed in early 1991 by a CDC committee (referred to as Committee 22.1) composed of PHS officials

Table 2.3.   Healthy People 2000: Surveillance and Data Systems Objectives

22.1	Develop a set of health status indicators appropriate for federal, state, and local health agencies, and establish use of the set in at least forty states
22.2	Identify, and create where necessary, national data sources to measure progress toward each of the Year 2000 national health objectives
22.2a	Identify, and create where necessary, state-level data for at least two-thirds of the objectives in at least thirty-five states
22.3	Develop and disseminate among federal, state, and local agencies procedures for collecting comparable data for each of the Year 2000 national health objectives and incorporate these into PHS data collection systems
22.4	Develop and implement a national process to identify significant gaps in the nation's disease prevention and health promotion data, including data for racial and ethnic minorities, people with low incomes, and people with disabilities, and establish mechanisms to meet these needs
22.5	Implement in all states periodic analysis and publication of data needed to measure progress toward objectives for at least ten of the priority areas of the national health objectives
22.5a	Implement in at least twenty-five states periodic analysis and publication of data needed to measure state progress toward the national health objectives for each racial or ethnic group that makes up at least 10 percent of the state population
22.6	Expand in all states systems for the transfer of health information related to the national health objectives among federal, state, and local agencies
22.7	Achieve timely release of national surveillance and survey data needed by health professionals and agencies to measure progress toward the national health objectives

Source: Data from National Center for Health Statistics, 1994.

and representatives of several national associations.[19] Included in this initial set were nine mortality indicators, four disease incidence rates, and five health risk factor indicators (Table 2.4). The consensus set is viewed as a beginning, a product developed within the constraints of available data. By 1992, forty-eight states were monitoring some of the indicator set, and thirty-six states were transferring the information to local health departments (USPHS, 1993).

According to a second progress review of the Year 2000 objectives, conducted by NCHS in 1992, 99 percent of the objectives could be measured by existing national data sources. However, the ability of states and communities to monitor and compare their progress toward these objectives remains a distant goal. Only 14 percent of the Year 2000 objectives can be tracked in a way that allows comparisons (USPHS, 1993). On average, states can monitor only 39 percent of the objectives; data on

Table 2.4.   Healthy People 2000 Objective 22.1: The Consensus Set of Health Status Indicators

---

 1. Race/ethnicity-specific infant mortality as measured by the rate (per 1,000 live births) of deaths among infants under one year of age

    White   Black

    American Indian   Chinese

    Japanese   Filipino

    Other Asian or Pacific Islander   Hispanic

 2. Total deaths per 100,000 population (ICD-9 nos. 0–E999)
 3. Motor vehicle crash deaths per 100,000 population (ICD-9 nos. E810–E825)
 4. Work-related injury deaths per 100,000 population
 5. Suicides per 100,000 population (ICD-9 nos. E950–E959)
 6. Homicides per 100,000 population (ICD-9 nos. E960–E978)
 7. Lung cancer deaths per 100,000 population (ICD-9 no. 162)
 8. Female breast cancer deaths per 100,000 women (ICD-9 no. 174)
 9. Cardiovascular disease deaths per 100,000 population (ICD-9 nos. 390–448)
10. Reported incidence (per 100,000 population) of acquired immunodeficiency syndrome
11. Reported incidence (per 100,000 population) of measles
12. Reported incidence (per 100,000 population) of tuberculosis
13. Reported incidence (per 100,000 population) of primary and secondary syphilis
14. Prevalence of low birthweight as measured by the percentage of live born infants weighing under 2,500 grams at birth
15. Births to adolescents (aged 10–17 years) as a percentage of total live births
16. Prenatal care as measured by the percentage of mothers delivering live infants who did not receive care during the first trimester of pregnancy
17. Childhood poverty, as measured by the proportion of children under 15 years of age living in families at or below the poverty level

    Under 18 years

    Under 15 years

    5–17 years

18. Proportion of persons living in counties exceeding U.S. Environmental Protection Agency standards for air quality during the previous year

---

Source: Data from National Center for Health Statistics, 1994.

racial and socioeconomic differentials are even more problematic (Stoto, 1992). Plans to change this situation are under way.

State assessment initiatives (funded by several sources, including the CDC) are now under way in twenty-six states.[20] The CDC-sponsored initiatives are intended to increase the assessment capacity of state and local health departments, so that by the year 2000, all states will be able to monitor at least 75 percent of the Year 2000 objectives and analyze the data, which can then be used for public health programing and health policy. States receive funding, technical assistance and training, and direct assistance from a CDC employee on long-term assignment, and they are to designate an assessment coordinator, identify data needs and barriers, and propose solutions. Training programs developed for the initiative are open to all states (National Committee on Vital and Health Statistics, 1993).

Several significant support systems for state and community agencies have been developed that pragmatically bolster the *Healthy People 2000* initiative. First, a series of three editions of *Model Standards* has been developed for local community use. The last edition was prepared to link the Year 2000 national objectives with community efforts and has been distributed to every local health department in the country.[21] It is intended to help mobilize a community by focusing resources, selecting pertinent objectives, and setting priorities. To serve as a guidebook, the national objectives are written in *Model Standards* with fill-in-the-blank targets, leaving communities to choose realistic goals for themselves. It is hoped that by making community objectives compatible with the national objectives, progress can be made toward a more uniform data set for comparing local and state data with those of other areas and the country as a whole (APHA, 1991). Preliminary results from a 1993 survey of local health departments indicated that roughly half are using the *Model Standards* in some way (J. Freedman, personal communication, June 30, 1994).

In addition, two CDC-sponsored planning processes support implementation of the *Model Standards*. The Assessment Protocol for Excellence in Public Health (APEXPH) targets the community's formal system of public health, outlining a stepped approach to organizational self-assessment and priority setting. On the other hand, the Planned Approach to Community Health (PATCH), which is geared toward chronic disease prevention and health promotion programs, is typically carried out by an agency's education/promotion arm or by an outside community organization. It is distinguished by its involvement of volunteer organizations, businesses, and individuals. Both community-level methods have been tested, modified, and proven successful (APHA, 1993).[22]

A major impediment to the work of public health, cited by the Institute of Medicine's (IOM) Committee for the Study of the Future of Public Health, is the inability of states and localities to carry out health assessment, an essential function for problem solving (IOM, 1988). Their thorough evaluation found that while federal agencies have contributed data, leadership, and intermittent technical assistance, health measurement activities have not been sufficiently supported by state and local health departments.[23] The IOM Committee (1988) recommended "that every public health agency regularly and systematically collect, assemble, analyze, and make available information on the health of the community, including statistics on health status, community health needs, and epidemiologic and other studies of health problems." Although the public health system has considerably more work to do to meet the recommendation proposed in the IOM's landmark report, awareness of the necessity for continuous vigilance of the public's health is focused and higher than ever, largely because of the *Healthy People* initiatives. As a framework for organizing health data collection by national objectives, the initiative is pragmatic and meaningful to all levels of public health planning. Through the process of setting state and community objectives, the inadequacy of health measures will be further exposed, moving agencies to collect better data.

Public Health Surveillance Today

Public health surveillance has changed dramatically since its beginnings in infectious disease control. As the CDC grew, it began to apply its epidemiological expertise in other areas. Today, surveillance activities cover a wide range of health concerns, including occupational health, injuries, health risk behaviors, and environmental conditions.

Chronic illnesses, however, do not lend themselves readily to traditional methods of surveillance through disease reporting. Many chronic illnesses have long latency periods between the exposure or precipitating event and the eventual disease or impairment. Often, chronic diseases have more than one cause, which confounds tracing relationships between exposure and outcomes. Finally, surveillance of the incidence of chronic disease alone is not sufficient, because chronic diseases often progress over many years of life, making monitoring the stages of disease equally important. For these reasons, other sources of information have been relied upon, including community studies of particular diseases (such as cardiovascular disease in Framingham, Massachusetts) and disease registries (Thacker & Berkelman, 1988, 175–76).

Disease Registries

Registries have been used to fill in the gaps about the incidence and prevalence of particular chronic conditions, usually tracking a single chronic illness or public health concern. Because registries systematically link health information about individuals over time from multiple sources, they provide the longitudinal data critical to determining treatment effectiveness, which is often lacking in other data systems. Although disease registries date back to the mid-1800s, they have proliferated over just the past thirty years, and their widespread use is a relatively new phenomenon. Stimulated by information about chronic disease from community surveys, state health departments became interested in estimating the extent of these problems in their states. The oldest population-based registry in the United States began in Connecticut (the Connecticut Tumor Registry) and has monitored cancer incidence rates for nearly fifty years (Stroup, Zack, & Wharton, 1994). In 1947, California also established a tumor registry that tracked cancer cases seen in selected hospitals, and by 1970, the registry covered the entire San Francisco Bay area (Berkman & Breslow, 1983).

Because registries attempt to identify all known cases of the condition being studied, the catchment area is commonly small, such as a community. Many begin as hospital-based registries focusing on a particular disease (e.g., heart disease and its treatment). Others originate in the public health sector. No comprehensive inventory of disease registries for the entire country is available; therefore, the full range of chronic conditions that have been or are currently being tracked is unknown. The surge of registry activity since the 1960s has occurred in response to several demands. First, a number of registries have been established to ensure that uniform data for CDC surveillance and research can be reported. In addition, advocates for persons with specific health conditions have lobbied for the development of distinct registries, ensuring an improved base of information, which can serve to highlight unmet needs. Finally, state health departments have developed additional registries to match their particular program needs. These are not insignificant forces. For example, a recent examination of public health registries in the state of Michigan identified forty-two separate registries partially or fully funded by the state's Department of Public Health (Solomon et al., 1991).

Cancers are, by far, the most common health condition tracked through registries. In fact, the largest chronic disease registry in the United States was established under the National Cancer Act of 1971, which mandated the Surveillance, Epidemiology, and End Results Program (SEER) to monitor the burden of cancer in the general population. Today, the program consists of eleven registries: five state-wide registries, five metropolitan areas, and a large four-county area. Twice a year, each local registry submits information to the National Cancer Institute, including patient demographics, diagnosed cancers, treatment, and follow-up. Roughly 120,000 cancers are registered annually by these centers. Trends in incidence, survival, and mortality, as well as the effectiveness of particular treatment modalities, are reported from these data (USPHS Task Force on State and Community Data, 1993).

Besides cancers, a wide range of other diseases and public health problems are being tracked through community and statewide registries. The epidemic of limb defects among children exposed prenatally to thalidomide, for example, spawned efforts to develop ongoing birth defects monitoring programs. Another example is the exposure registry. Workers exposed to high levels of potentially toxic agents are followed over many years to determine whether illnesses are associated with certain occupational risks and, if so, how to prevent them (Stroup et al., 1994).

While disease registries provide unique information about the prevalence of a chronic condition or a public health concern in a community, as well as about the effectiveness of certain kinds of treatment, the method has significant limitations. Registries require a long-term commitment of resources; therefore, only the more common chronic conditions can be practically studied. Additionally, because most registries begin the examination of a condition by identifying individuals already diagnosed, little can be learned about the precipitating risk factors, knowledge of which is necessary for improved prevention efforts. Finally, unlike surveys, registries may not be representative of the general population because only those who have access and have obtained medical care are identified (Berkman & Breslow, 1983).

Surveillance for Health Risk

As the role of personal health practices in both chronic illness and acute injuries became recognized, state programs grew interested in collecting more risk-factor information than was available in national surveys. An ongoing system of collecting population-based prevalence data was needed; in response, the CDC developed the Behavioral Risk Factor Surveillance System (BRFSS) in 1981. With CDC's training and coordination between 1981 and 1983, twenty-nine states began doing computer-assisted telephone interviews, using multistage sampling methods. State participation has grown yearly, and as of 1994, all states plus the District of Columbia now take part in the BRFSS. A fixed core of questions is covered consistently every year, and additional sets of core questions are rotated in alternate years. Examples of topics include smoking and physical activity behavior, injury prevention, and nutritional choices. Most recently, quality-of-life questions have been added to the fixed core of questions.

A large part of the BRFSS success can be attributed to two factors. First, the survey questionnaire itself is adaptable. While core questions must be asked, each state can add questions tailored to its own needs and modify them frequently. In 1994, all but six states added questions to the core survey for their own purposes. Secondly, states have directly applied the risk factor data to promote programmatic and policy changes. A 1987 CDC evaluation of BRFSS showed that 60 percent of participating states used the data to prepare health planning documents, set state health objectives, or plan specific programs. Nearly two-thirds used the data to support legislative initiatives, principally antismoking and seat belt use legislation (Remington et al., 1988).

The Computerization of Surveillance

Public health surveillance has been revolutionized by computers and their software applications. The National Electronic Telecommunications System for Surveillance (NETSS), initiated in 1984, now connects all state health departments for the routine collection, analysis, and dissemination of notifiable disease, injury, and some nonnotifiable disease data. The computerized system allows far more case detail and analytical capability. Instead of weekly telephone transmission of aggregated information, NETSS allows individual case records to be sent to CDC. Several software tools for public health officials have been developed by CDC to complement NETSS. For example, surveillance data from NETSS are made available through the CDC's Wide-Ranging Online Data for Epidemiologic Research software (WONDER/PC). The WONDER/PC program is designed to allow rapid acquisition, summary, and analysis of public health information, such as data on the *Healthy People 2000* objectives, BRFSS summaries, and CDC reports (CDC, 1991).

The success of computerized surveillance with NETSS is attributable to several factors. First, because of the software's flexibility, each state's epidemiology staff can customize it and adapt it to their own forms and procedures. Secondly, a standardized record format was adopted, so that records sent to CDC are recoded uniformly by the software program for ease of national aggregation and state comparisons (Dean, Fagan, &

Panter-Connah, 1994). While it is perhaps the most impressive national system of computerized data-gathering, NETSS is only the beginning of a whole new level of rapid surveillance that is technologically possible with the catalyst of computers.

DOMINANT FORCES SHAPING CONTEMPORARY HEALTH MEASUREMENT

The growing demands upon the health care system created by an aging society have generated difficult and persistent health policy problems. As life expectancy in the United States has continued to increase, so has the social burden associated with chronic conditions. The overall burden of chronic illness and disability is predicted to grow well into the next century, because the elderly are at much higher risk for chronic conditions, and their numbers are expected to increase. Today, roughly 35 million Americans are sixty-five years or older. By 2040, the number of elderly is expected to more than double, so that one in five Americans will be sixty-five years or older.

The dominant health care policy issues over the past three decades, shaped by the growth in chronic disease, have been inequities in access to care, the rapid escalation of costs, and concerns about the appropriateness and quality of care. These issues have driven most of the contemporary developments in health measurement.

Concerns for Health Care Equity

As technological developments in diagnosis and treatment of chronic illness increased and care became centered in the hospital, the costs of medical care to achieve a longer life became an expense the average American could not afford. In the late 1940s and early 1950s, private health insurance proved to be a significant safeguard for the middle class against increasing hospital costs. As competition in the health insurance industry grew, companies began to offer reduced premiums and broader plans for low-risk persons. "Experience rating" meant higher premiums for people with disabilities and the elderly, the groups most likely to have a chronic condition. Those most likely to need insurance were thus least able to afford it.

In the late 1950s, inequitable access to health care became an issue of social justice with political implications. Relieving the elderly of the high costs of medical treatments and hospitalization became a particular concern. While the retired elderly required considerably more hospital care than other age groups, fewer of them had insurance coverage, and because they lived on fixed incomes, most lacked the resources to pay for services out-of-pocket. Although the Kerr-Mills Act of 1960 intended to close the access gap for the medically indigent elderly through matching federal funds to states, the Social Security Administration's 1963 Survey of the Aged found that only 50 percent of the elderly had any form of health insurance. In the face of rapidly escalating hospital expenditures, this evidence was sufficient for Congress to enact the Medicare and Medicaid amendments in 1965, which provided direct coverage for the elderly and poor (Dobson & Bialek, 1985). These laws marked the beginning of a much stronger role for government in health care. The federal government became the largest health insurance payer in the country and, with this responsibility, needed far more information about its investment in health care to determine whether the gaps in access to care were being addressed.

In 1977, the first of several national surveys of personal health care costs was conducted. Referred to as the National Medical Care Expenditure Survey (NMCES) and conducted by the National Center for Health Services Research (currently known as the Agency for Health Care Policy and Research [AHCPR]), it was repeated a decade later.[24] Sources of access-to-care information in the intervening years included the NCHS's 1980 National Medical Care Utilization and Expenditure Survey (NMCUES) and the often-cited private-sector household surveys conducted by the Robert Wood Johnson Foundation in 1982 and 1986.

On a more regular basis, annual estimates of health insurance coverage for the entire population have been calculated from the Current Population Survey (CPS) every year since 1980. In addition, the NCHS administers a Health Insurance Supplement to the NHIS every few years (Brown, 1989). All these efforts have contributed information on personal health expenditures and/or sources of payment, subjects that quickly became and remain leading health policy concerns. Analysis of the data has been essential in documenting differences in insurance coverage, health status, and access to health care in this country.

Aday and Andersen made an important contribution to the understanding of access-to-care issues in the early 1970s. Funded initially by the Robert Wood Johnson Foundation, they explored and formulated indicators of access to health services that could be applied to a variety of health systems (Aday & Andersen, 1975). Besides developing process and outcome indicators to measure access (e.g., whether a person has a regular source of care, travel time to one's place of care), they conceptualized the dimensions of access to care, laying out relationships between characteristics of the individual, the health delivery system, utilization of services, and consumer satisfaction. Elements of this framework have been used to structure numerous large-scale national surveys. Aday and Andersen's concepts have substantially influenced the work of other researchers, and they remain the classic model for evaluating access to health care.

The Rising Costs of Health Care

By the early 1970s, health care costs had accelerated so dramatically that the dominant national concern about access to care was replaced by the urgent need to restrain health care inflation. Under a cost-based, retrospective payment system used by both private and government payers, the costs of new technology were absorbed by the insurer, insulating the consumer from the magnitude of the costs. Community hospitals were able to afford the latest innovations, and they competed to be the first to do so. Incentives to use less expensive forms of care that may have been more appropriate did not exist. While it was evident in congressional hearings in the early 1970s that access to health care and the availability of services in some locations were still problems, the most serious question was how to control costs.

Calculating U.S. Health Care Costs

The first estimate of total U.S. expenditures for health was probably made in 1929 by the Committee on the Costs of Medical Care; total expenditures were estimated at $4 billion, with the largest portion going for physician services (Committee on the Costs of Medical Care, 1932). In the late 1940s, the SSA began publishing annual accounts of health outlays in two series: one reporting private consumer expenditures and data relating to voluntary (private) health insurance, and the other addressing social welfare programs, including public health expenditures. In 1962, the SSA's Division of Research and Statistics combined elements from the two reports and, for the first time, reported national expenditures by type of service and source of funds for a calendar year. By 1962, the nation's tab for health care was $32 billion, three-fourths of it paid by the private sector, and hospitals had replaced physicians as the largest single expenditure item (Reed & Rice, 1964).

Following the creation of Medicare and Medicaid, the public sector share of the nation's health bill grew rapidly, and information about health expenditures was integral to evaluation of these new programs. Regular information from the SSA was distributed in many formats, including popular chart books, first produced in 1969. Well received by a diverse group of users, they simply portrayed how much was being spent and for what services, what changes were occurring over time, and who was paying for it. Background books, beginning with *Medical Care Costs and Prices: Background Book,* detailed such information and included short interpretations. These proved particularly useful to policymakers during and after the Economic Stabilization Period (1971 to 1974), as the health care sector's inflation rate far outpaced that of the general economy, and effects of the freezes could be evaluated.[25] While national figures were still being produced with calculators and attention to consistent methodology, trends in health care spending were becoming apparent to a wider population than policymakers alone. The country began to envision health care through a highly influential indicator—the size of its budget.

When the policy focus turned to costs, studies of particular diseases or health conditions began to include financial analyses within their measure of impact upon society. The President's Commission on Heart Disease, Cancer, and Stroke set a precedent in the mid-1960s by requesting a determination of the total costs (including the indirect costs to society) of these diseases—the foremost killers of Americans. The methodology used for this project was applied to all diseases in the 1966 PHS publication *Estimating the Cost of Illness* (Rice, 1966), which became the model for most of the economic analyses that have followed, many of which address chronic conditions.

Figures for total expenditures by programs and type of services continue to be produced regularly, chiefly by the Health Care Financing Administration (HCFA) since its establishment in 1978; however, the cost estimates have been shaped over the years by changing policy concerns. Expenditures have been disaggregated by age groups (distinguishing the aged from the nonaged and later separating children's costs), by states as their budgets grew unwieldy, and most recently, by businesses, households, or governments (Rice, Anderson, & Cooper, 1968; Cowan & McDonnell, 1993).

Health Information for Planning and Regulation

As the country grew increasingly aware of the high price being paid for health services, several government initiatives were applied to stem the escalating costs. One of these efforts held great potential for expanding the health information infrastructure at the same time. The National Health Planning and Resources Development Act (passed in early 1975) authorized a network of over two hundred areawide planning agencies, known as Health Systems Agencies (HSAs), to plan for the health care needs of a community and to regulate medical facility development and the use of new technology. Composed of both providers and consumers of health care services, HSAs were required by law to base their annual plans on data about the health status of their residents, information on health care delivery systems and their effectiveness, health resources in the area, utilization patterns, and environmental factors.[26] In addition, states were to designate a State Health Planning and Development Agency and establish a State Health Coordinating Council for HSAs. Local HSAs were the key organizations, however; they not only assessed and planned for the community, but also acted as regulators, determining the need for health facilities, reviewing hospital requests for major capital improvements, and making recommendations to the state (Larson, 1991).

Because HSA decisions were to be based on community-level data that were rarely available, the National Health Planning Act officially authorized HEW to help states develop a cooperative system for producing uniform and comparable health statistics for use by all levels of government. This was an endorsement of the already established Cooperative Health Statistics System (CHSS),[27] which NCHS had proposed in 1969 to meet the information needs of all levels of users. Because much of the information available at the time came from national surveys, the geographic detail required for planning at the state and local levels could not be attained. The need for small area data led to the idea of developing national statistics by aggregating data from the smallest levels up to the national level. The experience with vital statistics demonstrated that this was possible, but that it would take many years to achieve accurate and reliable data. The objectives of the CHSS included

1. development of uniform definitions and standards to permit comparison of data among states and local areas, and national aggregation of state data;

2. collection of data at the state level, although not necessarily by a state agency (these statistics could be used by all levels—local, state, and national);
3. one-time processing of data;
4. analysis and use of collected data for local health planning and development;
5. use of the Cooperative System by federal agencies needing health statistics;
6. national data collection at lower cost owing to decentralized operation (Moshman Associates, 1980, I-4).

The NCHS set up the system to capture a broad variety of health information, categorized into seven components. Besides vital statistics and health interview survey information, statistics were to be collected on health facilities, health manpower, hospital care, long-term care, and ambulatory care. States were contracted to collect specific minimum data sets and to submit data meeting quality standards with timely delivery. It was assumed that there would be adequate resources for the phased-in development of CHSS and that within a reasonable time, usable data for at least several data components would be available.

Until such data were available, states and local HSAs were faced with either using mortality data as a proxy for disease and disability prevalence or collecting richer data with local surveys. Recognizing that states and local HSAs would need considerable support to achieve the health assessment requirements of the act, NCHS advised the use of existing vital statistics, using mortality rates as proxies for serious deficiencies in the health care delivery system. NCHS also developed short-term training courses for planners in the use of health data and provided technical assistance to HSAs in the form of the regular publication *Statistical Notes for Health Planners.* If the goals of a coordinated health information system were to be achieved, however, considerably more was needed; therefore, the director of NCHS in the late 1970s called for strong, well-staffed state centers for health statistics in each state, to serve as centers for assembly and analysis of all health data, collection of primary data, and consultation with HSAs (Rice & Kleinman, 1977).

By 1979, NCHS had awarded contracts to forty-eight states for one or more of the seven components of health information, at a federal cost of roughly $8 million annually. A 1980 evaluation of the CHSS noted serious problems with the system, such as chronic underfunding at both the federal and state levels.[28] At the state level, legislatures were becoming skeptical about the benefit of federal dollars always accompanied by substantial federal requirements. In addition, state agencies were unable to ensure that federal monies flowed directly to the data programs rather than to general funds. At the federal level, proposed budgets were never fully funded, and some agencies that originally supported the program had stopped participating and shut off financial contribution. Questions arose as to whether the collection of national data and the development of state agencies to collect data were even compatible goals. Only vital statistics data seemed to have value to all users (Moshman Associates, 1980).

The expectations for the Cooperative Health Statistics System were extremely high. The 1980 CHSS evaluation panel stated in its final report:

> It was unrealistic to expect that national statistics for data components other than vital statistics could be developed in a short period through a bottom-up system of aggregation. A developmental period of considerable length is needed before data can be collected and compiled successfully and before benefits similar to those of the vital statistics program can be realized. . . . The NCHS emphasis on data component contracts has fostered unrealistic expectations about the availability of national data. Many observers assumed that implemented contracts with the States would result in a reliable product within a matter of months, not years, and that the products of these contracts would then be aggregated. (Moshman Associates, 1980, II-11)

The panel recommended development of a long-term funding plan to support state CHSS agencies with direct federal funding for purchasing data and building competence within the agencies. The panel further recommended that the collection of national data on health manpower and health facilities be turned over to the Bureau of Health Professions and HCFA, respectively, because the bottom-up approach of data collection had been particularly ineffective in producing usable national data for these components (Moshman Associates, 1980).

As states were assigned more responsibility for their destiny under the Reagan administration's concept of "new federalism," federal funding for health planning was decreased beginning in the early 1980s. NCHS activities in support of state data collection were either cut back or eliminated. By 1986, federal support for HSAs ended, and states were left to fund them; as a result, many closed. The HSAs relied on state measures of mortality and some morbidity figures, broken down by county. With even less money after 1986 to fund HSA activities, progress in data collection at the state and community level was set back seriously.

Despite the lack of financial support, the structure for better health data had been established and was spurred by the health planning efforts of the 1970s. By 1980, twenty-seven states had designated state CHSS Agencies, and today all fifty states have state centers for health statistics. Since the early 1980s, NCHS's support of state centers has been limited to biennial national meetings, periodic newsletters, and technical assistance when requested by the states themselves. Because no federal financial assistance has been available since the early 1980s, the level of development of each center is largely dependent on state funding. Thus, there is wide variation in the centers' capabilities, authority, and situation within state government. In some states, the centers play a pivotal role in information and policy development, while in others, their role is limited to the collection and analysis of vital statistics (National Committee on Vital and Health Statistics, 1993).

Administrative Databases: Another Source for Data

While government monies were being cut for state centers, the need for state-level information about health care expenditures continued to grow. Employers, business coalitions, organized labor, and consumer organizations pushed for public disclosure of comparable information, particularly concerning hospital costs. The era of health care consumerism had begun. Comparable information about the use and costs of services was needed to make meaningful distinctions among providers, to evaluate performance, and to purchase services wisely (Epstein, 1992).

Every encounter between a patient and a health care provider generates a record; clinical and administrative records, therefore, were obvious sources of readily available health information, particularly regarding utilization and costs. Because the largest health care expenditures were generated in hospitals, statewide hospital databases began to proliferate in the 1980s, with each state designing its own system. The power of hospital data as an analytical tool quickly became apparent, particularly patient-level discharge abstracts, which contain patient demographic information (e.g., age, sex, race), provider identification, clinical information (e.g., diagnoses and procedures), and billing and payer information. With these data, states have been able to study, compare, and in a few states, even regulate reimbursement rates based on their data sets.

Besides informing cost-control policy within states, hospital data sets continue to be used for at least four other purposes. First, they have enabled the population-based study of variation in medical practice. The finding that rates for particular procedures (e.g., hysterectomies) vary greatly depending on the geographic location where they are performed led to a new field of study in physician practice patterns. Furthermore, these studies revealed the need for national guidelines for medical practice based on medical effectiveness and outcomes studies. Hospital discharge databases can also be used as a surveillance system for certain public health objectives. Some health problems, such as severe injuries, can be monitored for incidence, treatment outcomes, and evaluation of prevention efforts, because the database contains 100 percent of severe injury events in the state. Health service researchers have also tapped hospital data to examine differences in access to hospital care among population subgroups. Finally, states have used hospital data to promote competition and prudent purchasing, by preparing periodic reports that compare hospital utilization, costs, and in at least one state, rudimentary information about the quality of care.

Twenty-eight states currently maintain hospital discharge database programs that collect patient-level data across all payers. Unfortunately, the methods that states use to collect and analyze data vary widely. One of three data collection means is generally used: HCFA's UB-82 (a uniform bill), the Uniform Hospital Discharge Data Set (a standard abstract form developed in the 1970s), or a tool unique to the state's system. Recognizing that the application of hospital data could be even broader if data collection methods were standardized, the National Association of Health Data Organizations was established in 1986. Its mission is to support public health data organizations and to promote uniformity of health data collection and dissemination among public and private users (Epstein, 1992).

Building on the richness of data on hospital cost and utilization available in state records, the federal government has developed a multistate hospital data system to be used for health services research and health policy analysis. Conducted by the AHCPR, the Healthcare Cost and Utilization Project (HCUP) is designed to produce national and state estimates based on comparable data obtained through statewide reporting systems. Data from the project span the period 1988–94 and include 20 percent of U.S. hospitals.[29] The primary goal of the project is to build a federal-state-industry partnership in health care data that will become a national resource for evaluating health system reforms (USPHS Task Force on State and Community Data, 1993).

Federal Claims Data

Through HCFA, the federal government has also created a rich source of health information for the elderly and disabled populations, based primarily on their computerized bills. As a prototype for the integration of data, the Medicare Provider Analysis and Review file (MEDPAR) links demographic information on individuals (e.g., age, gender, race, and residence), drawn from their eligibility files, to information on diagnoses and treatment from Part A (hospital) and Part B (physician and outpatient care) claims files. Building on the MEDPAR files, the National Claims History File includes not only claims data but additional clinical information abstracted from medical records; the result is a Uniform Clinical Data Set (UCDS)[30] for a random sample of beneficiaries. This data set can be further linked to the Medicare Beneficiary Health Status Registry and the Medicare Current Beneficiary Survey, as well as other beneficiary surveys as they are developed, to create the most integrated set of health care data in the country.

Such data integration is possible because a single payer, the federal government, administers the Medicare program. This level of standardization and data management is not possible in the Medicaid program (which is jointly administered and funded by the states and the federal governments) or in the private insurance sector. In the future, however, as private health insurers respond to provider and consumer demands for billing efficiency, health care data will become more fully computerized at all levels and may become increasingly standardized if managed care systems hope to compete on the basis of comparative performance.

Measuring Health Care Quality and Value

Cost containment is also a key force advancing the issue of health care quality and how it is measured. As the health care system's high costs became apparent, Americans began to question what they were getting for their health care dollars. Public health data helped substantiate the belief that the price being paid was no longer resulting in any significant difference in health benefits. Life expectancy and many disease mortality rates in the United States have been and still are no better (and in some cases are worse) than in other developed countries, where far less is spent for health care. For some time now, U.S. health expenditures have been the highest in the world; per capita costs were 50 percent higher than in Canada and, at over $2,800 per person in 1991, nearly three times as high as in Great Britain. Over 13 percent of the U.S. gross domestic product in 1991 was spent on health care, a larger proportion than in any other country in the world (NCHS, 1993). If U.S. health care is of better quality, it may be so in ways that have not yet been measured for health policy purposes.

Another impetus for quality measurement has been the growing body of health services research documenting the wide variation in medical practice. By establishing guidelines for care, unnecessary treatment could be avoided, costs reduced, and quality improved. Information gained from measuring the quality of health care delivery can also potentially be used to evaluate and compare providers. In addition, changes in how health care is paid for, in both the Medicare and Medicaid programs as well as the growth of prepaid health care systems, have heightened worries about incentives for underservice (Webber, 1988).

Public Sector Initiatives in Quality Assurance

With the introduction of Medicare and Medicaid in 1965, the federal government took the lead in monitoring health care quality and subsequently sponsored the largest programs in this area. Prior to this, few formal efforts at quality assurance had been made, other than the work of the Joint Commission on the Accreditation of Hospitals (JCAH, now JCAHO), the voluntary accreditation body that had established minimum hospital care standards. Under Medicare/Medicaid laws, providers were required to meet specific conditions of participation, many of which related to quality of care. A survey and certification program, modeled after the JCAH survey system, was begun to monitor compliance with standards. However, the survey process has only been able to measure whether a hospital was capable of providing the required level of care, with some attention to the actual process of care; patient outcomes have not been evaluated.

In the early 1970s, the National Center for Health Services Research (of the Department of Health and Human Services) sponsored programs of utilization review and quality assurance in experimental medical care review organizations (EMCROs). These voluntary associations of physicians reviewed hospital and outpatient services paid by Medicare or Medicaid, but they focused primarily on utilization review. Although no evaluations of EMCROs were ever conducted, their largest contribution perhaps consisted of demonstrating that monitoring could be achieved through local physician peer groups (Lohr & Brook, 1984).

Grappling with Medicare's rapid cost escalation as early as 1972, Congress established the Professional Standards Review Organization (PSRO) program. Its purpose was to ensure "1) that services were being provided economically and only when medically necessary; and 2) that services were of a quality that met professionally recognized standards of health care" (Webber, 1988). PSROs were nonprofit, locally based, and like EMCROs, run principally by physicians. At the peak of the program, 195 PSRO areas were identified, each covering about one million people, thirty-five hospitals, and two to three thousand physicians (Lohr & Brook, 1984). Quality standards were set locally, and the focus was hospital services; reviews were conducted by the hospitals themselves. PSROs developed a data management system that included demographic and hospitalization information for every Medicare and Medicaid hospital admission in their areas, from which provider profiles could be developed. In turn, these provider profiles were shared with the providers and practitioners in the area, as a means of effecting clinical practice changes. PSROs were also given the authority to recommend that specific practitioners and providers be excluded from participation in the Medicare program. They could also recommend denial of payment, but could not make the final determination; in practice, very few payments were rejected during the PSRO program.

During the 1970s, the PSRO program struggled to establish its contribution. It became a substantial element of the federal health budget and disbursed most of its resources on utilization review activities rather than quality assurance (Lohr & Brook, 1984). The physician community ceased supporting PSRO activities when the cost-containment emphasis overshadowed quality monitoring. Given the costs of the program itself, Congress called for evaluations and concluded that it was not cost effective. While the new Reagan administration called for PSROs to be phased out (just as it had done with the health planning program of the 1970s), Congress was not ready to eliminate them. The Utilization and Quality Control Peer Review Organization (PRO) program was established in

1982 to carry on the major objectives of PSROs, while reshaping their operations considerably.

Some of the major changes enacted included consolidating review areas (with roughly one PRO area per state), granting PROs final authority to deny payment, and precluding hospitals from performing their own utilization reviews (although many continue to do so as a preventive monitor). In addition, with the introduction of the prospective payment system (PPS) for hospital reimbursement, the functions of PROs were expanded in several ways, not only to monitor cost-containment concerns and overuse but also to assess for underservice related to the incentives of the new system. In fact, the PPS generated renewed support for PROs, particularly with regard to its function in quality monitoring.

While Congress clearly intended that PROs focus on cost containment, quality assurance features also evolved through PROs' two-year contracts, referred to as "Scopes of Work." PROs began to identify individual cases of poor care by using "generic quality screens." These screens helped nurse reviewers flag patient records for physician reviewers to determine whether a problem existed or not. However, neither the efforts to bolster quality assurance nor the structural changes that Congress intended to improve cost control have succeeded in making any substantial differences as evaluated through government performance reviews (Hayes, Lundber, & Ballard, 1994).

As early as 1986, Congress called for strategies to improve quality assurance in Medicare, legislating that the National Academy of Science appoint a committee to study the issue. The IOM released the committee's report in 1990 and recommended that Medicare costs be the responsibility of fiscal intermediaries, leaving PROs to work solely on quality assurance with hospital committees. HCFA instead chose to revamp the PRO program under the Health Care Quality Improvement Initiative (HCQII). The primary goals of the HCQII are to provide information to providers about the patterns and outcomes of care, to change practice behaviors and improve care for Medicare beneficiaries. Patterns of care are to be analyzed using small-area analysis, a method developed initially by Wennberg and Gittlesohn. However, to accomplish this effectively, PROs will need more sophisticated information.

HCFA provides the PROs with several data sets, including the MEDPAR analytic file, which consists of inpatient claims data, population data, practitioner data, and reference files such as the Area Resource

File. Recognizing the weaknesses of these databases, however, HCFA is developing the Uniform Clinical Data Set (UCDS), a rich set of abstracted clinical data from the patient record, which will allow far more objective and sophisticated quality review. However, the development of the UCDS for quality review purposes has been difficult and stormy, and currently it has been scaled back from its original broad application to condition-specific analyses (Hayes et al., 1994).

In addition to a more complete database, PROs will need professional staff with health services research skills and the ability to educate providers and practitioners and assist them in creating lasting changes in the way health care is delivered (Hayes et al., 1994). While focusing only on the Medicare population and for the most part on hospital care, the HCQII is another example of the current push for improved measures of quality and patient outcomes.

Public Sector Leadership in Standardizing Medical Practices

Policymakers, frustrated by the failure of many cost-containment efforts in the 1980s, grew interested in the potential of clinical practice guidelines.[31] For many years, professional and provider organizations in the private sector had been creating and disseminating practice guidelines with varying degrees of sophistication and adoption by health care providers. In 1989, federal legislation created the AHCPR in an effort to encourage private and public sector work in this area as part of a broader mission to enhance the quality, appropriateness, and effectiveness of health care services and access to these services. A significant part of the agency's charge included medical effectiveness research (e.g., studies in variation in clinical practice and patient outcomes research) and the development of clinical practice guidelines. It is hoped that "scientific evidence and clinical judgment can be systematically combined to produce clinically valid, operational recommendations for appropriate care that can and will be used to persuade clinicians, patients, and others to change their practices in ways that lead to better health outcomes and lower health care costs" (Field & Lohr, 1992).

Expectations for practice guidelines run high; however, success in achieving these goals depends upon fundamental conditions that currently do not exist. Perhaps the most basic of these is sufficient scientific evidence upon which to base guidelines, so that a significant number of practice changes can be made in the near future. Medical effectiveness research must accelerate. Because a broader conceptualization of out-comes is being used in this research (e.g., symptom states, functional sta-tus, emotional and cognitive states, and dissatisfaction with health care), the need grows for more and better methods of measuring health-related quality of life (Field & Lohr, 1992).

Quality Monitoring by the Private Sector

The need for better health-related quality-of-life indicators has also been stimulated by the total quality management (TQM) movement in the health care industry.[32] Corporate America began applying TQM principles in the late 1970s, significantly shifting Americans' quality ex-pectations by changing the management paradigm to one in which goods and services are produced to meet customers' needs and expectations and provide true value for the money. TQM was first adopted by the health care sector in 1985, when the John Hartford Foundation funded the Na-tional Demonstration Project on Quality Improvement in Health Care, testing whether the principles could be applied effectively. The results were positive, launching the TQM movement in hospitals (Widtfeldt & Widtfeldt, 1992).

The spread of the TQM process in hospitals has been rapid. A 1992 hospital survey found that of 781 responding hospitals, almost 60 per-cent had TQM programs running, and three-fourths of those without a program reported plans to initiate one in the next year. Survey projec-tions indicated that about 3,100 hospitals (with fifty or more beds) had TQM programs in place; however, most programs were less than two years old (Grayson, 1992). TQM has become a large and lucrative busi-ness, packaged as an educational program by consultants as well as by more seasoned hospitals and health care organizations, although not all with the same knowledge and experience base (Burda, 1991).

The basic elements of the TQM process involve

1. efforts to know the customer ever more deeply and to link that knowledge ever more closely to the day-to-day activities of the or-ganization;
2. efforts to mold the culture of the organization, largely through deeds of leaders, to foster pride, joy, collaboration, and scientific thinking;
3. efforts to continuously increase knowledge of and control over variation in the processes of work through the widespread use of

scientific methods of data collection and analysis and action on data. (Berwick, 1991)

It is the use of scientific methods (i.e., the ability to quantify variation in practice and outcomes in particular) that further underscores the need for more refined indicators of patient outcomes and methods of measurement.

Consumerism and "Health Report Cards"

Demands for accessible health outcome measures are also being made by many consumers, particularly large business employers. The concept of a "report card" for health plans emerged from this rising consumerism. While the idea that health plans produce comparable summaries of the quality of care they provide appears modest on the surface, some estimate that it will take even the most advanced organizations five, ten, or even fifteen years to produce valid and reliable health report cards (Zimmerman, 1994).

Nevertheless, many initiatives have begun in the face of a daunting challenge. Development of the Health Plan Employer Data and Information Set (HEDIS), for example, was begun in 1989. Initiated by several employers and managed care organizations, it is designed to be a tool for large purchasers to use in evaluating competing health plans. The data set focuses on clinical quality, access, patient satisfaction, utilization, and financial management evaluations. In 1993, Kaiser Permanente of Northern California produced its first Quality Report Card; it contained one hundred health indicators, thirty-two of which were indicators commonly associated with public health assessment, such as low birthweight and immunization rates. While it is debatable whether such indicators are the most appropriate ones for evaluating the care delivered by a health plan, using public health assessment for quality assurance for the health care delivery system represents an interesting development.

Many diverse approaches to health report cards are now emerging. While they vary considerably, they all are fraught with similar problems, largely because of the enormous variability of existing data and information technology within and among health systems. Before health report cards are usable, sizable obstacles must be overcome, such as variations in the way conditions, procedures, and patient disposition are coded; the questionable validity of the "grades," given the ease of manipulation in many cases; resistance from practitioners and providers concerned with growing external control over practices; and lack of consistency in the kinds of data being requested by consumers (Zimmerman, 1994).

As the decision makers for Medicare and Medicaid payment, federal lawmakers agree that the current state of health information is inadequate for the consumer-like decisions before them. Most health care reform bills introduced in 1993 and 1994 called for improvements in the country's health information system; many addressed the need for better data on health costs, utilization, and quality of care, but few identified the means of accomplishing it.

Whether these efforts to simplify health system evaluation with report cards will ultimately be integrated into national health care policy remains to be seen. Policymakers will need to address the many barriers precluding a quick solution, including the costs of supplementing the current national data infrastructure. However, current efforts to measure health status and interventions accurately, even within the smallest private sector organizations, strengthen support for improved health indicators and can only serve to advance the field of health measurement.

Quality Monitoring and the Future of Health Indicators

The wave of quality monitoring exemplified by medical effectiveness research, practice guidelines development, the Medicare program's PRO activities, and by the TQM movement and health report cards in the private sector imposes formidable health information demands. Patrick and Bergner (1990) believe that these forces, as well as the need for better information for health policy decisions, will direct the development or adaptation of health indicators by demanding

1. Short, reliable, self-administered, comprehensive measures that are sensitive to variations in health care organization and medical practice
2. Specific measures to supplement generic measures of health-related quality of life
3. Measures that assess the health outcome of preventive services, health promotion, and health protection
4. Measures that combine quantity and quality of life so that remaining years of life are adjusted for some measure of positive or negative health
5. The application of instruments in effectiveness studies to measure change over time

The measurement of health status has advanced considerably over the past forty years, producing a wide variety of health-related quality-of-life measures. Entire texts are now available that cover the breadth of the subject.[33] Many of the newer indicators measure the separate domains of health status as articulated in the WHO definition of health. While the WHO definition seemed impractical and unmeasurable when it was first introduced, methods of measuring physical, mental, and social well-being have subsequently been developed, and the definition in turn has become more meaningful (McDowell & Newell, 1987). Other health indicators combine different components of health or mortality and morbidity data to produce an aggregated index of health. Still others have been designed to allow comparison among diverse health interventions. For example, the Quality of Well-Being Scale, developed by Kaplan and associates, ascribes a social preference to a specific health state (described by morbidity, functional status, and prognosis), resulting in numerical expressions for all health states, which are preference weighted and can therefore be ranked according to their relative importance (Kaplan, 1988).

While all these health indicators measure aspects of health in a far more comprehensive and meaningful way than simple mortality and morbidity data, they are often complex and lengthy, difficult to interpret, and potentially costly to administer (Steinwachs, 1989). The application of health-related quality-of-life measures to today's health policy questions will depend on the availability of valid and reliable tools and on whether they are efficient methods that can be integrated into existing health data collection efforts and coupled with data on health care use and costs (Steinwachs, 1989). Unfortunately, many methodological issues remain to be resolved.

CONCLUSION: LESSONS FROM THE PAST

In light of the attention currently focused on health care reform and the associated surge of interest in health measurement, a look back at the history of health indicators in the United States provides many useful insights. While some health indicators and information systems have successfully endured social reform, political change, and even lean budget years, others have not. Lessons can be learned from them all.

Health indicators, like social indicators in general, should serve an ultimate goal (Mootz, 1988). Careful analyses are important to the interpretation and usefulness of indicators, because collections of statistics by themselves are far less likely to survive budget cuts and social change. A good example is the series of three *Social Indicators* reports produced in the 1970s. Their strength lies in the appearance of being an impartial rendering of the facts of the situation, but their weakness is in leaving the reader to determine their meaning. In reality, choices about selection and reporting of data have been made: either the statistician has relied on previous methods, which does not advance general understanding, or has applied his or her personal perspective to organize the facts without openly sharing the interpretation.

Innes (1975) contends that "the way we measure things does make a difference to the way we think about things" and that by understanding and controlling the choice of indicators, better public decision making is possible. She proposes several criteria of good social indicators, i.e., those that will further public decisions. An indicator should be pertinent to questions of concern and be understood and accepted by all its users. An indicator needs to be trusted as reliably produced and capable of measuring what it says it does without hidden bias. Furthermore, the concepts underlying the indicator should be clear, and it should relate to a more complex theoretical framework.

Institutionalization of Health Indicators

Innes (1975) also formulated a short list of factors that are associated with successful indicators, those that have become institutionalized. When several of these factors are present, the chances are increased that the indicator will establish itself as a mainstay in public decision making. The term "institutionalization" as applied to social indicators means "the establishment of procedures and practices to ensure the continuing existence of an indicator and which legitimizes and formalizes its methods and concepts" (180). While Innes's work focused on single social measures, such as the unemployment rate, it seems applicable to the success or failure of health measurement systems as well.

According to Innes, an important factor in the institutionalization of social measures is the reputation of the agency that collects and manipulates the data; it must be respected and not subject to immediate political control. Such was not the case in the 1970s, when HSAs were authorized to take a larger role in local data collection and use. There was little confidence in the ability of the small, newly organized planning units to accomplish the necessary assessment, particularly since realistic funding levels were never achieved (another important factor in successful institutionalization). The lack of objective local data no doubt contributed to the inability of HSAs to insulate themselves from local interests and in turn to control technological expansion. Furthermore, the planning and data infrastructures were tied to the belief that health care needed to be more carefully regulated; thus, when political doctrine shifted to the "new federalism" of the 1980s, there was little to sustain the sophisticated plans for integrated local, state, and national data.

Data also need to be presented in a nonpolitical context. Those who use the information provided annually in the *Health, United States* compendium have come to rely on its sources, which include vital statistics and NHIS results. Such data are perceived as unbiased and as such are also used by the media, further securing these indicators' roles in monitoring health trends.

Today's vital statistics system is perhaps the best example of cooperatively generated data that can be used by all levels of government: local, state, and federal. Responsibility for registration remains vested in the state and specific registration areas (such as metropolitan areas). Local registrars send vital records to the state agency, which in turn transmits the data to NCHS. Many states have adopted the standardized registration certificates developed by NCHS, but others have modified them to meet their own needs (Stroup et al., 1994). Given that all levels benefit from the information, costs are shared; the federal government purchases the data, while each state's general revenues cover the operating costs. National standards for data quality are set, and compliance is monitored by verifying random certificates. Greater accuracy is anticipated as the registration process itself becomes more fully computerized.

States recognize the value of collecting data at the local level and of being able to make interstate comparisons. While the usefulness of any set of health indicators must be apparent to secure initial support, such awareness may not suffice to maintain a monitoring system. It took over seventy-five years, for example, to recruit all states for vital registration, when the value of such information was evident. In the mid and late 1900s, it seemed unlikely that states would be able to coordinate efforts sufficiently to allow comparisons of national figures, even though some states had demonstrated the will. Complete participation in a uniform system may never have occurred had the federal government not interceded with standardized forms, training, and funds for data sharing. Finally, unlike other health indicators, the system of vital registration is sustained by the variety of uses it serves in addition to producing health information. Copies of birth and death certificates generate revenue for local and state departments, thereby creating a broader base of financial and user support than any other current health measure.

Health indicators are also likely to be sustained when arrangements exist to use the information in connection with specific policies. For example, the CDC's state-based BRFSS has fulfilled the need for data required to plan, support, and evaluate health promotion programs. By 1987, only five years after the system was pilot tested, well over half of the states had established BRFSS; by 1993, all states were participating, as the value of such data became apparent to state health promotion activities. Simple, flexible, and policy-relevant survey designs have enabled most states participating in BRFSS to apply their findings directly to state health program and policy decisions, including support for legislation to decrease smoking risk and increase seatbelt use. Statewide systems of hospital discharge data have also grown rapidly, because they too meet specific policy needs—in this case, for local health care cost and utilization statistics. Until such data are available in a more accessible form, hospital discharge abstract data will continue to be refined and relied upon as proxy information to understand broader health policy issues.

The Need for a Conceptual Framework

Another important criterion for the success of any indicator is that it relate to a larger concept or theory of social concern. Herein lies a significant shortcoming of many health measurement efforts to date. Beyond describing health phenomena, the purpose of indicators should be to explain relationships between health needs, the health care delivery system, the care process, and health outcomes. Much of the renewed interest in health measurement today is focused on the need for better outcome indicators, such as health-related quality-of-life and functional status. Outcome data are critical, because they permit broader study of the effectiveness of health interventions. However, outcome data alone do not suffice for health decisions. Indicators of health risk, as well as indicators of the process (interventions) of health care, are equally necessary if valid conclusions are to be drawn. Measures of the health system's structure, process, and outcomes need to fit into a framework, knitting individual pieces of information together, so that relationships can be constructed and interpreted. Also critical to the usefulness (and survival) of health indicators and any other conceptual model that may be applied in the future is the possibility that some of what is measured can be changed or manipulated through health policy to effect improvements in the system and better health outcomes.

The overview of health measurement provided here demonstrates that progress in health measurement has not been impeded severely by the lack of a unifying framework; however, the maturation of the field would likely be accelerated if one existed. For example, both measurement and health services research on access to care, a singular aspect of health, have been catalyzed considerably by the conceptual work of Aday and Andersen. Their framework embodies elements of structure and process (as potential barriers to care) and outcomes of health care. In addition, they identify those health system or health promotion indicators that are or are not manipulable through policy (Aday, Andersen, & Fleming, 1980). Partial health system models like this one or those that rely on available data are useful, because by applying them, health indicators become refined and fuller models are eventually reached.

WHO's *Health for All* targets and the U.S. *Healthy People 2000* objectives have contributed substantially to the conceptualization of health—first, by defining health goals and secondly, by articulating indicators that suggest both factors and strategic solutions believed to relate to the goal. These sets of health indicators are not all-inclusive, but they serve as a reasonable starting point. Recognizing the limits of these national goals (and corresponding indicators), however, is critical. While they are useful for purposes of comparison (e.g., comparing the health status of individuals in urban and rural communities), by themselves, they only begin to describe the relationships between health processes and health outcomes, which are critical to understanding why differences exist (Mootz, 1988).

In conclusion, growth in the field of health measurement has been particularly rapid since the 1960s, largely because of expanding health policy needs. Given the vigor of current political forces behind improved health measurement and the need for a better information infrastructure, the field has never been supported more broadly. Now it is being pressed to contribute to solving the country's financial crisis. Interpreting health trends is at least as important, if not more so, as devising new indicators, particularly those related to healthy aging and the management of chronic conditions. As partial models of chronic conditions—the nation's number one public health concern—begin to coalesce, work in the field of health indicators will become more efficiently focused and responsive to public policy needs.

Notes

1. The Massachusetts State Board of Health in 1874 was first to establish a voluntary plan for weekly physician reporting (by postcard) of prevalent diseases (Chorba et al., 1989).

2. *Public Health Reports* continued to publish weekly morbidity reports until the late 1940s, when the National Office of Vital Statistics assumed responsibility. In 1952, mortality data were added to the published summaries, which would eventually mature into the *Morbidity and Mortality Weekly Report (MMWR)* (Thacker & Berkelman, 1988).

3. Efforts to control malaria included ditch draining, use of diesel oil, and use of the newly formulated insecticide DDT. Officials agreed later that malaria had probably disappeared before the massive efforts to control it got under way.

4. As the unit grew and changed its internal structure over the years, the acronym CDC has stood for many similar but different terms.

5. At times when continued federal support for surveillance could have been decreased, several events occurred that reinforced the value of ongoing CDC surveillance activities: the Cutter incident of 1955 (where surveillance efforts revealed that live virus had been introduced accidentally into polio vaccine), the epidemic of Asian influenza in 1957, and the eradication of smallpox worldwide in the 1960s, led by the CDC (Thacker & Berkelman, 1988).

6. Notifiable disease surveillance relies primarily on case reports received from physicians, laboratories, and other health care providers. Practitioners are required by state law to mail a case report form for notifiable diseases (most of which are infectious diseases) to the state health department. Such data are usually incomplete and unrepresentative; completeness of reporting has been estimated to vary from 6 to 90 percent for many of the common diseases. Penalties exist for not reporting fully, but they are rarely imposed (Thacker & Berkelman, 1988; Chorba et al., 1989). Problems with this system are well known and stem from lack of knowledge on the part of physicians as to what is required, concerns for patient confidentiality, and perceptions that the list of conditions is too extensive. Further computerization of the system may alleviate many of the major barriers to a fully accurate and reliable system for monitoring infectious diseases and may allow tracking of a broader set of health conditions.

7. Sydenstricker cited findings from the Life Extension Institute survey, for which 100,000 men underwent health examinations conducted by general practitioners (results reported in 1930), and from the Metropolitan Life Insurance Company survey of industrial policy holders and their families, conducted in 1915–17.

8. Besides providing contributory, non-means-tested pensions, which would help pay for health care in retirement, Title I of the Social Security Act of 1935

established a "transitional" federal program of old age assistance (OAA), a non-contributory, means-tested pension, which would fill in the gaps until social security could be funded by contributions. OAA stipulated that benefits were not to be paid to those living in public institutions. However, OAA benefits could be used for the purchase of long-term care services provided in charitable and private nursing homes, which effectively shifted elderly long-term care from public almshouses into private-sector rest and convalescent homes.

9. Among the major contributors to the commission's operating expenses were the AMA (the largest private benefactor), the National Foundation for Infantile Paralysis, and the American Cancer Society. The special studies and surveys conducted by the commission were largely supported by the PHS and the Commonwealth Fund.

10. While the state health department provided personnel assistance and services, funding for the survey was provided by the commission and the Commonwealth Fund.

11. See appendix A for listing of all NCHS data sets discussed in this chapter.

12. In addition to these three national health surveys, many European countries today have continuing health surveys, most of which began in the 1970s (Armitage, 1976).

13. For those impatient with the state of health indicator knowledge and its application, it is important to note that economic indicators (the general prototype for social indicators) were being measured as early as the 1920s. The Bureau of Economic Research in the United States began accumulating and tracking hundreds of economic indices prior to the Great Depression, which eventually led to the development of theories that could predict changes in the economy based on a sophisticated subset of these indicators (Innes [de Neufville], 1975).

14. A new statistic, called the "expectancy of healthy life," was derived for the report, to recognize the impact of serious disability; it was calculated simply as life expectancy minus expected years of bed-disability and institutionalization.

15. A recent inventory of PHS data projects and systems identified seventy-six periodic general purpose surveys or supplements containing health data either currently available or planned for the near future (see the appendixes for a listing of all governmental and nongovernmental data sets discussed in this chapter). Most of these address chronic conditions, either broadly, as in the Longitudinal Studies of Aging (1984–90 and 1994–2000) (LSOAI and LSOAII) and the Access to Care Survey (ACS) (1994), or specifically, as in the Cancer Risk Factors Supplement of the NHIS and the Hispanic Health and Aging Studies (HHAS) (USPHS, 1993).

With the vast amount of information collected in large-scale surveys, it is unfortunate that no national health survey has sample sizes large enough to yield reliable state- and community-level estimates. Synthetic estimates can be derived from some of the largest surveys by using statistical models, and NCHS is working to improve these techniques. Another approach being taken by NCHS is to redesign the 1995 NHIS by stratifying within states. Still in its early development, this method could potentially yield estimates for fifteen to twenty-five states. In addition, NCHS is investigating the possibility of adding a telephone survey, which would enable estimates to be made for all states. The feasibility and costs for both projects have yet to be tested (National Committee on Vital and Health Statistics, 1993).

16. Meanwhile, Canada had already detailed a prevention policy, called *A New Perspective on the Health of Canadians,* which emphasized healthy life-styles.

17. The plan broadly framed fifteen national health strategies by identifying risk factors for the leading causes of morbidity and mortality among different age groups. These strategies were categorized further into three groups: preventive services, health protection, and health promotion objectives. To achieve a broad-based consensus, the process of developing the strategic plan was purposefully inclusive. A group of over 150 experts from the private sector was convened by the PHS; working from background papers prepared by several federal agencies, the experts were charged with developing the public drafts of objectives for the fifteen strategies. Over two thousand groups and individuals were then invited to provide feedback on the objectives before the final 1980 publication, in which 226 objectives were identified with target goals for 1990.

18. Like the earlier decade's strategies, the *Healthy People 2000* objectives (three hundred plus subobjectives) were the product of a broadly inclusive national process, and the same basic framework was applied to develop objectives for the year 2000. Facilitated by the Institute of Medicine (IOM), a consortium of nearly three hundred national organizations and all the state health departments came together with the PHS. The consortium convened regional hearings to gather testimony for use by working groups of experts, who then prepared the Year 2000 objectives.

19. Associations involved in defining the eighteen indicators included the Association of State and Territorial Health Officials, the National Association of County Health Officers, the U.S. Conference of Local Health Officers, the APHA, and the Public Health Foundation.

20. Seven states have State Assessment Initiatives funded by CDC/NCHS, ten states have planning grants from the Robert Wood Johnson Foundation, and eleven are funded by the Maternal and Child Health Bureau of the Health Resources and Services Administration (USPHS, 1993).

21. The original *Model Standards* was developed in 1976 through discussions between the CDC and several national associations. In 1977, Congress mandated the development of standards for community preventive health services, supporting this preliminary work by the collaborating associations (APHA, 1991).

22. Marshall Kreuter has written an informative history of the PATCH process, which describes how the concept emerged in 1983 as a CDC response to the federal policy shift on block grants to states. Consolidation of several grants into one "Prevention Block" coupled with decreased funding eliminated the CDC support function for state-level health education activities; however, two central components of earlier efforts were maintained: *(a)* the assessment dimension, which grew into the BRFSS, and *(b)* PATCH (Kreuter, 1992).

23. Reasons for this include competition with highly visible public health projects within departments, fragmentation of assessment efforts among state envi-

ronmental and mental health agencies when separate from the larger health department, and insufficient direct federal assistance to the states. According to the IOM report (1988), nearly 75 percent of state and local expenditures go for personal health care services, and this diversion of funds from other public health functions is worsened by the growing problem of medical indigence.

24. The 1987 version is referred to as the National Medical Expenditure Survey (NMES). The design of the two surveys was somewhat unique in that questions were asked about affective well-being and health perceptions along with extensive questions about health problems and activity limitations (Patrick & Erickson, 1993).

25. To control serious problems in inflation in the late 1960s, President Nixon froze wages and prices in the entire economy. Given the higher inflation rates within the health care sector, the economic freeze on hospitals was extended beyond that on other sectors; it was eventually lifted when its continuance would have required legislation.

26. Although the HSA framework still exists, it is no longer supported by federal funding.

27. Between 1970 and 1980, six federal laws reaffirmed the role of a cooperative system of health statistics spanning local, state, and federal levels in collecting information for health planning, health manpower reporting, and health care facilities reporting. The CHSS was not officially recognized as the system until a 1978 act directed each state to designate an agency for the administration of statistical activities.

28. While the total fiscal year 1977 appropriation for planning was $125 million, the entire national health planning effort represented less than 0.001 percent of total health care expenditures. Concerns were expressed early on that the potential for the regulatory system would be thwarted and that its effectiveness needed to be judged within these fiscal constraints (Cain & Thornberry, 1977).

29. The HCUP is the third in a series that began in 1970. The HCUP-1 and HCUP-2 databases were smaller samples drawn directly from hospital data, as opposed to data derived from statewide databases. The comparable data enabled nearly 150 different studies to be undertaken (USPHS, 1993).

30. See appendix B for listing of all HCFA data sets discussed in this chapter.

31. "Practice guidelines" is a broad term used to describe various types of statements about appropriate clinical care, for example, practice standards, protocols, and algorithms. They are systematically developed statements to assist practitioner and patient decisions about appropriate health care for specific clinical circumstances.

32. Total quality management is also known as continuous quality improvement (CQI), the quality improvement process (QIP), and perhaps more rudimentarily, industrial quality management science (IQMS).

33. Two books—McDowell and Newell (1987) and Patrick and Erickson (1993)—are particularly useful and comprehensive guides to health-related quality-of-life instruments and their applications.

References

Aday, L. A., & Andersen, R. 1975. *Development of Indices of Access to Medical Care.* Ann Arbor, Mich.: Health Administration Press.

Aday, L. A., Andersen, R., & Fleming, G. 1980. *Health Care in the U.S.: Equitable for Whom?* Beverly Hills, Calif.: Sage Publications.

American Public Health Association. 1991. *Healthy Communities 2000 Model Standards.* Washington, D.C.: APHA.

American Public Health Association. 1993. *The Guide To Implementing Model Standards.* Washington, D.C.: APHA.

Armitage, P. 1976. National health survey systems in the European Community. *International Journal of Epidemiology 5:* 321–26.

Bauer, R. A. 1966. *Social Indicators.* Cambridge, Mass.: MIT Press.

Berkman, L., & Breslow, L. 1983. *Health and Ways of Living, The Alameda County Study* (pp. 3–60). New York: Oxford University Press.

Berwick, D. M. 1991. Controlling variation in health care: A consultation from Walter Shewhart. *Medical Care 29:* 1212–25.

Brown, E. R. 1989. Access to health insurance in the United States. *Medical Care Review 46:* 349–85.

Burda, D. 1991. Total quality management becomes big business. *Modern Healthcare* (January 28, 1991): 25–29.

Bureau of the Census, U.S. Department of Commerce. 1980. *Social Indicators III.* Washington, D.C.: Government Printing Office.

Cain, H., & Thornberry, H. 1977. Health planning in the Unites States: Where we stand today. In *Health Goals and Health Indicators: Policy, Planning, and Evaluation.* Boulder, Colo.: Westview Press.

Caplan, N., & Barton, E. 1978. The potential of social indicators: minimum conditions for impact at the national level as suggested by a study of the use of "social indicators" 73. *Social Indicators Research 5:* 427–56.

Centers for Disease Control and Prevention. 1991. National electronic telecommunications system for surveillance—United States, 1990–1991. *Morbidity and Mortality Weekly Report 400:* 02–03.

Chorba, T., Berkelman, R., Safford, S., Gibbs, N., & Hall, H. 1989. Mandatory reporting of infectious diseases by clinicians. *Journal of the American Medical Association 262:* 3018–26.

Commission on Chronic Illness. 1957. *Chronic Illness in the United States, Prevention of Chronic Illness* (pp. 285–311). Cambridge, Mass.: Harvard University Press.

Committee on the Costs of Medical Care. 1932. *Medical Care for the American People; The Final Report of the Committee on the Costs of Medical Care.* Chicago: University of Chicago Press.

Cowan, C., & McDonnell, P. 1993. Business, households, and governments: Health spending, 1991. *Health Care Financing Review 14:* 227–48.

Culyer, A. J. 1983. *Health Indicators—An International Study for the European Science Foundation* (pp. 1–22). New York: St. Martin's Press.

Dean, A. G., Fagan, R. F., & Panter-Connah, B. J. 1994. Computerizing public health surveillance systems. In S. M. Teutsch & R. E. Churchill (eds.), *Principles and Practice of Public Health Surveillance* (pp. 200–17). New York: Oxford University Press.

Department of Health, Education, and Welfare (DHEW). Series for 1960–66. *Health, Education, and Welfare Indicators*. Washington, D.C.: Government Printing Office.

Department of Health, Education, and Welfare. Series Supplements for 1960–1963. *Health, Education, and Welfare Trends*. Washington, D.C.: Government Printing Office.

Department of Health, Education, and Welfare. 1977. *Health, United States, 1976–1977*. (Foreword). Washington, D.C.: Government Printing Office.

Dobson, A., & Bialek, R. 1985. Shaping public policy from the perspective of a data builder. *Health Care Financing Review 6*: 117–34.

Duncan, J. W., & Shelton, W. C. 1978. *Revolution in United States Government Statistics 1926–1976* (pp. 200–13). U.S. Department of Commerce—Office of Federal Statistical Policy and Standards. Washington, D.C.: Government Printing Office.

Epstein, M. 1992. Guest alliance: Uses of state-level hospital discharge databases. *Journal of AHIMA 63*: 32–37.

Etheridge, E. 1992. *Sentinel for Health—A History of the Centers for Disease Control* (pp. xv–xix; 276–87). Berkeley, Calif.: University of California Press.

Ferriss, A. L. 1979. The U.S. federal effort in developing social indicators. *Social Indicators Research 6*: 129–52.

Field, M. J., & Lohr, K. N. (eds.) 1992. *Guidelines for Clinical Practice—From Development to Use. Institute of Medicine—Committee on Clinical Practice Guidelines*. Washington, D.C.: National Academy Press.

Fox, D. 1989. Policy and epidemiology: Financing health services for the chronically ill and disabled, 1930–1990. *The Milbank Quarterly 67* (suppl. 2, pt. 2): 57–87.

Grayson, M. A. 1992. Benchmark TQM survey tracks a new management era in administration. *Hospitals* (June 5, 1992): 36.

Hayes, R. P., Lundber, M. T., & Ballard, D. J. 1994. Peer review organizations: Scientific challenges in HCFA's health care quality improvement initiative. *Medical Care Review 51*: 39–60.

Innes (de Neufville), J. 1975. *Social Indicators and Public Policy* (pp. 40–56; 57–59; 180–95). New York: Elsevier Scientific Publishing Company.

Institute of Medicine, Committee for the Study of the Future of Public Health. 1988. *The Future of Public Health*. Washington, D.C.: National Academy Press.

Kaplan, R. 1988. New health promotion indicators: The general health policy model. *Health Promotion 3*: 35–49.

Kreuter, M. 1992. PATCH: Its origin, basic concepts, and links to contemporary public health policy. *Journal of Health Education 23*: 135–39.

Land, K., & Spilerman, S. 1975. *Social Indicator Models* (pp. 5–14). New York: Russell Sage Foundation.

Larson, J. 1991. *The Measurement of Health—Concepts and Indicators* (pp. 77–86). New York: Greenwood Press.

Lawrence, P. 1976. The health record of the American people. In *Health in America 1776–1976* (pp. 16–21). Compiled by the Health Resources Administration of the U.S. Public Health Service. Washington, D.C.: Government Printing Office.

Lohr, K. N., & Brook, R. H. 1984. *Quality Assurance in Medicine.* Santa Monica, Calif.: The Rand Corporation.

McDowell, I., & Newell, C. 1987. The theoretical and technical foundations of health measurement. In *Measuring Health: A Guide to Rating Scales and Questionnaires* (pp. 12–35). New York: Oxford University Press.

Mootz, M. 1988. Health (promotion) indicators: realistic and unrealistic expectations. *Health Promotion 3:* 79–84.

Moshman Associates, Inc. 1980. *Directions for the '80s—Final Report of the Panel to Evaluate the Cooperative Health Statistics System.* Washington, D.C.: Moshman Associates.

National Center for Health Statistics. 1993. *Health, United States 1992* (Table 115, p. 161). Hyattsville, MD: Public Health Service.

National Center for Health Statistics. 1994. *Healthy People 2000 Review, 1993* (p. 150). Hyattsville, MD: Public Health Service.

National Committee on Vital and Health Statistics. 1993. *Report of the Subcommittee on State and Community Health Statistics* (appendix D, pp. 9–12). Washington, D.C.

Office of Disease Prevention and Health Promotion, Department of Health and Human Services. 1986. *The 1990 Health Objectives for the Nation: A Midcourse Review.* Washington, D.C.: Government Printing Office.

Patrick, D., & Bergner, M. 1990. Measurement of Health Status in the 1990s. *Annual Review of Public Health 11:* 165–83.

Patrick, D., & Erickson, P. 1993. *Health Status and Health Policy—Allocating Resources to Health Care* (pp. 216–21). New York: Oxford University Press.

Pihlbland, C. T. 1937. *National Health Survey: Preliminary Results.* Washington, D.C.: National Institute of Health and the U.S. Public Health Service.

Reed, L., & Rice, D. 1964. National health expenditures: Object of expenditures and source of funds, 1962. *Social Security Bulletin* (August): 11–21.

Remington, P., Smith, M., Williamson, D., Anda, R., Gentry, E., & Hogelin, G. 1988. Design, characteristics, and usefulness of state-based behavioral risk factor surveillance: 1981–87. *Public Health Reports 103:* 366–75.

Rice, D. 1966. *Estimating the Cost of Illness.* Division of Medical Care Administration, Public Health Service. Washington, D.C.: Government Printing Office. May.

Rice, D., Anderson, A., & Cooper, B. 1968. Personal health care expenditures of the aged and non-aged, fiscal years 1966 and 1967. *Research and Statistics Note.* Washington, D.C.: Department of Health, Education, and Welfare. Note no. 11, June 14.

Rice, D., & Kleinman, J. 1977. National health data for policy and planning. In

J. Elinson, A. Mooney, & A. Siegmann (eds.), *Health Goals and Health Indicators: Policy, Planning, and Evaluation*. Boulder, Colo.: Westview Press.

Solomon, D., Henry, R., Hogan, J., Van Amburg, G., & Taylor, J. 1991. Evaluation and implementation of public health registries. *Public Health Reports* 106: 142–50.

Steinwachs, D. 1989. Application of health status assessment measures in policy research. *Medical Care 27* (Suppl.): S12–S26.

Stoto, M. 1992. Public health assessment in the 1990s. *Annual Review of Public Health 13:* 59–78.

Stroup, N., Zack, M., & Wharton, M. 1994. Sources of routinely collected data for surveillance. In *Principles and Practice of Public Health Surveillance*. New York: Oxford University Press.

Sydenstricker, E. 1933. The vitality of the American people. In *Recent Social Trends in the United States.* New York: McGraw-Hill.

Thacker, S., & Berkelman, R. 1988. Public health surveillance in the United States. *Epidemiologic Reviews 10:* 64–90.

U.S. Public Health Service; U.S. Department of Health, Education, and Welfare. 1979. *Healthy People: The Surgeon General's Report on Health Promotion and Disease Prevention.* Washington, D.C.: Government Printing Office.

U.S. Public Health Service; U.S. Department of Health and Human Services. 1980. *Promoting Health/Preventing Disease: Objectives for the Nation.* Washington, D.C.: Government Printing Office.

U.S. Public Health Service; U.S. Department of Health and Human Services. 1990. *Healthy People 2000: National Health Promotion and Disease Prevention Objectives.* Washington, D.C.: Government Printing Office.

U.S. Public Health Service; U.S. Department of Health and Human Services. 1992. *Healthy People 2000: National Health Promotion and Disease Prevention Objectives.* Washington, D.C.: Government Printing Office.

U.S. Public Health Service; U.S. Department of Health and Human Services. 1993. *A Public Health Service Progress Report on Healthy People 2000: Surveillance and Data Systems.* Washington, D.C.: Government Printing Office.

U.S. Public Health Service Task Force on State and Community Data. 1993. *Inventory of Public Health Data Projects and Systems.* (Draft document).

Webber, A. 1988. History and mission of quality assurance in the public sector. In *Perspectives on Quality in American Health Care*. Washington, D.C.: McGraw-Hill's Healthcare Information Center.

Widtfeldt, A. K., & Widtfeldt, J. R. 1992. Total quality management in American industry. *AAOHN Journal 40:* 311–18.

World Health Organization. 1981. *Development of Indicators for Monitoring Progress Towards Health for All by the Year 2000.* Geneva: World Health Organization.

World Health Organization—European Regional Office. 1985. *Targets for Health for All.* Copenhagen: World Health Organization.

Zimmerman, D. 1994. Grading the graders: Using "report cards" to enhance the quality of care under health care reform. Washington, D.C.: National Health Policy Forum Issue Brief, no. 642.

3/ CHILDREN WITH CHRONIC HEALTH CONDITIONS

James Perrin

The long-term illnesses of childhood encompass a very wide variety of conditions, most of which are rare to extremely rare (a different situation from that for adults, who face a relatively small number of generally common chronic conditions). Examples of severe childhood conditions include arthritis, diabetes, hemophilia, leukemia, chromosome disorders, spina bifida, craniofacial anomalies, and congenital heart disease. Table 3.1 indicates rates for the more common diagnostic groups. Asthma is the most common severe chronic illness. Even among children with asthma, however, most have relatively mild disease, requiring little treatment, except during occasional seasonal attacks, and rarely requiring hospitalization. About 10 percent of children with asthma have a severe variety that interferes regularly with their activities and requires ongoing health care services.

Childhood chronic illnesses vary substantially with respect to their impact on mobility, cognitive abilities, visibility, frequency, and need for treatment. Despite differences in prognoses, modes of therapy, and complications, caring for a child creates a series of tasks for the family that relates more to having a child with a chronic illness than to the specific illness itself (Hobbs, Perrin, & Ireys, 1985). These generic issues include relatively high costs of care, extensive home caretaking by parents and other family members, interference with education, the need to interact with many and diverse health professionals, and additional stress on the family in daily life. It is striking how frequently each of these issues recurs in any discussion of family response or adjustment to chronic illness, regardless of the specific diagnosis.

Table 3.1. Major Categories of More Prevalent Chronic Health Conditions (Rates per 100)

	Newacheck & Taylor, 1992	Cadman et al., 1986	Pless & Roghmann, 1971*			Newacheck, 1989	McManus, Newacheck, & Greaney, 1990
			a	b	c		
Respiratory (asthma and respiratory allergies)	13.0	3.2	2.3	1.6	4.6	1.3	0.6
Neurological (cerebral palsy, epilepsy)	0.4	1.3	1.6	1.8	0.8	0.4	0.5
Surgery (deafness, hearing loss; blindness, vision impairment)	2.8	2.5	2.0	0.3	2.4		
Musculoskeletal	1.5	2.7	1.3	0.2	0.4	0.9	2.1
Speech	2.6	3.5					
Frequent and repeated ear infections	8.3					0.3	0.2
Eczema, skin allergies	3.3		0.8	0.6	1.6		
Digestive allergies; diarrhea, bowel trouble	3.9						
Heart disease	1.5	1.9					
Frequent, severe headaches	2.5						
Mental disorders						2.0	0.7

*a, U.K. National Health and Development Survey; b, Isle of Wight (U.K.); c, Rochester (N.Y.) Child Health Studies.

PREVALENCE

Studies of chronic health conditions among children and adolescents provide a wide range of prevalence estimates, varying from about 7 percent to 35 percent (Table 3.2) (Gortmaker, 1985; Newacheck, 1989; Newacheck & Taylor, 1992; Pless & Roghmann, 1971). The sizable differences in the prevalence estimates mainly reflect differences in definition, source of data (medical records vs. interview), and respondent providing the data. Furthermore, some of the National Health Interview Survey (NHIS)[1] studies include children or young adults only when limitation of activity accompanies a chronic condition (McManus, Newacheck, & Greaney, 1990), and several studies suggest that only about 20 percent of children with chronic health conditions have much activity limitation. Most chronic illnesses among children are mild, requiring few special services and having little impact on the child's daily life. Estimates from the NHIS indicate that about 7–10 percent of children face *some* limitations from a chronic health condition; however, severe conditions likely to interfere with daily functioning and require frequent medical care affect only 2–5 percent of children (Newacheck & Taylor, 1992).

RATIONALE

In this chapter, three conditions are used as examples of the broader category of long-term illness in childhood: spina bifida, severe asthma, and leukemia. Although each condition raises issues specific to it, most family and child concerns arise more from the chronic nature of spina bifida, asthma, or leukemia than from the specific condition. Spina bifida is a birth defect resulting from incomplete closure of the spinal column and cord during fetal life (Myers & Millsap, 1985). The spinal defect causes problems in muscular control, especially of the lower extremities; urinary tract disease, because of incomplete innervation of the urinary tract system; and often other abnormalities of the central nervous system. Some, but not all, children with spina bifida have significant impairments of cognitive function. Severe asthma is a chronic condition with a variable prognosis, which becomes increasingly well managed with appropriate pharmacological and preventive therapies. Nevertheless, it still accounts for some childhood and adolescent deaths, and it is notable for racial disparities in prevalence and impact (Weitzman et al., 1992). Acute

Table 3.2. Prevalence of Chronic Physical Disorders in Childhood and Adolescence

Study	Sample	Definitions	Age (years)	Prevalence	Main Categories
Newacheck & Taylor, 1992	1988 NHIS, CHS (N = 17,110)	Any chronic health condition (detailed checklist)	0–18	31%	20% mild; 9% moderate; 2% severe
Cadman et al., 1986	Ontario Child Health Studies (random household survey) (N = 3,294)		4–16	19.6%	14.0% chronic illness only; 1.9% limitation of function only; 3.7% both
Pless & Roghmann, 1971	(a) U.K. National Health and Development Survey, 1971 (N = 5,362)		0–15	11.4%	
	(b) Isle of Wight (U.K.), 1970 (N = 3,271)	Handicapping physical disorders	10–12	5.7%	
	(c) Rochester (N.Y.) Child Health Studies (N = 1,756)	Condition list (like NHIS, CHS Supplement)	6–16	11.9%	
Weitzman, Walker, & Gortmaker, 1986	Berkshire County (Mass.) (N = 573) (random household telephone survey)	Basic NHIS questions	6–17	35%	
Gortmaker et al., 1990	1981 NHIS, CHS (N = 11,699)	Condition list, but excluded less serious conditions	4–17	8.9%	
Haggerty, Roghmann, & Pless, 1975	Rochester Child Health Studies (N = 1,520)	Condition list (like NHIS CHS Supplement	7–18	13.8%	
Newacheck, 1989	1984 NHIS (N = 15,181)	Limitation of activity by chronic condition	10–18	6.2%	0.5% unable to perform major activity; 3.7% limited in major activity; 2.0% limited in other activities
McManus et al., 1990	1984 NHIS (N = 10,394)	Limitation of activity by chronic condition	19–24	5.7%	1.8% unable to do major activity; 2.2% limited in major activity; 1.7% limited in other activities
Westbom & Kornfält, 1987	Swedish district medical records, 1981 (N = 6,080)	WHO criteria	0–15	8.4%	5.9% mild; 1.8% moderate; 0.7% severe

Table 3.3.   Children Assisted by Technology

Technology Categories*	Lower Limit Estimate	Upper Limit Estimate
Ventilator dependent	680	2,000
Parenteral nutrition	350	700
Intravenous therapies	270	8,275
Other respiratory or nutritional device	1,000	6,000
Renal dialysis	1,000	6,000
Other (e.g., urinary catheters, colostomies)	?	30,000
Total	(30,000)	52,975

Source: Data from Office of Technology Assessment, 1987.
*Excludes apnea monitoring in first half-year of life.

leukemia, the most common cancer of childhood, was almost uniformly fatal only a quarter of a century ago. As with many other childhood cancers, leukemia currently has a high rate of long-term survival and apparent cure, although long-lasting secondary health consequences sometimes result.

Current estimates are that the large majority (over 90 percent) of children with severe chronic health impairments survive to young adulthood (Gortmaker & Sappenfield, 1984), even though the lay belief may be that many of these children are doomed to an early death. Similarly, a common view holds that most children with chronic illnesses depend on major technologies, requiring substantial and expensive home care. In reality, children assisted by technology, although a sizable group, account for only a small proportion of children with severe long-term illnesses. In 1987, about fifty thousand children were estimated to be assisted by technology (Table 3.3). Even with twice this number, only about 5 percent of children with severe long-term illnesses fit the category of assisted by technology. Their very high rates of survival give chronically ill children and adolescents an increasingly prominent role, with approximately one in twenty U.S. children having a moderate or severe chronic health condition. Furthermore, increasing evidence supports the notion that early intervention and preventive services improve long-term outcomes. A small proportion of children with severe illnesses may have significant disability that impairs their ability to become independent young adults (Perrin, Guyer, & Lawrence, 1992). Yet with proper support, most children and adolescents with severe illnesses can be employed and educated, enter into significant relationships, and have little long-term dependence on public institutions.

COMORBIDITIES

Some children have both significant *developmental* and *physical* disabilities. Nevertheless, most children with chronic physical disability do not have associated cognitive impairments. Adding children and adolescents with developmental disabilities to those with chronic illnesses approximately doubles the rates of childhood disability noted above (Perrin, Guyer, & Lawrence, 1992). That is, 3–5 percent of children have severe chronic physical health conditions, and 6–10 percent of children have significant developmental disability or physical disability or both. Children with mainly developmental disabilities generally need far fewer high technology medical services and less medical care than do children with most physical disabilities. In other respects, however, their use of services and demands on the system of care have many similarities. Although this chapter deals primarily with children with chronic physical disorders, many of the issues raised affect families with children with developmental disabilities as well. This latter group is considered separately in chapter 4.

Two comorbidities particularly affect children with chronic health conditions and have implications for planning services: educational dysfunction and its impact on behavior, and psychological status. Chronic health conditions interfere frequently with a child's performance in school (Fowler, Johnson, & Atkinson, 1985; Walker & Jacobs, 1985). Part of this impact reflects increased absence due to fatigue, episodes of illness, or needed medical care often available only during the school day. Certain in-school therapies (e.g., physical therapy) may remove some children from the school room frequently. Other children face educational barriers through lack of in-school services, such as a child who needs medication in a school unable to store or distribute medications. Schools may have physical barriers for a child in a wheelchair, who otherwise needs no special services.

The cognitive impact of long-term physical disorders in children has not been studied satisfactorily (Mearig, 1985). Although most chronic physical conditions have no apparent major impact on cognitive performance, some may change cognitive functioning in subtle ways. For example, the teenager with diabetes has diminished cognitive functioning when her blood sugar is particularly high. Many medications have known or unstudied cognitive effects. Medications used in asthma affect cognitive functioning, although typically in subtle or limited ways. The degree to which these illnesses and treatments affect children and methods of addressing them in educational planning has not had sufficient attention.

Children with chronic physical conditions have approximately twice the risk of apparently able-bodied children of having significant psychiatric or behavioral problems (Cadman et al., 1987; Pless & Roghmann, 1971). Surprisingly, this increased risk seems to be affected neither by the severity of the condition nor by the specific condition, with one exception: children with primary central nervous system disease (mainly seizure disorders) appear to have a much higher risk for behavioral problems than do other children (Gortmaker et al., 1990; MacLean et al., 1992; Stein & Jessop, 1989). Recent work on mechanisms that lead to increased risk suggests that key predictive factors relate to response to the stress of illness among both children and their parents, changed patterns of parenting, and mental health problems among parents of children with chronic illnesses.

NEEDED SERVICES

Services needed by children with chronic illnesses and their families fall into five main categories: medical care (primary and specialty), nursing, educational planning, social services, and mental health services. These five main groups are often supplemented by other specialized therapies, such as occupational and physical therapy, respiratory therapy, nutrition, and speech and hearing services (Hobbs, Perrin, & Ireys, 1985). Services needed by children and families change over time, both as the child grows and develops and as the family adjusts to a child's chronic health condition. Thus, the service plan for an individual family must be monitored and reviewed on a regular basis, with adjustments made, under the family's direction, as needs change. Furthermore, families may need help with coordinating these multiple services, dealing with conflicting demands, or balancing various needs and services.

Children and adolescents with chronic health conditions require both primary and specialty medical and surgical care. While most children receive almost all of their medical care from a community-based physician or nurse, children with chronic physical conditions typically need ongoing care from health centers providing highly specialized and centralized services, often at a distance from their homes. Despite their need for usual preventive services, children with chronic illnesses are at higher risk of being underimmunized and of lacking other basic elements of primary pediatric care (Palfrey, Levy & Gilbert, 1980; Raddish et al., 1993). This lack of primary care partly reflects the tendency for these children and their families to link more with specialty physicians than with primary care physicians. In addition, frequent episodes of illness or surgery during the earlier years when most children receive basic immunizations may hinder attention to preventive care.

Data from the 1970s suggested that poor children with chronic illnesses had higher rates of uninsurance than did poor children without chronic illness (Butler et al., 1985). Recent major expansions in Medicaid and the Supplemental Security Income Program (SSI) for children (which brings Medicaid coverage in most states) have likely brought children with chronic illnesses to the same rates of uninsurance and underinsurance as all other children in the United States (Perrin & Stein, 1991). When insured, families typically have access to specialized medical and surgical care, hospital care, pharmaceuticals, and durable medical equipment. Other main services, however, are less well supported and thus relatively less available to most families.

Most families provide substantial amounts of home and community care for their child, regardless of the specific diagnosis. Although families themselves provide most of this care, there is only limited support for nursing or training services to help families hone their skills and learn home and self-care. Families also need help with educational planning, mainly around issues of integration into educational programs, special accommodations for children with physical disabilities, access to medications when needed, handling of emergency situations, and (at times) special instruction. Needed social services help families gain access to other appropriate services, and preventive mental health services help diminish the risk of long-term psychiatric or behavioral consequences of chronic illness in the child and the parents. The relatively few families whose children have severe conditions and are assisted by major technology rarely have access to additional services, such as specialized babysitting or respite care (Perrin, Shayne, & Bloom, 1993), yet families face barriers to most of these educational, social, and mental health services.

Parents consistently report difficulty in coordinating these multiple services. A child with spina bifida may receive care from an orthopedist, urologist, neurosurgeon, pediatrician, and occupational and physical therapist. She may require a wheelchair for mobility. She may work with a psychologist for a learning disorder and with a nurse to learn clean intermittent catheterization. This child and family may have ten professionals on the care "team." Families receive conflicting recommendations from different members of the team, who may disagree with each other about needs for therapy or the relative tradeoffs among different treatment approaches. Service systems rarely have anyone to help families cope with conflicting advice and competing services. Over time, most families coordinate their own services, but (especially in the early months of a child's health condition) they may need substantial help from outside agencies to help coordinate care and learn to make informed decisions involving their child's daily life. Coordination services, however, although likely cost-effective when provided in appropriate ways, are available to relatively few families.

The three conditions chosen as examples demonstrate some issues in prevention, diagnosis, treatment, management, and habilitation. Spina bifida, a condition acquired early in fetal life, increasingly can be prevented. Substantial new evidence indicates that dietary supplementation with folic acid markedly decreases the risk of having an infant with spina bifida (Milunsky et al., 1989). Work is ongoing to increase the availability of folic acid in the diet of women of childbearing age through supplementing commonly used food products. Previously, the main forms of prevention included avoidance of pregnancy among couples at high risk (a very difficult prediction) or termination of pregnancy when the fetus had been identified as likely to have spina bifida. This latter approach, using α-fetoprotein screening, leads to a highly accurate but not perfect method of identifying such fetuses. The possibility of terminating a fully normal pregnancy, coupled with the concern of many people with spina bifida, made this approach controversial. Before nutritional supplementation, the frequency of spina bifida varied from about 1 in 2,000 live births to 1 in 750, with wide variations based on ethnic origin, poverty, and family diet.

Although the initial diagnosis is not difficult, initial treatment and management of spina bifida require a neurosurgeon capable of managing small infants (a service available only in specialized facilities). Long-term care requires many other medical and surgical providers, and children usually undergo numerous surgical procedures in the first two years of life, including neurological, orthopedic, and urological surgery. Current rates of long-term survival of children with spina bifida are well over 50 percent, with the major threats being overwhelming infection in the perinatal period and renal failure due to frequent kidney infections.

Many children with spina bifida have associated malformations of the brain and midbrain, which may cause hydrocephalus, cognitive impairments, and deficits in sensory functions. Children with spina bifida have varied levels of mobility impairment, and some require wheelchairs.

Despite these multiple issues, the large majority of children with spina bifida who survive can be educated well and become increasingly independent as they mature. Thus, management must be directed both to preventing medical complications and to improving functioning, so that these young people can become productive adults. They will need the full array of services listed above as well as specialized therapies, especially occupational and physical therapy.

Children and adolescents with severe asthma face somewhat different service patterns. Causes of asthma are multifactorial (Leffert, 1985). Much evidence points to the role of parental smoking as one key factor (Weitzman et al., 1990). Preventive activities for asthma include diminishing exposure to inciting toxins or events, especially ambient smoke. Similarly, children must learn techniques of avoiding triggers, even when faced with peer pressure to have contact with the trigger. Although the onset of asthma can be at any age, many children with severe asthma develop the condition before school age, often in the first two years of life. Children with milder forms often stop having asthma during early to midadolescence, but many children with severe asthma continue to have it in adulthood. Asthma accounts for a significant and increasing amount of hospitalization of children, and for a small but growing number of child and adolescent deaths (Gergen & Weiss, 1990). Increasingly effective medications can prevent many asthma attacks, although there is concern regarding distribution of information about these newer therapeutic options. Frequent hospital use in asthma may reflect inadequate access to up-to-date outpatient care. Self-care programs for children with asthma and their families teach how best to manage asthma and diminish the anxiety that often surrounds an attack (Lewis et al., 1984; Perrin et al., 1992). Despite mounting evidence of their efficacy, self-care programs are not widely distributed and are poorly supported by third-party payments. Children with asthma also face special school problems, insofar as their frequent but brief attacks may cause repeated short absences that can hinder their progress but which are not long enough to justify home tutoring to help keep them on track with their classmates. Many children with asthma need chronic or acute medications in school. Although most children with asthma should learn to administer their own medications in school, many schools have policies against self-administration of drugs. Asthma, like most other chronic illnesses, is associated with approximately double the risk of psychological problems in the child.

Childhood leukemia presents similar complex, multidisciplinary issues. An uncommon condition (occurring in about 4 in 100,000 children per year), little is known about prevention, except for the association of leukemia with significant radiation exposure (Pendergrass, Chard, & Hartmann, 1985). Leukemia can present with a variety of symptoms (e.g., arthritis, bruising, fatigue, or swollen glands). Many children have these symptoms, and distinguishing the rare child with leukemia from this larger group can take time and be difficult. Once diagnosed, several physiological and epidemiological parameters influence the prognosis and help direct the specific medical therapies used.

Extensive and exciting work by multiinstitutional child oncology groups has led to extraordinary improvements in the outcome of childhood leukemia. Combinations of chemotherapy and radiation have led to the survival of most children with acute lymphocytic leukemia, the most common form in children. Survivors face several problems, however, including the risks of secondary cancers (usually as young adults), cognitive impairments from central nervous system irradiation, or infertility from testicular irradiation. Treatment can also have acute side effects, including infection, bleeding, and extreme fatigue. Treatment interferes with the child's daily activities (and those of the family), and these children also need the full range of medical, nursing, educational, social, and mental health services. Particularly important issues include reintegration into school, appropriate testing for cognitive disabilities, mental health services to prevent child and family psychological problems, and nursing education to diminish risks of infection. Much of the initial care takes place in specialty medical centers, with little involvement of community services. For many children, this centralization requires significant travel. In an important experiment in Iowa, the care of children with leukemia was decentralized to community physicians with apparently equally good clinical results, diminished costs, and increased satisfaction among families (Kisker et al., 1980; Strayer, Kisker, & Fethke, 1980).

ORGANIZATION OF SERVICES FOR CHILDREN AND FAMILIES

The service system for children with chronic illnesses and their families is best described as fragmented and out of joint (Milunsky et al., 1989;

Myers & Millsap, 1985). Although the needs of children and families call for comprehensive services, access to specific services varies, and comprehensiveness is typically a function of whimsy, geography, and third-party coverage. Generally, specialized medical and surgical care is available almost entirely through centralized health centers, such as children's hospitals or departments of pediatrics in academic health centers. Specialty services for adults are available through community internal medicine practices, but little specialized care for children occurs in community settings. The main exceptions are in large multispecialty group practices, where the number of children enrolled may justify having pediatric subspecialists available. The rarity of most individual conditions makes the hiring of pediatric subspecialists unattractive to all but the largest groups. Some larger groups manage children's specialty care through referral to adult specialists who have a variable knowledge of pediatric issues. An adult rheumatologist who specializes in low back pain and degenerative arthritis will know relatively little about the vagaries of juvenile arthritis in a ten-year-old but may be asked to provide this specialized care.

Lack of coordination between primary and specialty medical care creates ongoing problems for children with chronic health conditions. Once an unusual condition is diagnosed, the primary care physician is often out of the loop, because cystic fibrosis or leukemia is believed to be too rare, complex, and specialized for generalist physicians. Main sources of primary care for children with chronic illnesses are generally the same as those for children without apparent illness (Liptak & Revell, 1989). They include community pediatricians, nurse practitioners, community health centers, hospital outpatient departments, and rural and migrant health centers.

The lack of connection provides families with a dilemma. When the child with spina bifida has a fever, likely associated with a urinary tract infection, should the parents call their community physician a few blocks away or take the child to an academic health center emergency room for care at night? Whom should the family of a child with asthma call at night when the child begins to wheeze? The fever in a child with leukemia could herald a mild cold or a far more severe infection. Yet again, the family may be unsure whom to contact to manage the fever. At the least, this lack of clarity increases family anxiety, but it also likely leads to inappropriate medical care in many circumstances. Furthermore, for such services as genetic counseling, both the primary and the specialty physician may believe that the other is providing the service; lack of communication often leaves gaps in service.

A few important experiments have succeeded in integrating primary and specialty care and providing increasing amounts of service at the community level, but for most families the lack of connection between primary and tertiary care services remains a significant problem. Not knowing whom to call when their child has a fever, the family may drive long distances to a specialty center and receive an extensive but not necessarily appropriate evaluation. This reliance on specialized services may lead to unnecessary hospitalization or excessive use of technologies, when less expensive sites and sources might well be used. Furthermore, the emphasis on tertiary care forces many families to travel great distances to seek health services at distant and less user-friendly sites, causing parents to be absent from work and children to be absent from school. The growth of managed care, with primary care providers as gatekeepers, may lead to more (or at least different) collaboration between primary and tertiary care providers.

The joint federal-state Title V programs for children with special health care needs have a legislative mandate to develop community-based systems of care for chronically ill children and their families, providing as much care as possible in or near home communities and diminishing the need for travel (Guyer, 1990). These programs are part of the maternal and child activities supported largely by federal appropriations under Title V of the Social Security Act (Lesser, 1985), but state Title V efforts vary tremendously. Some invest increasingly in services to coordinate care and help families advocate for needed services, when in the past, Title V often supported specialty medical or surgical clinics and some hospital care for children with specified chronic health conditions (Ireys & Eichler, 1988; Ireys, Hauck, & Perrin, 1985). It is too early to say whether the new Title V mandate will lead to coordinated systems of care integrating primary and tertiary medical services and broadening the comprehensive base of services for families.

Title V programs have a mixed history of meeting the needs of sizable numbers of children with severe long-term illnesses. Although the enabling legislation has not required limiting services to poor families, most state programs have done so, and only a relatively small proportion of children with chronic illnesses receives services from their state's Title V programs. The current Title V legislation requires that 30 percent of funds be expended on children with special health needs.

The relatively small number of children assisted by technology receives significant amounts of in-home or community health services (Perrin, Shayne, & Bloom, 1993), often from home care agencies. Some agencies provide a wide range of services including home nursing, occupational and physical therapy, and educational services. Other agencies provide nursing care only. Benefits supporting nursing care and personal care attendants for young people with disabilities may limit their use in school settings. For example, some insurance policies allow care only at home and not elsewhere in the community, even though providing that care would allow a child to participate in school.

The school system also helps children with chronic health conditions. Many children require specialized educational programs. Others have physical disabilities requiring adapted educational or physical education programs. For children with cognitive impairments, traditional special educational services may be appropriate. For many other children, with physical but without significant cognitive impairments, access to needed school services may come only from their being labeled as special education students, where they may receive services under the "other health impaired" category. Most of these school efforts are supported by the federal Individuals with Disabilities Education Act (IDEA). This act also supports preschool and early intervention programs for children with disabilities or "at risk" of having disabilities. The at-risk category may be particularly pertinent to young children with chronic health conditions.

Children who are tired because of illness may need a shortened school day or opportunities for breaks during it; others may need access to specialized therapies or diets, to specialized care during school hours (e.g., clean intermittent catheterization for children with spina bifida), or to medications. The educational system, central to the lives of children, must work with the family and health providers to ensure access to the best, most appropriate, and least restrictive educational program for a child with a physical illness (American Academy of Pediatrics, 1990). A few school systems have developed specific programs for children with chronic illness without requiring entry into the special educational system. Most school districts provide home tutoring only after an absence of one or two consecutive weeks, whereas many childhood chronic illnesses cause frequent acute exacerbations and frequent short absences.

The SSI program is a key public program for children with disabilities, which has undergone significant expansion in the last few years (Perrin, Shayne, & Bloom, 1993). This program, designed to supplement the income of low-income people with disabilities, expanded dramatically after a Supreme Court decision *(Sullivan v. Zebley)* changed the rules for determining childhood disability. The Court ruled that the Social Security Administration (SSA) had unfairly limited the disability evaluation that children received, had no way of accounting for multiple conditions, and was unwilling to assess functioning of children beyond specific diagnostic criteria. Since the 1990 decision, the number of children and adolescents receiving SSI benefits has increased from approximately 280,000 recipients to almost 800,000 in 1994 (SSA, Office of Disability Statistics, personal communication, December 1993). SSI brings Medicaid coverage in almost all states, even when the family's income is higher than the usual Medicaid eligibility level. This program thus provides many families whose children have significant disabilities with both additional income through a monthly cash benefit and access to health care, which would otherwise be unavailable or very costly.

Despite the need for coordinated and comprehensive community services to enable children to participate in school and families to participate in community life, the reality typically does not meet the ideal. Families face highly fragmented services; they often need care from numerous providers, who may only be available on certain days of the week, sometimes in different locations, and who may not communicate effectively among themselves. Many specialty care centers provide comprehensive multidisciplinary services in their central locations, including medicine, nursing, and social services. Yet the availability of these services depends on the whimsy of the providers in that institution, such that a hospital may have a strong arthritis program but a weak oncology program. Few centers have developed comprehensive programs based on a generic model that recognizes the common issues faced by families with a child with a chronic health impairment. The centralized nature of specialty services also limits coordination with community efforts. Again, examples abound of excellent programs that have decentralized the care of children to the community, such as the regional Title V program in Iowa (MacQueen, 1986); the program to decentralize the care of children with leukemia and other cancers in Iowa (Liptak & Revell, 1989; Strayer, Kisker, & Fethke, 1980); the programs of Project REACH in north Florida, now expanded statewide through that state's Title V program (Pierce & Freedman, 1983); the work of the Pediatric Home Care Team at Albert Einstein College of Medicine in the Bronx (Stein, 1983); and community efforts based at LaRabida Hospital in Chicago (Hochstadt &

Yost, 1991). Nevertheless, these experiments are too scarce, leaving most children with fragmented services that are rarely well coordinated.

The two key advances that have improved the lives of children with chronic illnesses and their families have been *(a)* the tremendous strides in medical and surgical technology that have markedly improved survival over the last three decades and *(b)* developments that have come from growing parental competence and empowerment in taking responsibility for their own children. This latter phenomenon developed primarily from self-help groups for parents whose children had chronic health conditions; these groups often formed around specific conditions. Parents have become an increasingly powerful voice for change regarding care for their children with chronic illnesses. They have developed community groups in many cities, which now train parents, help them find resources, teach them ways of working the system, and advocate for change in public state and federal programs. Forging a link between the parents of a child newly diagnosed and effective parents from these community organizations may be one of the more important therapeutic efforts that clinicians undertake.

In the ideal situation, Joan, a seven-year-old girl with spina bifida, receives specialized care from a team of surgeons, pediatricians, nurses, and therapists, who meet together in a specialized health center and regularly monitor her care and progress. The team works together efficiently so that conflicts among types of advice are worked out and the evaluation proceeds smoothly, not requiring multiple trips to the specialty center. Both Joan and her parents are actively involved in the assessment process, and they also participate in recommendations for further evaluation, treatment, and home and community care. The assessment leads to an interim plan agreed to by the family, shared with community health providers and other agencies, and communicated to the school to help Joan's integration into regular classes. The community physician is involved and knowledgeable about her care, accessible in emergencies, and particularly attuned to making arrangements in the home community for management of urinary tract infections, so that she will not have to return to the specialty center for any recurrence. The school has worked with this family for several years, having assessed whether Joan has any learning problems (she has none). Initially, Joan needed an adult to provide catheterization to diminish the risk of urinary tract infections, but now she can do it by herself. Occasionally, the visiting school nurse supervises her, mainly to help with questions and provide positive reinforcement for

Joan's self-care. Occasionally, Joan needs medications to prevent or treat urinary tract infections, and the school has a system for storage and distribution that does not interfere with her being in the classroom. She ambulates with crutches that prevent her participation in some but not all physical education activities, and she can play in some recess games. In second grade, she usually has no classroom changes during the day, but a couple of classmates have agreed to carry her books during the few times she must move quickly. Joan gets physical therapy twice a week after school, so she does not have to miss class. Her stable condition has meant that she missed only a few days of school this year, and her visits to the specialty health center are now typically scheduled during vacation or summertime. Visits to her community physician, as with other school-age children, take place after school or on Saturdays.

Home care for Joan is currently straightforward. Despite her spina bifida, she is toilet trained for both bowel and bladder, although she occasionally has accidents. Her family's home is mainly on one floor, so accessibility is not a great problem. Her parents know parents of many other children with spina bifida and have learned about the risks and complications of this condition and the likely issues for Joan as she grows up.

This ideal situation happens too infrequently. More commonly, the health care system and coordination among the specialty center, community services, and the school work less well, and families learn too little about their child's condition. Thus, John, an eight-year-old with severe asthma, sees an allergist in a suburban practice, a pulmonary specialist in a specialty health care center, and a community-based family practitioner. Each physician tends to focus on his or her own special area of interest, sharing assessments and recommendations with each other by letter, but not working out a coordinated program of care for John. The pulmonologist has prescribed medication, including a home nebulizer, but has not addressed the problems the family faces with the safety and management of the equipment in their crowded home. The allergist recommended that John receive allergy shots to try to diminish the severity of his symptoms, so he must now travel to that office for an hour once a week to get the shots and then wait to make sure that he has no serious reaction. The community physician has been involved in keeping John up to date on immunizations but tends to assume that the other two physicians take care of the asthma. John uses an inhaler when he has early signs of an asthma attack. The school, fearful of allowing anyone to carry around medications or other drugs, requires that the medicine be locked in the school medicine cabinet. The school is a small elementary school with nursing care just two hours a week. At other times, the principal's secretary dispenses medication. Thus, John must be excused to the principal's office when he needs medication. The secretary, unfortunately, is not always available to help him, and he may have to wait as his asthma worsens. The secretary finds asthma a frightening condition, and her anxiety often spills over to John, who has twice needed to be taken to a hospital emergency room during the school day.

John has been hospitalized four times this year. Each occasion seemed to represent a failure of preventive care in the few days before hospitalization. When John was first diagnosed with asthma three years ago, his parents were given a book about it, but they have had little further education about asthma and its treatment. If John gets sick in the evening, his parents are never sure whom to call. Usually, they first call his family practitioner, who is the most available of the three, but she often refers the child directly to the pulmonary specialist. That referral commonly leads to an emergency room visit, where John is seen by physicians-in-training, almost always different from the ones who saw him previously, and each of whom has a slightly different approach to treating an acute attack of asthma. Unfortunately, even when John has been hospitalized, his physicians and nurses have not taken the opportunity to improve the family's education about preventive and self-care, which represents a lost opportunity.

INDICATORS OF SUCCESS

The unit of observation for determining the success of community programs should include the child in the context of the rest of the child's household. Child-specific process indicators include measuring access to or use of the range of comprehensive services important for improving child and family functioning. Specific indicators are a comprehensive plan in place, access to all needed services, and services coordinated and provided in a way that enables the child to be at home or in the community as much as possible. Most work regarding child outcomes has focused on disease-specific physiological status measures, such as mortality and morbidity; the degree of fixed disability; the status of the condition (whether it is quiescent or severe); and the presence of long-term complications (Stein et al., 1987). For example, measures of physiological status for a child with spina bifida include orthopedic and physical therapy assessments, levels of bowel and bladder functioning, renal function, and measures of central nervous system functioning, including neuropsychological assessment. For asthma, several measures of severity take into account the frequency of attacks, the use of preventive and treatment medications, and indicators of functioning, such as school days missed or days in bed (Perrin, MacLean, & Perrin, 1989). Pulmonary function tests, especially carried out between attacks, may also have some benefit in monitoring a child's asthma status, but they have little relationship to most other aspects of a child's functioning. Outcomes for a child with leukemia relate primarily to death versus apparent disease-free state after five years, along with assessment of secondary consequences, such as infertility, central nervous system functioning, and other side effects of chemotherapy and radiation.

Physiological status measures a narrow set of parameters relating to the child's outcome in the context of the chronic illness. Although activities-of-daily-living measures have been developed for adults, few exist for children. Most work in this area has focused on developmental assessment as a way of understanding a child's intelligence and developmental abilities. Much less work has examined measurement of a child's physical functioning. Stein and Jessop (1990) have developed a measure of functional status (FS-IIR), designed to examine children's activity status across disease states, which has had increasingly promising use. Starfield and colleagues at Johns Hopkins are currently working on a broad measure of childhood functioning that they expect will have applicability across different chronic health conditions. Nevertheless, important work needs to be done to strengthen the measurement of functional status in a developmentally appropriate way for children as a way of assessing the success of programs for children with different chronic health conditions.

A third area of measurement assesses the integration of the child (and the family) into the community and its services. Here, simple measures include educational achievement and school attendance. These typically available measures have had modest success in their application to children with chronic illnesses. More sophisticated but less used approaches examine broad participation in other community activities. For example, a measure of community participation might be the degree to which a child using a wheelchair can participate in community recreation activities, the library reading hour, and the many other clubs and community activities that most other children can join.

Psychological functioning of children with chronic illnesses should also be considered an outcome. As noted above, a chronic illness in childhood approximately doubles the risk of having a significant behavioral or psychiatric consequence. Measurement in this field has been confounded because some commonly used assessments of childhood psychological functioning probe for symptoms associated with a long-term illness, which are interpreted as indicating psychological dysfunction (Perrin, Stein, & Drotar, 1991). Thus, "frequent allergies" may count as an indicator of behavioral dysfunction, even though many parents report allergies in their children with asthma; likewise, fatigue caused by an illness or its treatment may affect a score on a behavioral measure. Some measures are less affected by this problem, carefully avoiding this potential for confounding (Walker et al., 1990).

Long-term outcome measures for children and adolescents with chronic illness include physiological and psychological status and adult activities of daily living. Broader assessments include securing of independent employment, the success of marriage or other important relationships, and the degree of independence and level of education attained. A few recent studies have examined these issues, although the availability of longitudinal data is limited. Most importantly, recent work does indicate that most young people with chronic health conditions can achieve most of these common accomplishments of the transition to adulthood (Gortmaker et al., 1993; Pless & Wadsworth, 1989).

Finally, measures of success for the family include assessment of the developmental, educational, and psychological status of siblings and the work force participation, mental health, and household marital status of the adult members of the household. Parents of children with chronic illness frequently miss work because of their child's condition or treatment. Many European countries recognize that having a child with a disability causes increased parental need for time away from work and provide additional job leave benefits, which allow more parents to maintain employment. Parents of a child with a chronic illness are significantly less likely to both be employed than are parents of same-aged children without a chronic illness (Breslau, Salkever, & Staruch, 1982). Thus, these children who engender high costs of care are also associated with decreased family resources, because both parents cannot work outside the home. Work force participation by parents in single-parent households seems less affected by the presence of chronic illness in a child, although the tasks can be extraordinarily difficult for a single parent.

Rates of depression appear to be higher among parents of children with major disability than among parents of apparently able-bodied children. Problems in parental mental health also increase the risks of mental health problems among their children with a disability. Depressed parents generally do less well in managing the normal tasks of bringing up a child. Thus, rates of mental health problems and depression among parents of these children are additional program indicators.

Whether having a child with a chronic illness increases rates of household breakup or divorce remains controversial (Sabbeth & Leventhal, 1984). Given the current relatively high rates of divorce in American families, the impact of a child with a chronic illness is relatively marginal. On the other hand, abundant evidence indicates that having a child with a chronic illness creates tremendous stress on the parental relationship and significantly increases parental work. Thus, assessment of family functioning is an additional criterion.

Most evaluations cannot use the full list of indicators above, and typically, programs must select among them on the basis of the main areas of program focus (Perrin et al., 1993). Any program monitoring, however, should attempt a broader approach than measurement of physiological state or functioning, including at a minimum physical, psychological, and social functioning (choosing among the indicators described). For children, elements of family functioning should be measured as well (likely emphasizing mental health and community/workplace participation of adult family members). Table 3.4 (see p. 94) lists the main groups of indicators and potential data sources for them.

CURRENT MONITORING SYSTEMS

Current federal programs have remarkably few satisfactory means of monitoring the numbers of children and adolescents with disabilities, much less the types of services children receive or their outcomes. The SSA has limited diagnostic information for childhood SSI recipients. However, the coding scheme used mainly reflects the diagnosis for which the child or adolescent receives SSI benefits. Thus, a child with multiple congenital anomalies who also happens to have mental retardation might be listed as the latter insofar as it is easier to adjudicate and less open to clinical judgment about severity. Current estimates from the SSA are that approximately two-thirds of recipients under age eighteen have primary developmental retardation, primary mental health disorders, or primary disorders of the central nervous system. The other one-third have all other types of physical disabilities. Beyond diagnostic information, the SSA primarily gathers data on reassessment of eligibility and the actual cash benefit received. No other data about services used, use of cash benefits, or status of child or family are gathered. It is possible to link a specific file of SSI recipients with Medicaid data tapes,[2] potentially achieving a richer understanding of service use and multiple diagnosis issues affecting SSI recipients, although this is not done on any regular basis.

Medicaid files, especially at the state level, could provide some opportunity to understand utilization patterns and, to a degree, needs of children and adolescents with a variety of chronic illnesses. Here too there is wide state-to-state variation in the quality of Medicaid data and their availability for monitoring purposes. Maryland, New Jersey, California, Georgia, and New Hampshire have Medicaid data sets that are reasonably clean and robust in data elements useful for monitoring the health status of children. In addition, Medicaid claims data are typically based on incomplete diagnostic information at the time of each visit, although work by a group at Johns Hopkins may develop mechanisms of profiling to distinguish children with chronic illness from other children and examine their patterns of use (Starfield et al., 1991). Ellwood (1990) has used the four-state tape-to-tape Medicaid data set to examine patterns of use by children with disabilities and other high-cost conditions in the mid-1980s, but there has been little other systematic examination of Medicaid data.

The Title V program, despite a legislative mandate for over half a century to provide services for children with special health care needs (formerly called Crippled Children's Services), has never developed a systematic approach to estimating the numbers of children with long-term illnesses or special health care needs. Currently funded at about $1.1 billion in combined federal and state funding, the Maternal and Child Health Programs spend about one-third of their resources on children with special health needs, mainly those with chronic health and developmental conditions. When the program attempts to define numbers of potentially eligible children, it typically relies on external sources of data such as the NHIS to develop synthetic estimates.

States that have attempted similarly to develop measures of numbers of children with chronic health conditions usually estimate them by multiplying calculated national rates by the childhood population in the state. No states have developed satisfactory childhood disability registers based on birth data and later ascertainment of chronic conditions. Some states monitor their population of children covered by the Title V program, although few do more than catalogue enrollment with some diagnostic information. (Remarkably, after more than half a century of targeted public investment in this population, there are no satisfactory data to determine its prevalence nationwide nor to distinguish important regional or state differences in the prevalence of conditions, which have importance for program development.)

To a degree, state and federal special education programs collect data on children enrolled and must do so to determine the amount of assistance that each state receives from the federal program, although these rosters have limited information on service patterns or any process and outcome measurement. This enrollment approach provides information mainly on numbers of children enrolled and some categorization of the types of problems they have.

Several federal surveys have potential applicability to monitoring the success of programs for children with chronic illnesses and their families. The questions that have been used and some of the techniques of data collection could also be applied to community settings to understand the impact of programs over time. The NHIS and its occasional Child Health Supplements have had significant application to studying the prevalence, consequences, and predictors of chronic illness and disability among children and adolescents. Data available through the NHIS include diagnostic information, information on use of health services, and measures of child and family functioning. Psychological data are also available on the child. The planned disability supplement for the NHIS may provide substantially more data about the interaction of health, disability, and functioning. The National Longitudinal Survey of Labor Market Experience of Youth (NLSY)[3] is another national data set that allows examination of the impact of chronic health conditions on the functioning of youth and young adults. Here, the diagnostic data are limited (having diagnostic coding only for health conditions considered to be job limiting by the respondent), but the survey provides extensive data on work force participation, education, psychological status, marital status, and support by public programs. Other national data sets have been used to examine issues of child health and disability, including the National Medical Care Utilization and Expenditure Survey (NMCUES) and the National Health and Nutrition Examination Surveys (NHANES).

Community special education programs are mandated to develop an individualized educational plan for each child enrolled. This multidisciplinary plan, developed in conjunction with the family and with their approval, specifies measurable goals for the child and a time frame for achieving them. Plans are to be reviewed at least yearly to assess achievement and revise goals. Although the data from these plans generally have not been well collated, they offer potential for monitoring and evaluating program services over time. If applied more broadly to long-term illness in childhood, the use of individualized family service plans (IFSP) holds similar opportunity. Most programs that provide comprehensive services to children with long-term illnesses and their families have similar mechanisms for oversight of the child's care plan. Thus, its addition to program operation is not difficult. Such a plan, however, provides no evidence about households that do not participate in the program or receive services. Thus, it is not a community-based scheme but rather a program-based one. Monitoring of community-based efforts creates a surveillance system that integrates the NHIS sampling model and questions with additional questions that are typically part of the IFSP development.

CONCLUSIONS AND RECOMMENDATIONS

One in twenty U.S. children and adolescents has a serious, long-lasting chronic health condition. As a group, they and their families need access to a broad range of coordinated multidisciplinary services, including medicine, nursing, social work, mental health, and educational planning. Although a few examples exist of coordinated services designed to improve the long-term outcome for families, most households face fragmented services and important gaps in needed services. The need to remedy their situation reflects in part that the large majority of these children with serious illnesses survive to adulthood and can be participatory members of U.S. society.

Current means of monitoring care for these children and their families are limited largely to diagnostic information, with some information about services provided occasionally, but with little monitoring of broader outcomes for the child or family. Recommendations for these families include providing the appropriate range of comprehensive, coordinated, multidisciplinary services and developing schemes for monitoring outcomes on the basis of a broad and generic view of a child's functioning. Furthermore, the index of examination should include the family as a whole, specifically the functioning of siblings and parents.

As much as possible, the community and its residents should be the unit of observation. All other approaches provide some bias of enrollment or use of services, excluding infrequent users or nonenrolled populations. Beyond population-based surveys, four main sources identifying children with chronic conditions may be considered in any state or community:

1. Children enrolled in SSI
2. Children receiving services through the state Title V Program for Children with Special Health Care Needs
3. Children enrolled in early intervention programs
4. Children receiving care for their chronic conditions at tertiary care institutions

Birth registries of children with major congenital anomalies, significantly low birth weight, or major complications in the neonatal period may also serve as a source for enrollment in a community study. On the other hand, although these children are at moderately high risk of developing long-term chronic health conditions, the attributable risk (of chronic conditions) due to perinatal conditions is quite low.

Insofar as most children with chronic physical conditions receive a substantial portion of their medical and surgical care in pediatric specialty institutions, those sites may be a source of enrollment or identification. Managed care, however, especially to the degree that it limits access of children with chronic conditions to pediatric specialty services, may make it less likely that all children with chronic conditions will pass through such specialty services. Many children, especially in smaller communities and rural areas, will receive specialty services at a site distant from their home communities, making that source of identification or enrollment more difficult. Nevertheless, even in those circumstances, the number of specialty sources used is limited, and it is generally not difficult to identify them for any population. The use of SSI enrollment will also identify a population of children with relatively severe chronic conditions, although the SSI program limits recipients to relatively low-income families, excluding most children with chronic conditions. Each of these sources will include only certain segments of the population of children and adolescents with chronic conditions, but they likely reflect the widest spectrum available.

As indicated in Table 3.4, the main sources of data include surveys of

Table 3.4.   Child and Family Indicators and Potential Data Sources

Child Indicators	Potential Data Sources or Survey Measures
Process	
Comprehensive plan in place	Survey, agency reports (e.g., special education or early intervention programs; health or social service agencies)
Access to and use of all needed services	Survey, claims data
Coordination of services	Agency reports
Outcome (health status)	
Physiological	
Mortality	
Condition-specific measures (e.g., frequency of attacks, pulmonary function tests, use of preventive medications, all in asthma)	Survey, claims data
Complications	Survey
Functional	
Disability	Survey (e.g., WEEFIM; FS-IIR), SSI files
Developmental capacity	Survey, agency files (esp. school or early intervention)
Psychological status	Survey (e.g., PARS, CBCL)
Integration into community	
Schooling	School records, survey
Other participation	Survey
Long-term outcomes	All likely from survey
Employment	
Income	
Educational attainment	
Social adjustment	
Family assessment	
Parental mental health	Survey (e.g., CES-D)
Parental work force participation	Survey
Sibling mental health, related measures	Survey

enrolled, randomly selected populations, selected claims files (mainly from public and private health insurance programs), and certain community or state agency file data. Developing state monitoring systems, potentially linked to federal agency data (especially SSI enrollment and disability data) could serve as a base for a reasonable monitoring system. Nevertheless, certain family data and many of the items recommended here for consideration related to children's functioning and outcomes can come only from survey techniques.

Notes

1. See appendix A for listings of NCHS data sets referred to in this chapter.

2. See appendix B for listings of the HCFA data sets referred to in this chapter.

3. See appendix C for listings of selected governmental and nongovernmental data sets referred to in this chapter.

References

American Academy of Pediatrics, Committees on Children with Disabilities and School Health. 1990. Children with health impairments in schools. *Pediatrics* 86: 636–38.

Breslau, N., Salkever, D, & Staruch, K. S. 1982. Women's labor force activity and responsibility for disabled dependents. *Journal of Health and Social Behavior 23:* 169–83.

Butler, J. A., Budetti, P., McManus, M. A., Stenmark, S., & Newacheck P. W. 1985. Health care expenditures for children with chronic illness. In N. Hobbs & J. M. Perrin (eds.), *Issues in the Care of Children with Chronic Illness* (pp. 827–63). San Francisco: Jossey-Bass.

Cadman, D., Boyle, M., Szatmari, P., & Offord, D. R. 1987. Chronic illness, disability, and mental and social well-being. *Pediatrics 79:* 805–13.

Cadman, D., Boyle, M. H., Offord, D. R., Szatmari, P., Rae-Grant, N. I., Crawford, J., & Byles, J. 1986. Chronic illness and functional limitation in Ontario children. *Canadian Medical Association Journal 135:* 761–67.

Ellwood, M. R. 1990. SSI-related disabled children and Medicaid. Report for the Office of the Deputy Assistant Secretary for Social Services Policy, DHHS; mimeograph, Systemetrics/McGraw-Hill, June 1990.

Fowler, M., Johnson, M., & Atkinson, S. 1985. School achievement and absence in children with chronic health conditions. *Journal of Pediatrics 106:* 683–87.

Gergen, P. J., & Weiss, K. B. 1990. Changing patterns of asthma hospitalization among children: 1979 to 1987. *Journal of the American Medical Association 264:* 1688–92.

Gortmaker, S. L. 1985. Demography of chronic childhood diseases. In N. Hobbs & J. M. Perrin (eds.), *Issues in the Care of Children with Chronic Illness* (pp. 135–54). San Francisco: Jossey-Bass.

Gortmaker, S. L., Perrin, J. M., Weitzman, M., & Homer, C. J. 1993. An unexpected success story: Transition to adulthood of youth with chronic physical health conditions. *Journal of Research on Adolescence 3:* 317–36.

Gortmaker, S., & Sappenfield, W. 1984. Chronic childhood disorders: Prevalence and impact. *Pediatric Clinics of North America 31:* 3–18.

Gortmaker, S. L., Walker, D. K., Weitzman, M., & Sobol, A. M. 1990. Chronic conditions, socioeconomic risks, and behavioral problems in children and adolescents. *Pediatrics 85:* 267–76.

Guyer, B. 1990. Title V: An overview of its evolution and future role. In M. Schlesinger & L. Eisenberg (eds.), *Children in a Changing Health Care System.*

Assessments and Proposals for Reform. Baltimore: Johns Hopkins University Press.

Haggerty, R. J., Roghmann, K. J., & Pless, I. B. 1975. *Child Health and the Community*. New York: Wiley.

Hobbs, N., Perrin, J. M., & Ireys, H. T. 1985. *Chronically Ill Children and Their Families*. San Francisco: Jossey-Bass.

Hochstadt, N. J., & Yost, D. M. (eds.). 1991. *The Medically Complex Child: The Transition to Home Care*. Chur, Switzerland: Harwood Academic Publishers, 1991.

Ireys, H., & Eichler, R. 1988. Correlates of Variation among State Programs for Children with Special Health Care Needs: Report of a Survey and Six Case Studies. MCJ-360479. National Technical Information Service, U.S. Department of Commerce, Springfield, Va. 22161.

Ireys, H. T., Hauck, R. J. P., & Perrin, J. M. 1985. Variability among state Crippled Children's Service programs: Pluralism thrives. *American Journal of Public Health 75*: 375–81.

Kisker, C. T., Strayer, F., Wong, K., Clarke, W., Strauss, R., Tannous, R., Jance, R., & Spevack, J. 1980. Health outcomes of a community-based therapy program for children with cancer. *Pediatrics 66*: 900–906.

Leffert, F. 1985. Asthma. In N. Hobbs & J. M. Perrin (eds.), *Issues in the Care of Children with Chronic Illness* (pp. 366–79). San Francisco: Jossey-Bass.

Lesser, A.J. 1985. The origin and development of maternal and child health programs in the United States. *American Journal of Public Health 75*: 590–98.

Lewis, C. E., Rachelefsky, G., Lewis, M. A., De la Sota, A., & Kaplan, M. 1984. A randomized trial of ACT. (Asthma Care Training) for kids. *Pediatrics 74*: 478–86.

Liptak, G. S., & Revell, G. M. 1989. Community physician's role in case management of children with chronic illnesses. *Pediatrics 84*: 465–71.

MacLean, W. E., Perrin, J. M., Gortmaker, S. L., & Pierre, C. B. 1992. Psychological adjustment of children with asthma: Effects of illness severity and recent life events. *Journal of Pediatric Psychology 17*: 159–71.

MacQueen, J. 1986. Iowa's Mobile and Regional Clinics. Iowa City: State of Iowas, Department of Health, Division of Maternal and Child Health.

McManus, M. A., Newacheck, P. W., & Greaney, A. M. 1990. Young adults with special health care needs. *Pediatrics 86*: 674–82.

Mearig, J. S. 1985. Cognitive development of chronically ill children. In N. Hobbs & J. M. Perrin (eds.), *Issues in the Care of Children with Chronic Illness* (pp. 672–97). San Francisco: Jossey-Bass.

Milunsky, A., Jick, H., Jick, S. S., Bruell, C. L., MacLaughlin, D. S., Rothman, K. J., & Willett, W. 1989. Multivitamin/folic acid supplementation in early pregnancy reduces the prevalence of neural tube defects. *Journal of the American Medical Association 262*: 2847–52.

Myers, G. J., & Millsap, M. 1985. Spina bifida. In N. Hobbs & J. M. Perrin (eds.), *Issues in the Care of Children with Chronic Illness* (pp. 214–35). San Francisco: Jossey-Bass.

Newacheck, P.W. 1989. Adolescents with special health needs: Prevalence, severity, and access to health services. *Pediatrics 84:* 872–81.

Newacheck, P. W., & Taylor, W. R. 1992. Childhood chronic illness: Prevalence,
severity, and impact. *American Journal of Public Health 82:* 364–71.

Office of Technology Assistance (OTA), U.S. Congress. (May 1987). *Technology-
Dependent Children: Hospital vs. Home Care.* Washington, D.C.: OTA.

Palfrey, J. S., Levy, J. C., & Gilbert, K. L. 1980. Use of primary care facilities by
patients attending specialty clinics. *Pediatrics 65:* 567–72.

Pendergrass, T. W., Chard, R. L., Jr., & Hartmann, J. R. 1985. Leukemia. In N.
Hobbs & J. M. Perrin (eds.), *Issues in the Care of Children with Chronic
Illness* (pp. 324–43). San Francisco: Jossey-Bass.

Perrin, J. M., Guyer, B., & Lawrence, J. 1992. Health care services for children
and adolescents. *Futures of Children 2:* 58–77.

Perrin, J. M., MacLean, W. E., Gortmaker, S. L., & Asher, K. N. 1992. Improving the psychological status of children with asthma: A randomized controlled
trial. *Journal of Developmental and Behavioral Pediatrics 13:* 241–47.

Perrin, J. M., Maclean, W. E., & Perrin, E. C. 1989. Parents' perception of health
status and psychological adjustment of children with asthma. *Pediatrics 83:*
26–30.

Perrin, E. C., Newacheck, P., Pless, I. B., Drotar, D., Gortmaker, S. L., Leventhal,
J., Perrin. J. M., Stein, R. E. K., Walker, D. K., & Weitzman, M. 1993. Issues
involved in the definition and classification of chronic health conditions. *Pediatrics 91:* 787–93.

Perrin, J. M., Shayne, M. W., & Bloom, S. R. 1993. *Home and Community Care
for Chronically Ill Children.* New York: Oxford University Press.

Perrin, J. M., & Stein, R. E. K. 1991. Reinterpreting disability: Changes in SSI
for children. *Pediatrics 88:* 1047–51.

Perrin, E. C., Stein, R. E., & Drotar, D. 1991. Cautions in using the Child Behavior Checklist: Observations based on research about children with a chronic
illness. *Journal of Pediatric Psychology 16:* 411–21.

Pierce, P. M., & Freedman, S. A. 1983. The REACH Program: An innovative
delivery model for medically dependent children. *Children's Health Care 12
(2):* 86–89.

Pless, I. B., & Roghmann, K. J. 1971. Chronic illness and its consequences: Observations based on three epidemiologic surveys. *Journal of Pediatrics 79:*
351–59.

Pless, I. B., & Wadsworth, M. E. J. 1989. Long-term effects of chronic illness on
young adults. In R. E. K. Stein (ed.), *Caring for Children with Chronic Illness*
(pp. 147–58). New York: Springer Publications.

Raddish, M., Goldmann, D. A., Kaplan, L. C., & Perrin, J. M. 1993. The immunization status of children with spina bifida. *American Journal of Diseases of
Childhood 147:* 849–53.

Sabbeth, B. F., & Leventhal, J. M. 1984. Marital adjustment to chronic childhood
illness. *Pediatrics 73:* 762.

Starfield, B. H., Weiner, J., Mumford, L., & Steinwachs, D. 1991. Ambulatory care groups: A categorization of diagnoses for research and management. *Health Services Research 26:* 53–74.

Stein, R. E. K. 1983. A home care program for children with chronic illness. *Children's Health Care 12:* 90–92.

Stein, R. E. K., & Jessop, D. J. 1989. What diagnosis does not tell: The case for a noncategorical approach to chronic illness in children. *Social Science and Medicine 29:* 769–78.

Stein, R. E. K., & Jessop, D. J. 1990. Functional Status II(R). *Medical Care 28:* 1041–55.

Stein, R. E. K., Perrin, E. C., Pless, I. B., Gortmaker, S. L., Perrin, J. M., Walker, D. K., & Weitzman, M. 1987. Severity of illness: Concepts and measurements. *Lancet 2:* 1506–9.

Strayer, F., Kisker, C. T., & Fethke, C. 1980. Cost-effectiveness of a shared-management delivery system for the care of children with cancer. *Pediatrics 66:* 907–11.

Walker, D. K., & Jacobs, F. H. 1985. Public school programs for chronically ill children. In N. Hobbs & J. M. Perrin (eds.), *Issues in the Care of Children with Chronic Illness* (pp. 615–55). San Francisco: Jossey-Bass.

Walker, D. K., Stein, R. E. K., Perrin, E. C., & Jessop, D. J. 1990. Assessing psychosocial adjustment of children with chronic illnesses: A review of the technical properties of PARS III. *Journal of Developmental and Behavioral Pediatrics 11:* 116–21.

Weitzman, M., Gortmaker, S. L., Sobol, A. M., & Perrin, J. M. 1992. Recent trends in the prevalence and severity of childhood asthma. *Journal of the American Medical Association 268:* 2673–77.

Weitzman, M., Gortmaker, S., Walker, D. K., & Sobol, A. 1990. Maternal smoking and childhood asthma. *Pediatrics 85:* 505–11.

Weitzman, M., Walker, D. K., & Gortmaker, S. L. 1986. Chronic illness, psychosocial problems, and school absences. *Clinical Pediatrics 25:* 137–41.

Westbom, L., & Kornfalt, R. 1987. Chronic illness among children in a total population. *Scandinavian Journal of Social Medicine 15:* 87–97.

4/ PERSONS WITH DEVELOPMENTAL DISABILITIES
Mental Retardation As an Exemplar

K. Charlie Lakin

The Developmental Disabilities Assistance and Bill of Rights Act defines developmental disabilities as a severe chronic condition that is attributable to a mental or physical impairment or a combination of mental or physical impairments, manifested before a person attains age twenty-two, and likely to continue indefinitely. This condition results in substantial functional limitations in three or more of the following areas of major life activity: self-care, receptive and expressive language, learning, mobility, self-direction, capacity for independent living, and economic self-sufficiency.

This "functional" definition reflects the findings of a task force (Gollay, 1980), which suggested that services and programs focus on the specific needs and abilities of persons rather than on underlying conditions. Previously, a categorical definition prevailed, which identified mental retardation, epilepsy, cerebral palsy, spina bifida, and/or autism as developmental disabilities.

The preceding chapter addressed the question of medical and other specialty services appropriated to children with identified chronic conditions, including those introduced here under the label of developmental disabilities. This chapter extends that discussion into two other areas: the prevention of childhood disability and the tracking of those with developmental disability after they enter adult age.

To determine whether a person meets the functional definition of developmental disabilities, the substantiality of his or her limitations and the age at which they are manifested need to be assessed. Substantiality relates to the extent to which limitations in functioning imply an inability to perform the activities of major aspects of daily living with age-

99

appropriate independence. No objective standard for the extent of limitations that constitute developmental disabilities has been established in legislation, planning, or advocacy, even though the term is used widely as the general descriptor of persons with severe chronic impairments of lifelong significance. The primary reasons for this are that no major national entitlement program uses developmental disabilities per se as its eligibility criterion, and no reliable system of individual assessment has been developed to diagnose a developmental disability. While no such standards exist, they will likely be forthcoming. Currently, most states identify programs that once served persons with mental retardation as being for persons with developmental disabilities or mental retardation/ developmental disabilities. A few states (e.g., Ohio) are studying the mechanisms and implications of using functional assessment as a primary determinant of service eligibility. The 1994–95 Disability Supplement to the National Health Interview Survey (NHIS)[1] was initiated to provide information on prevalence, health, and community service use of individuals who meet the functional definition of developmental disabilities. Although the scope of that survey has widened, it retains a significant focus on developmental disabilities. Service eligibility for persons with developmental disabilities retains primarily categorical disability distinction. Among the conditions comprising developmental disabilities, mental retardation is the most prevalent.

The standard definition of mental retardation used most widely for diagnostic and service eligibility purposes is "significantly subaverage general intellectual functioning (IQ of less than 70 or 2 or more standard deviations below average) existing concurrently with deficits in adaptive behavior (i.e., functional skills), manifested during the developmental period." This definition is reasonably congruent with that of developmental disabilities, except for the IQ component. For purposes of specificity, this chapter uses the term mental retardation.

PREVALENCE AND POPULATIONS OF PERSONS WITH MENTAL RETARDATION

There are three primary methods for estimating the prevalence of mental retardation. One method is to establish a statistical or behavioral standard that permits a group of a certain size or with certain characteristics to be defined on the basis of measured performance. A second method involves surveying service agencies within a catchment area to obtain an unduplicated count of all persons identified as receiving or qualifying for services as a member of the target population. This method, however, looks specifically at "treated" prevalence and potentially overlooks eligible persons who are not receiving services. Another problem is that many persons receive services for generic reasons related to their mental retardation (e.g., food stamps, housing subsidies, and other services related to poverty). A third method involves surveying households to obtain information on the diagnostic and/or functional characteristics of the household members. Historically, the problem with this approach has been respondents' reluctance to report mental disability among family members. Although some report more readily today, disability is usually defined by service organizations rather than by functional standards, which may result in the same shortcomings as the incidence of treated prevalence methodology.

Statistical Estimations of Prevalence

Standardized measures of intelligence (IQ) are used universally as part of the diagnosis and definition of mental retardation. A theoretical normal distribution of intelligence shows that 2.3 percent of the population will hypothetically score in the range of mental retardation on an IQ test. Acute neurological conditions and injuries, however, create a bulge in the normal distribution of IQs at the very low end. Therefore, advocacy groups often cite 3 percent as the prevalence of mental retardation, although this estimate has no objective support.

To contend that the estimated 3 percent of the population who would score below 70 on an IQ test have mental retardation assumes that they all would be significantly deficient in age-appropriate adaptive behavior and would remain so throughout their lives. In reality, many individuals whose IQs are below 70 do not exhibit difficulties in adaptive behavior. Mental retardation is not always a permanent condition—people can and do "cure" themselves by living relatively independent lives. Individuals are typically identified as having mental retardation during the school years, when academic problems bring attention to them; most are not officially recognized as having mental retardation beyond the school years (Grossman, 1973; President's Committee on Mental Retardation, 1970). A wide variation thus exists between the number of people who will at some point in their lifetimes be labeled as having mental retardation and the number who at any one time are treated as having retardation.

The primary reason for the wide variance in expected prevalence and the number of people actually identified may derive from this confusion over incidence and prevalence (MacMillan, 1977; Tarjan, 1964). While 2–3 percent of the population may be identified as having mental retardation at some point, closer to 1 percent of the population is identified at any one time (Birch et al., 1970; Dingman & Tarjan, 1960; Farber, 1968; MacMillan, 1977; Mercer, 1973; Tarjan et al., 1973). This considerably lower prevalence indicates that mental retardation is a permanently recognized condition for only about 0.5 percent of the population ("the stable population of persons with mental retardation").

The Stable Population of Persons with Mental Retardation

The functional characteristics and associated needs of adults with moderate to profound retardation (IQs of 50 or below) are such that relatively few achieve full independence, even though some may develop a range of self-care and employment skills.[2] Currently, a number of health, social, and demographic factors may be affecting the prevalence of this level of disability, including a sharp drop in infant mortality in the United States, resulting in high-risk premature babies surviving with severe developmental defects, and increased life expectancy of persons with mental retardation. On the preventive side, prevalence is being reduced by improved access to genetic screening, pre- and perinatal health and medical care, immunizations, and abortions. In combination, these factors may well have lowered the incidence of moderate to profound mental retardation while maintaining or slightly increasing its prevalence, causing a trend toward a generally older population of persons with moderate to profound mental retardation. The primary locus of social responses to the needs of persons with moderate to profound mental retardation will continue to shift from home and school (currently available through age twenty-one) to a full range of much more costly adult services.

The Transitory Population of Persons with Mental Retardation

Most persons identified as having mental retardation retain that label for only a limited portion of their lives. When identified, the vast majority are classified as having mild retardation, with IQs ranging roughly from 51 to 69. A sizable majority are identified as having mental retardation only while they are in school settings, although this number has been decreasing as less stigmatizing categories (especially learning disabilities) have been used to authorize and provide specialized educational services (U.S. Department of Education, 1980, 1985, 1992).

Schools play a substantial role in creating and treating the active prevalence of mental retardation: approximately 75 percent of the people identified at any one time as having mental retardation are children or adolescents (Lemkau, Tietze, & Cooper, 1941, 1942; Mercer, 1973; Tarjan et al., 1973). Virtually all persons identified as having mental retardation are identified before age twenty-one, and two-thirds do not retain that label in adulthood. Therefore, most mental retardation and almost all mild retardation is not a permanent state, but most often a transitory artifact of the social and academic expectation of schools. The combined prevalence of active mild retardation and stable (moderate to profound) retardation supports the estimate of only a 0.8–0.9 percent prevalence of active mental retardation at any one time.

Variations in Active Prevalence by Age Groupings

The severity of disability and the varying size of this population at different points in the life span are of particular importance to service systems. Infancy and early childhood are periods when the prevalence of identified mental retardation is low (less than 0.5 percent) but the severity is high. During the school years (ages six to twenty-six), the identified prevalence is high (about 1.4 percent reported by school districts to the Department of Education), but the severity is lowest. Prevalence again decreases in the adult years (returning to about 0.5 percent), but the severity of impairment is again relatively high.

Table 4.1 summarizes NHIS data on the primary cause of major activity limitations within a three-year sample of the U.S. population. It shows the prevalence of mental retardation per se and four conditions with which mental retardation is coinvolved when there are major activity limitations.

CORE SERVICE NEEDS

Mental retardation relates directly to the discrepancies between an individual's behavior and the expected behavior of a person of that age and culture. The most effective way to reduce those discrepancies is by

Table 4.1. Estimated Prevalence of Persons with Mental Retardation as Identified for Persons with Major Activity Limitations with "Main Cause" Indicated, 1985

	Under 18 Years[1]		All Ages	
	Number	% Population	Number	% Population
Noninstitutionalized population[2]				
Mental retardation	573,000	0.91	947,000	0.40
Cerebral palsy	74,000	0.12	151,000	0.06
Epilepsy	60,000	0.10	325,000	0.14
Schizophrenia/psychosis (evident				
in childhood)	18,000	0.03	69,000[3]	0.03[3]
Total	725,000	1.16	1,492,000	0.63
Institutionalized population				
MR/DD settings[4]	48,500		252,000	
Nursing homes[5]	500		47,500	
Psychiatric facilities	NA		4,500	
Total	49,000	0.07	304,000	0.13
Total estimated MR population	774,000	1.23	1,796,000	0.76
1985 Population base	62,992,000	26.33	239,283,000	100.00

Note: The statistics on noninstitutionalized populations (LaPlante, 1988) represent the prevalence of mental retardation among persons for whom chronic impairments are identified to be the main cause of limitations in major activities (kind or amount of work, housekeeping, or schooling). Institutionalized populations represent populations of persons identified as having the conditions above within institutional populations in 1985 (1986 in case of MR/DD facilities). In addition to conditions that represent the main cause of limitations in major activities, NHIS included identification of specific conditions within general classes for 1/6 of the sample regardless of limitations that might result. For the three major conditions causing limitations, the following number of cases and prevalences were estimated for noninstitutionalized populations, regardless of major activity limitations: mental retardation—1,086,000, or 0.45%; cerebral palsy—262,000, or 0.11%; and epilepsy—1,043,000, or 0.44%. NA means that data were not available.
1. Under 18 years of age for the noninstitutional population, under 21 years of age for the institutional population.
2. LaPlante, 1988.
3. Populations aged 18 and over with limiting condition estimated from the prevalence of impairments in the under 18 population because of inability to infer whether adults' condition of this type occurred in the developmental period.
4. Data from Center for Residential Services and Community Living, University of Minnesota (excludes generic foster care covered in survey of noninstitutionalized populations).
5. Data from analyses of 1985 National Nursing Home Survey by Center for Residential Services and Community Living, University of Minnesota. Includes primary diagnosis mental retardation and cerebral palsy.

providing opportunities to learn and practice age- and culturally appropriate behavior and skills. A number of emerging approaches in the "ideal" system of supportive care are being discussed. To avoid redundancy with chapter 3, the emphasis here is on nonmedical care. The issue of access to medical care and the development of other chronic conditions is common to many chronic conditions among children and is well covered by other chapters in this book. Before the core service needs of adults with mental retardation are addressed, however, prevention of mental retardation must be considered. Minimizing the number of persons identified as having mental retardation has important implications, because the resources and opportunities available for persons with mental retardation are finite.

Prevention of Mental Retardation

Community efforts have recently focused on prevention in response to the challenges of chronic conditions and disability. Evidence of this focus can be found in the Preventive Health Amendments of 1992; the publication of *Healthy People 2000: National Health Promotion and Disease Prevention Objectives* (U.S. Public Health Service, 1990) and *The Prevention of Primary and Secondary Conditions* (Centers for Disease Control, 1991); and in the emphasis on prevention of illness and disability in the ongoing discussion of health care reform. While prevention program expenditures are arguably the most cost-effective use of resources related to mental retardation, their costs and effects are difficult to define and measure, because they do not relate specifically to preventing mental retardation, but generally to supporting the birth and development of healthy, full-term children. This section describes a number of crucial areas in the prevention of mental retardation. Effective programs in each of these areas will have an important direct role in reducing mental retardation.

Prenatal Care and Monitoring

Prenatal care is generally acknowledged to be a significant predictor of favorable birth outcome (Institute of Medicine, 1985). Studies have shown that good prenatal care is associated with lower infant mortality rates (Gold, Kenney & Singh, 1987) and that lack of care is associated with preterm deliveries and low birthweight, which are significant predictors of developmental disabilities, including mental retardation (e.g., Buescher et al., 1988). Despite evidence supporting the benefits of prenatal care, providing access to services for poor and uninsured individuals remains a major challenge in this country, which is clearly associated with racial/ethnic differences and highlights the importance of culturally sensitive, specifically targeted efforts (Brown, 1988; Poland, Ager, & Olson, 1987). Evidence also suggests that many of those least likely to obtain prenatal care are at greatest social and environmental risk (e.g., persons who live or work in hazardous environments, have poor nutrition, or engage in adverse health behaviors). Programs and services that improve prenatal care and monitoring appear likely to make significant contributions to preventing mental retardation.

Reducing Low Birthweight

Infants of low birthweight (less than 2500 grams) are approximately three times as likely to experience developmental disabilities, including mental retardation, cerebral palsy, and autism (IOM, 1985). The evidence is clear that reducing the rate of low-weight births will make a significant contribution to reducing the number of children and adults with mental retardation.

Adolescent Pregnancy

Teenage pregnancies are significantly related to low birthweight. In 1988, 13 percent of mothers aged 14 and younger gave birth to low-birthweight babies, compared with 9 percent of mothers aged 15–19 and 7 percent of mothers aged 20–39 (NCHS, 1990). In addition, a number of social, economic, and educational factors associated with teenage pregnancy are associated with mental retardation, particularly mild transitory mental retardation evident primarily in the school years. Responding to teenage pregnancy is a huge challenge, with 70 percent of teenagers sexually active and birthrates for unwed teenage mothers increasing (CDC, 1992).

Nutritional Supplementation

Proper nutrition is critically important to prenatal development and to the development of children, particularly in the first three years of life. Inadequate nutrition is associated with vulnerability to illnesses and environmental toxins related to mental retardation (Committee on Environmental Hazards, 1987). The Supplemental Food Program for Women, Infants and Children (WIC) is dedicated to proper nutrition for pregnant women and children; its nutritional supplements are also supported with prenatal care services. The U.S. General Accounting Office (GAO) (1990) analyzed existing studies comparing the birthweights of children of WIC participants with those of nonparticipating control groups and concluded that WIC program participation is associated with higher birthweight and with cost-benefit ratios ranging from $1.92 to $4.21 for every $1.00 invested in WIC. Other federal programs that have been developed to support adequate nutrition for children include the Food Stamp program and the National School Lunch and Breakfast programs.[3]

Environmental Exposures

Pre- and postnatal exposure to harmful chemicals significantly affects fetal and postnatal development, exhibited in reduced birthweight, congenital malformations of the heart, and cognitive and other developmental limitations. The four chemical exposures of greatest known significance are fetal exposure to alcohol, smoking, and drugs, and child exposure to lead.

Fetal alcohol syndrome (FAS), now a well-recognized national health problem, is associated with a number of chronic behavioral and intellectual outcomes, including mild mental retardation and related congenital conditions. FAS affects approximately forty thousand (about 1.4 in 1,000) newborns each year, with rates among minorities being several times higher than for whites (Chavez, Cordero, & Becerra, 1988). Maternal smoking has been shown to have negative effects on prenatal development, including twice the rate of low birthweight as that of children born to nonsmoking mothers. Drug-exposed newborns make up about 11 percent of newborn children, a number believed to be growing rapidly (Select Committee on Children, Youth and Families, 1989). A 1990 report titled *A Generation at Risk* (U.S. GAO) concluded that while definitive information does not yet exist, "recent studies and surveys of neonatal programs suggest that some infants will suffer from central nervous system effects including neurobehavioral deficiencies." The report cited analyses indicating that 25 percent of drug-exposed children had developmental delays, 40 percent experienced neurological abnormalities, and 42–52 percent required special education. High lead levels have been found to be particularly damaging to central nervous system development and are linked to delayed physical and mental development (Bellinger et al., 1987). The U.S. Public Health Service (1988) estimated that in 1984 approximately three million children under six years of age had potentially harmful blood lead levels.

Table 4.2. Traditional Continua of Care in Residential and Habilitation/Vocational Programs for Persons with Mental Retardation

Residential Services	Habilitation/Vocational Services		Support Services
	Children	Adult	
Public MR/MI institution	No education	No day activity	Health-related services
Private institutions (residential schools)	Homebound (tutoring in living unit)	Day activity center	Therapy services
Nursing homes	School program in residential institution	Work activity center	Counseling and behavioral interventions
Community ICF-MRs	Day program in special school	Sheltered workshop	Transportation
Group homes	FT special class regular school	Supported work	Advocacy services
Personal care homes	PT regular/PT special class/resource room	Subsidized work	Social/leisure recreation
Foster care homes			Parent/care provider training
Boarding and care homes	Regular class with personal assistance, tutoring, and other assistance as needed		Other specialized services
Semi-independent living (adult)			
Supported independent living (adult)			
Respite care			
Independent (adults)	Regular classroom	Competitive employment	Generic community services
Nat/adopt. family (child)			

Early Intervention

Early intervention programs are intended to provide early life stimulation to children who have or are at risk for developmental delays. Early intervention includes infant and child assessment; developmental stimulation and teaching programs; family training and counseling; physical, speech, and other therapies; respite care; adaptive equipment; and a wide array of other services to assist the family in meeting the developmental needs of its children. The best programs provide training and support to parents to promote stimulation and learning in the child's natural settings throughout the day. Increasingly, early intervention includes support to sustain family involvement in the child's development. Early intervention programs serving very young children of low birthweight have shown positive benefits in reducing developmental delay and increasing measured intelligence (Infant Health and Development Program, 1990). Further evidence suggests that participation in Head Start, which is focused on at-risk three- and four-year-old children from low-income families, specifically reduces the number of children identified as having mild mental retardation during the school years (Lazar et al., 1984). A U.S. GAO report (1992) concluded that "Investments in effective early intervention programs that improve children's health and development benefit society as a whole. Effective early interventions can decrease federal, state and local government expenditures. Some early intervention programs, like WIC, pay back the investment rapidly, while others may not show results for many years" (38).

Community Services for Adults with Mental Retardation

Traditionally, services for persons with mental retardation were conceptualized as program models of increasing/decreasing intensity (and generally segregation) within major areas of daily life. In the area of housing (residential services), for example, residents of a particular community were provided with a continuum of service that ranged from large public institutions to independent living (Table 4.2). Such continua tacitly acknowledged that each component had a place in the system and that certain types of people were appropriately assigned to certain types of settings. Today's service system is more likely to accept the premise that individual outcomes rather than program models should be the focus of community services.

Persons with mental retardation have had substantially increased access to community services in recent years. Given documented associations between living in the community and desired personal outcomes, it is useful to look at broad indicators of changes in community service delivery as reflective of emerging concepts of the ideal care. Significant progress has been made in providing opportunities for persons with mental retardation to live in their own communities. In 1977, for example, only 8 percent of the 247,796 persons receiving residential services outside their homes were in places of six or fewer residents, compared with 51 percent (out of 314,503) in 1995. Because of rapidly declining populations, states have recently begun to close their institutions at unprecedented rates. Since 1988 three states and the District of Columbia have closed all their state mental retardation/developmental disabilities (MR/DD) institutions, and several states have plans to do so by the end of the century. Another indicator of changing patterns of residential care is the average number of people with mental retardation living in each residential setting and receiving residential services. That average decreased from 22.5 residents in 1977 to 3.7 residents in 1995.

Community living, however, must be seen as more than simple shifts among service models; it must be tied directly to the concept of community and to the goals people have for their lives. Most definitions of community focus on aspects of mutuality and reciprocity, as reflected in shared interests, interpersonal relationships, interdependent roles and involvement, and common expectations. The goals of community living for persons with mental retardation and the indicators of its benefits must be linked to definitions of a satisfying quality of life as people define it within their respective communities. Most definitions of this general goal include at least the following broad aspects of community life.

Presence in the Community

Presence is the sine qua non of community membership and is therefore an important indicator of community accomplishment in services for persons with mental retardation. Although the United States has experienced a quarter century of deinstitutionalization, great variation is found across states in the extent of community services development. Early efforts to reduce the populations of large public institutions resulted in the development of many large private institutions, and tens of thousands of persons with mental retardation were transferred to nursing homes (Prouty & Lakin, 1996). In 1982, about 6,000 persons with profound mental retardation lived in community residential settings; by 1990, there were approximately three times that number (Hayden, Lakin, Bruininks, & Chen, 1992; Lakin, Bruininks, & Larson, 1991; Lakin et al., 1989).

Progress in developing community services for current institution residents depends on focusing on services that meet the needs of persons with profound mental retardation, which often presents a challenge. The approximately 143,800 people with mental retardation living in residential institutions and nursing homes in 1994 were primarily people with severe intellectual, medical, and behavioral disabilities (Prouty & Lakin, 1995).[4] In 1994, 66 percent of residents of state institutions were reported to have profound mental retardation (Prouty & Lakin, 1995); similar patterns exist for persons with medical or behavioral impairments. Substantial and growing community presence for these persons currently exists, but institutional placement still prevails (Lakin et al., 1989). Systematic discrimination continues to be common practice against persons with severe impairments, despite evidence that they greatly benefit from community living (Larson & Lakin, 1989).

Supported community living is a new concept that is having major effects on the goals and desired indicators of quality of life for citizens with mental retardation. Supported community living includes several basic premises (O'Brien & O'Brien, 1991; Racino et al., 1992; Skarnulis & Lakin, 1990):

- All persons need and deserve a home of their own.
- Funding for housing should be separate from funding for services.
- Services should be planned around personal preferences and desired life styles.
- The natural supports and relationships available through family, community, and friends should be fostered.
- People should have a choice in the type and source of services they receive.
- Services should be deliverable in varied ways.
- Service providers should seek less intrusive ways to deliver services and be more sensitive to being in a person's home.
- Service providers must adjust to a "market" in which "clients" and revenues are determined by demand for specific services rather than a total number of people to be provided comprehensive care.

Each of these premises implies significant change from the traditional facility-based system of service delivery. A relatively small fraction of persons with mental retardation currently participates in supported living,[5] but the concept contributes to the personalization of community services, focusing heightened attention on basic aspects of the quality of life.

Health, Safety, and Basic Comfort

As people with mental retardation test and extend their abilities to live independently in their communities, they must be assured of appropriate attention to their health. People who depend on Medicaid to finance their medical care are reported to have problems obtaining medical care and related services. Like many other persons with disabilities, people with mental retardation who have modest incomes that exclude them from qualifying for Medicaid are frequently without health insurance; are excluded from private insurance because of preexisting condition exclusions, high premiums, and copayments; or are provided benefit packages that limit specific benefits they need (Consortium for Citizens with Disabilities, Health Task Force, 1991). People from rural areas who need specialized medical services are also likely to have difficulty accessing needed services. Providing community membership for all persons with mental retardation (i.e., enabling a large proportion of those in nursing homes to live in the community) will require that medical service delivery systems better accommodate the access limitations and specific health care needs of people with mental retardation.

The three methods typically used to ensure the basic safety and well-being of persons with mental retardation living outside nursing homes or state institutions are (a) training family and personal assistants, (b) providing technical assistance, and (c) monitoring. Ensuring safety and well-being is a growing challenge for several reasons. The first is the rapid multiplication of community residential services (Prouty & Lakin, 1996). Second, although living arrangements with less than full-time supervision permit people to enjoy their greatest possible liberty, they reduce monitoring of their well-being. Third, caseloads for service coordinators (case managers) are often too large (thirty to seventy service recipients per case manager) (Prouty & Lakin, 1991), and most licensing and survey programs provide for only annual or semiannual visits. Current systems will need to expand by multiples of three or more to accommodate the shift of populations from nursing homes and other institutional settings into community settings.

Responding to the challenges of ensuring safety in a dispersed service delivery system requires new ways of thinking about quality assurance and related quality-enhancement activities. While quality assurance will continue to focus attention on basic health and safety, it is being increasingly defined around quality-of-life outcomes, with health and safety being just one component (Blake et al., 1994). Establishing and maintaining relationships and commitments among persons with mental retardation, their families, friends, neighbors, and advocates is recognized as playing a critical role in protecting people's well-being (O'Brien & O'Brien, 1993).

Basic protection also means assurances regarding basic rights and freedom from abuse, exploitation, and neglect. The low expectations and high degree of stigma faced by persons with mental retardation represent substantial barriers to their ability to benefit fully from the Americans with Disabilities Act (Lakin & Jones, 1993). Being accepted and valued as a full member of the community is an important protection of rights for all people.

The basic right of children in this culture to live in a family is generally recognized and respected. The Adoption Assistance and Child Welfare Act of 1980 requires that states make initial efforts to prevent out-of-home placements through support and services to natural families. When out-of-home placement is unavoidable, plans must be developed to return the child promptly; when return home is no longer viable, adoption or permanent foster family placement must be secured. The United States has made great strides in reducing the number of children with mental retardation living outside natural or adoptive homes, from about 91,000 in 1977 to 48,500 in 1988 (Taylor, Lakin & Hill, 1989). While permanency planning is a guarantee for children served in child welfare/social service systems, however, it is not mandated for those whose services are funded by Medicaid and education programs. Significant challenges remain in providing equal opportunities for typical family living for all children and youth, including providing supplemental income and medical assistance; extending adherence to the permanency planning process to children with mental retardation, regardless of how services are funded; and prohibiting the admission of children to congregate-care settings (Taylor et al., 1989).

Basic protection should include freedom from discrimination based on severity of impairment in opportunities for community living (Taylor, 1988), standards for guardianship (Flower, 1994), and freedom from repressive environments (O'Brien, 1989; Reichle & Light, 1992). Progress has been made in recognizing the rights of persons with challenging behavior to enjoy less restricted lives in community environments (Reichle & Light, 1992). As services to persons with challenging behavior become more dispersed across community settings, there is a critical need to establish, expand, and integrate ongoing training, technical assistance, and crisis support activities for families and community agencies. Such efforts are often cost-effective alternatives to institution services (Rudolph & Lakin, 1994).

Opportunity for Personal Growth and Development

Persons with mental retardation need to learn new skills that add to their competence and fulfill their interests, and these functional skills are developed better through community living than through institutional living (Larson & Lakin, 1991). More and more, the focus of instruction and supported participation for persons with mental retardation is being derived from the interests of individuals and from analyses of what these individuals need to know to fulfill their personal goals and desires. Personalized individual planning models (e.g., personal futures planning, lifestyle planning) are being used to identify personally valued outcomes in such areas as housing, family involvement, social relationships, leisure activities, employment, and other central components of typical daily life (Mount & Zwernik, 1988; Smull & Harrison, 1992). As a result, persons with mental retardation have achieved levels of independence, inclusion, and self-determination that were rare ten to fifteen years ago (Lakin, Burwell, Hayden, & Jackson, 1992; Reichle, York, & Sigafoos, 1991; Schleien et al., 1993).

The quality of community experiences of persons with mental retardation largely depends on the persons providing support and instruction to them. Developing and improving systematic approaches to the recruitment, training, and retention of community personnel, particularly direct care/personal assistance staff, will be a great challenge in the next decade (Larson, Hewitt, & Lakin, 1994). Annual turnover of staff in community residential settings averages 55–75 percent nationwide (Braddock & Mitchell, 1992). A minority of staff have had any specialized training other than that provided by the agencies for which they work (Hill et al.,

1989), yet these individuals have greater responsibility and less direct supervision than people in similar roles in institutions.

Social Relationships

Social relationships, especially those with family members, are a key to quality of life. Frequently, family involvement, which is notably greater when the person with mental retardation resides in the community, provides important protection, monitoring, and individual advocacy (Lutfiyya, 1991). Many families, however, express dissatisfaction with the quality of communication with community service providers and with the lack of facilitation of family involvement (Larson & Lakin, 1991).

Establishing and sustaining social relationships represent major challenges for persons with mental retardation in the community, who are sometimes as isolated as their counterparts living in institutions (Bercovici, 1983).[6] Persons with mental retardation tend to be less socially integrated than the general population (Hill et al., 1989). Researchers have begun to document the methods that individuals and agencies use to promote and sustain meaningful social relationships (Green & Schleien, 1991; Taylor & Bogdan, 1989). Many of these methods can be subsumed under the following broad areas:

1. Sustaining the family social network after a child has left home
2. Participating in churches, schools, civic organizations, and other local institutions
3. Becoming involved in organizations that are typical sources of social relationships and friendships
4. Participating in community improvement projects

Efforts to sustain interactions over prolonged periods appear particularly important, since programs of pairing simply for peer interaction (buddy programs) tend to have few lasting effects (Hirsch & DuBois, 1989; Meyer & Putnam, 1988).

Valued Community Participation

Nothing is more important to persons with mental retardation than being valued community members. Because of years of segregation and discrimination, recognition of people's full citizenship often requires proactive involvement. Actively using the resources of a community (libraries, theaters, parks, restaurants, stores, etc.) is an important way of communicating one's membership. Compared with people in institutions, people living in the community are more likely to use community resources (Hayden, Lakin, Hill, Bruininks, & Copher, 1992; Hill et al., 1989).

Work is the simplest, most valued, and most cost-effective way for adults with mental retardation to contribute to their communities. Supported employment has been the most visible and rapidly growing method of assisting people to contribute to their community, but these opportunities remain relatively uncommon for persons with mental retardation.[7] Persons with severe and profound mental retardation are even less likely to have access to work opportunities. Competitive and supported employment opportunities need to be not only substantially expanded but better designed to include more direct interaction between the persons with mental retardation and coworkers; the use of work-site employees as providers of support is among the innovations for accomplishing this. Opportunities for people with mental retardation to contribute to their communities through work lag far behind their opportunities to reside in communities. An important factor in this discrepancy is the continued disallowance under Medicaid long-term care programs of funding for vocationally oriented services, while funding for segregated day habilitation programs remains unlimited.

Involving persons with mental retardation in the selection and maintenance of their home environments engages them in a valued social role, increases their skills in independent living, and marks them (not an agency) as the one paying for housing and thus contributing to the local economy. Persons in community settings tend to participate more in household tasks than those in institutional settings, although considerable variation exists within community settings, with family care settings being least likely to involve people in domestic duties (Hill et al., 1989). Domestic involvement is also particularly low among persons with more severe impairments, although research shows that greater participation is associated with higher expectations of participation, more opportunities for partial or assisted participation in tasks, and increased staff training (Hill et al., 1989).

People with mental retardation can be visible not only as workers and householders but also as consumers of goods and services, volunteers, representatives on boards and committees, spokespersons and political activists, participants in community organizations and recreation/leisure activities, and so forth (Abery, 1994; Rynders & Schleien, 1991). These efforts are critical to having people with mental retardation valued by their community.

Personal Autonomy and Self-determination

Supporting and enhancing self-determination are essential parts of providing the opportunities for people to benefit fully from community living. Unfortunately, denial of personal control for persons with mental retardation is often taken for granted. Assisting people in developing their full potential and exercising their full rights of citizenship requires providing them with opportunities to make and act on choices in all aspects of daily life (Abery, 1994). Local, state, and national self-advocacy organizations have created more pervasive general expectations that people with mental retardation must be included in making program and policy decisions that affect their lives (Hayden & Shoultz, 1991a, 1991b).

SERVICE SYSTEM ISSUES

Services for persons with mental retardation are evolving from a system in which most people lived in large congregate settings, particularly state institutions, to one in which people live in typical community housing with varying levels of staff supervision and support. This transformation often puts traditional service systems in conflict with what people with mental retardation need to support community lifestyles; these conflicts begin with financing.

Intermediate Care Facilities for Persons with Mental Retardation (ICFs-MR)

Forty-three percent of all persons with mental retardation who are receiving services while living outside their family homes reside in ICF-MR-certified congregate-care settings of four or more residents.[8] Under this program, these facilities and their services are treated in much the same manner as nursing facilities. The federal Medicaid program cost-shares from 50 to 80 percent (depending on a state's per capita income) of a comprehensive daily rate for Medicaid-eligible residents. ICFs-MR must comply with specifically designed, highly detailed administrative, environmental, personnel, and treatment requirements.

ICF-MR care is expensive. In 1995, the average annual cost to the Medicaid program of an ICF-MR recipient was about $70,900. The costs of large public ICFs-MR ($85,800 per resident per year) are also much higher than the costs of other ICFs-MR and range dramatically from state to state (from a low of about $136 a day to over $465 a day). ICF-MR expenditures have increased at an annual rate of approximately 10 percent since 1987.[9] In 1992, over half of the estimated $17.1 billion for noneducational services for persons with mental retardation and related conditions (excluding direct cash payments such as Supplemental Security Income (SSI) or Social Security Disability Insurance (SSDI), generic services like Medicaid physician services, or generic subsidies like food stamps) went to ICFs-MR (Braddock et al., 1994). Medicaid is essentially the sole payer for all care provided within an ICF-MR, since nearly every resident is a Medicaid enrollee. Typically, individuals who live in ICFs-MR participate in one of three types of day programs, either on or off site: *(a)* developmental or day habilitation programs, in which individuals are taught various developmental and daily living skills; *(b)* sheltered workshops; and *(c)* supported employment programs. Only the first of these is reimbursable as an ICF-MR service, with off-site day habilitation programs typically reimbursed as an active treatment subcontractor of the ICF-MR.

As can be inferred, the ICF-MR program is considerably out of step with the evolving approaches to community services. It provides little flexibility, requires people to live in congregate-care homes to receive services, and establishes incentives for nonwork day activities. Despite this, ICF-MR populations remained stable between 1982 and 1993 (total population, 144,000 ± 4,000) because of the favorable federal cost-share they provide to states. However, since 1993, ICF-MR populations have begun to fall, decreasing from 147,729 residents in June 1993 to 134,384 in June 1995.

Medicaid Home and Community-Based Services (HCBS)

Since 1981, states have had the option of providing HCBS to persons with mental retardation and related conditions. Under this option, certain existing Medicaid requirements are waived, and states are allowed to finance designated noninstitutional services for Medicaid-eligible individuals who would otherwise remain in or be placed in a Medicaid institution (i.e., a nursing facility or an ICF-MR). Noninstitutional services allowed under the HCBS program include case management, personal care services, adult day health services, habilitation services, respite care, or any other service that will lead to stable or decreased costs for Medicaid-funded long-term care. Although not allowed to use HCBS reimbursements to pay for room and board, virtually all states offering HCBS do provide services in the home under the categories of personal care, habilitation, and homemaker services and, in most instances, use cash assistance from other Social Security Act programs to fund the room and board portion of the residential program. Given its flexibility and its potential for promoting the goal of community-based care and habilitation, the HCBS program has been beneficial to states in providing community services. In applying to provide HCBS, however, states must document that should the application be approved, the total state Medicaid expenditures and the total number of ICF-MR plus HCBS recipients would not exceed the expenditures and total recipients that would have resulted without the HCBS authorization. For most of the history of the HCBS program, these restrictions limited states' ability to use the HCBS alternative as fully they would have wished.[10] But since 1992, the Health Care Financing Administration has allowed far greater flexibility in approving state plans for HCBS programs, and as a result, both the number of HCBS recipients and expenditures grew by more than 130 percent from June 1992 to June 1995.

Medicaid long-term care services for persons with mental retardation and related conditions were long criticized for their institutional orientation. The HCBS program and, to a much lesser extent, the development of ICF-MR services in homes of four to fifteen residents have dramatically reduced the statistical substantiation for such criticisms. The HCBS program provides the opportunity to help people live in their own homes, but it cannot ensure that they will be able to do so.[11] An important difference between the HCBS and ICF-MR programs is the remarkably reduced number and specificity of federal standards for the former, which require only that states make and document appropriate procedures for the protection of the basic health and safety of recipients.

Medicaid Community-Supported Living Arrangements (CSLA)

Although Medicaid HCBS programs now exist in all states to provide services to persons who would otherwise be at risk of ICF-MR or nursing home care, states have wanted continued expansion of Medicaid community service benefits, for example, increasing the number of people who can be served in the community beyond the total number of authorized HCBS recipients. States have also had an interest in receiving federal assistance to serve persons who would not necessarily be ICF-MR eligible (i.e., do not require twenty-four-hour plans of care and/or active treatment). In 1990 Congress enacted legislation to allow up to eight states to provide CSLA to Medicaid-eligible persons with mental retardation and related conditions. CSLA provided greater flexibility in service provision, permitted specific targeting of services to eligible groups and geographic areas within a state, did not require demonstration of a need for care at the ICF-MR or nursing home level for eligibility, and allowed each state to develop its own quality assurance plan within defined federal standards. Total cost of the CSLA program was capped on an annual basis in each of the program's five years and at a five-year total of $100 million.

Proposals among the eight states[12] selected to provide CSLA varied in target populations, projected numbers of recipients, services to be included, cost per recipient, and other aspects. The CSLA program offered the potential of enhancing the quality of services by integrating a number of elements long viewed as necessary to such an effort, including variety and personalization of services, choice of services and vendors, and consumer involvement in quality assurance. Program development as defined by the number of individuals served was considerably slower than originally projected. In 1992, only 265 individuals were being served, and in 1995, the final year of the CSLA program, approximately 3,500 individuals were being served, at a total expenditure of $20.8 million. The CSLA program ended in September 1995 with virtually all CSLA participants being enrolled in state HCBS programs. The legacy of the CSLA programs is evident in how most of the HCBS programs in the CSLA states were modified toward the end of the CSLA "experiment" to reflect the goals and principles of "community-supported living."

Medicaid Nursing Facilities (NFs)

In 1995, approximately 34,000 persons with mental retardation were residing in Medicaid NFs. This number has been steadily declining as a result of the 1987 Omnibus Reconciliation Act, which stipulated that states must screen persons with mental retardation in nursing homes for the appropriateness of their placement and then submit "Alternative Disposition Plans" regarding the findings of those reviews. Both Medicaid

HCBS financing and institutional ICF-MR placements are available to individuals leaving nursing homes.

Other Services

In addition to the specific programs for persons with mental retardation described above, Medicaid finances twelve mandatory services, including physician services, inpatient and outpatient hospital services, laboratory services, home health services, NF services, and others. Most states also offer (at the state's option) dental services, physical therapy, optometrist services, eyeglasses, prescribed drugs, speech and language services, personal care services, and other services used by people with mental retardation who live in community settings. For example, most service recipients with mental retardation have a designated case manager/service coordinator, which may be a Medicaid-financed service through a Medicaid targeted case management program, an HCBS service, or a state- and local-funded service. Most ICF-MR and HCBS recipients also receive transportation services, whose costs are often included within the per diem rate for the day or residential program.

Other Programs

The two primary payment sources for non-Medicaid services for persons with mental retardation are Supplemental Security Income/State Supplemental Payment benefits (SSI/SSP), and state and local MR/DD agency funds (including the federal Social Services Title XX Block Grant). Unlike persons in ICFs-MR, individuals in community non-ICF-MR living arrangements (including HCBS recipients) are entitled to retain their full SSI/SSP benefits. Non-ICF-MR residents in residential settings, including most HCBS recipients, are usually required to finance their own room and board, which usually means signing over their SSI/SSP benefit checks to the provider, keeping a small monthly amount as personal spending money. The SSI/SSP payment is treated as a voucher to cover the costs of room and board. In many cases, the residential provider is the representative payee for the resident, so that SSI/SSP is sent directly to the provider. This system, however, raises concerns, because SSI/SSP is supposed to be a benefit paid to an individual with a disability for basic necessities, not a residential program payment controlled by others.

State MR/DD agencies are the primary payment source for non-

Medicaid services. These funds are made available from state revenues and certain federal flow-through programs, most notable the Social Services Block Grant. Although the largest single state expenditure for services to persons with mental retardation is usually the Medicaid match, other state funds contribute to a wide range of residential, vocational, and other day programs. In many states, MR/DD agencies distribute funds to regional or county human service agencies, which in turn contract for residential programs from service providers. County revenues may be used to augment state funds. On the individual level, many state and local housing authority benefits may be tapped to assist in financing a residence, for example, HUD Section 8 housing subsidies. A number of other HUD programs have also assisted service providers in financing group homes.

State funds are also the principle sources of financing for services related to employment. While vocational rehabilitation programs are technically committed by law to giving priority in services to the most severely impaired (among whom are persons with mental retardation), they have played a relatively limited role in supporting vocational services for persons with mental retardation. The eighteen-month limit on supported employment services means that many persons with mental retardation who have permanent needs for support are excluded from vocational rehabilitation services.

FACTORS LIMITING ACCESS AND USE

Currently, many people with mental retardation cannot obtain community residential, vocational, and day habilitation services, resulting in growing waiting lists for community services (Davis, 1987; Hayden & DePaepe, 1993; Ward & Halloran, 1989). Adult children who have remained at home appear to have the most serious problems with access to services and other programs. Two periods are notable: (a) early adulthood, when children typically leave the family home and special education entitlements end, and (b) middle age, as aged parents are no longer able to care for a child still living in the family home (Hayden, Spicer, et al., 1992). Among factors that contribute to the limited access to community services is the competition for these services, which comes from individuals leaving institutions and results in much less being available for those requesting services for the first time. States are attempting to reduce their institutional costs, particularly by closing existing state institutions (82 state institutions were closed between 1988 and 1995), but they often fail to use the saved resources for financing community services to absorb the case load.

As community service goals and financing are redefined, an important related policy issue concerns the development of new quality assurance systems. The ICF-MR program evolved as a heavily regulated program to respond to the abuses of many large institutions. The pendulum is now swinging back to less regulated systems of care, in which people with mental retardation have more control over where and how they choose to live. A number of states, local governments, and agencies have begun to experiment with new approaches to quality assurance and enhancement (Blake et al., 1994). The Accreditation Council on Services for People with Disabilities (1993) has totally redesigned its accreditation process around outcome objectives and indicators of value to the recipients of services. Consumer choice and self-determination must be balanced, however, with the requirements of publicly financed programs to protect the health and safety of individuals receiving services.

COMMUNITY OUTCOMES AND INDICATORS

Paralleling the balance of this chapter, this section is divided into two general parts: *(a)* prevention of mental retardation and *(b)* community services for persons with mental retardation.

Prevention Activities

Because measurement of the prevalence of mental retardation and other developmental disorders is expensive, this section focuses on more readily available risk factors (e.g., reductions in the rate of low-birthweight infants) and service system responses presented earlier as preventive. The suggested community-level indicators are shown in Table 4.3. These often parallel the indicators of access to care proposed by the Institute of Medicine (Millman, 1993) and *Healthy People 2000* (U.S. Public Health Service, 1990). Most of these indicators are best obtained using a survey, with persons identified at the time of delivery of care as being in a high-risk or other target group. These "follow-back" surveys are recommended over population-based community surveys because they are substantially less expensive. Medicaid claims data might also be used to quantify the frequency of medical care visits and the procedures received.

Table 4.3. Preventive Activities Indicators

Indicator	Data Source
Prenatal care and monitoring	
• Proportion of pregnant women in all socioeconomic and racial/ethnic groups who have at least one physician or prenatal specialist visit in each trimester	• Follow-back survey or Medicaid claims review
• Proportion of pregnant women and women in pregnancy "risk" groups who participate in prenatal education	• Follow-back survey
• Proportion of participating women who retain key information on prenatal care and health practices.	• Program participant survey
Reducing low birthweight	
• Proportion of individuals from populations at risk for low birthweight who are aware of factors associated with low birthweight	• Community survey or high school survey
• Proportion of eligible pregnant women and women at highest probability of pregnancy who are enrolled in nutritional support programs	• Follow-back survey
• Proportion of women who are aware of the dangers and signs of preterm labor and of actions to prevent preterm delivery	• Follow-back or community survey of all births
• Proportion of low-birthweight births generally and among different groups in the community	• Hospital discharge abstracts
Adolescent pregnancies	
• Proportion of teenage births among all births	• Hospital discharge abstracts
• Proportion of the total adolescent population and at-risk subgroups who are reached by pregnancy prevention programs.	• Synthetic estimates compared with program encounters
• Percentage of all community members who have knowledge of and access to family planning clinics and contraceptives	• Community survey
• Proportion of teenage mothers and fathers receiving instruction in health, safety, and staying in school	• Follow-back survey
• Proportion of teenage parents who have access to ongoing medical care services for their children, and the proportion who use them	• Follow-back survey or Medicaid claims
Nutrition	
• Proportion of pregnant and at-risk women, children, and youth who are identified as needing nutritional support, and the proportion who are enrolled in nutritional support programs	• Follow-back survey
• Proportion of pregnant women or those in high-probability groups who have access to meal programs in the schools or the community	• Follow-back survey
• Proportion of pregnant women and parents from all racial/ethnic and socioeconomic groups who are aware of the nutritional needs of infants and young children	• Follow-back survey

(continued)

Table 4.3.   *(continued)*

Environmental factors

• Measurement of smoking and drug and alcohol use among pregnant women and women at the highest probability of pregnancy	• Follow-back survey or community survey
• Proportion of pregnant women and women in the childbearing years who smoke, drink, or use drugs and who are enrolled in treatment	• Follow-back survey
• Number of public programs in place (including disincentives such as taxes and fines) to reduce exposure to toxins in the environment, with evaluation systems set up to measure progress	• Survey of public agencies

Early intervention

• Proportion of parents participating in parenting classes within various communities	• Follow-back survey
• Proportion of infants and children receiving medical and developmental evaluations	• Follow-back survey or Medicaid claims
• Proportion of children who have been identified and recruited for early education programs within various communities	• Follow-back survey
• Proportion of developmentally delayed and at-risk children participating in early education programs	

Indicators for Community Services for Adults with Mental Retardation

The guiding principles of services for mental retardation have shifted significantly. Beyond the commitment to community services, careful consideration has been given to how services can be used and evaluated for their contributions to improving the quality of life for persons with mental retardation. Although these indicators of progress are somewhat new elements in monitoring the quality and effectiveness of community services, they are available in at least one or more states.

The emphasis is on two basic types of indicators: those concerned with access to care and those associated with client perspectives on the appropriateness, quality, and functional outcomes from this care. The indicators are shown in Table 4.4. Given the relatively low prevalence of developmental disability in the general population, the suggested sources for most of the proposed measures are either synthetic estimates of prevalence compared with agency encounter–based estimates of the target groups or surveys of service recipients.

Table 4.4. Adult Service Indicators

Indicator	Data Source
Community presence	
• Proportion of target population living in community settings as opposed to institutions	• Synthetic estimates or community survey and provider encounters
• Percentage of financial allocations for services going to people living in the community	• Agency survey
• Proportion of individuals with severe target disabilities living in community settings	• Synthetic estimates or community survey and provider encounters
• Number of people on lists waiting for services	• Agency survey
Health, safety, and comfort	
• Proportion of community residents who have access to key health and related services, and the proportion for whom these services are judged adequate	• Recipient survey or Medicaid claims
• Proportion of community residents who have their safety and well-being monitored on a frequent basis by government agencies, case managers, family members, etc.	• Recipient survey
• Proportion of individuals able to benefit from appropriate technology who have access to it	
• Proportion of people who have chosen the place where they live and/or who hold the lease on it, and the proportion who have private and personalized spaces that they control	• Recipient survey
• Proportion of families with children with mental retardation who receive various family cash subsidies and supports (e.g., respite care, home health care, home modifications, etc.)	• Recipient survey
Personal growth and development	
• Proportion of individuals increasing their functional daily living skills and the proportion decreasing challenging behavior	• Recipient survey
• Proportion of people engaging in activities and instruction directly related to their own expressed desires, and the proportion satisfied with those activities and instruction	• Recipient survey
• Proportion of direct care staff leaving their positions each year, and the proportion expressing satisfaction with the relevance and utility of their training	• Provider survey
Social relationships	
• Proportion of individuals with weekly (or more frequent) visits from family and friends of the family	• Recipient survey
• Proportion of people who have friends among neighbors and other community numbers, with whom they are involved on a weekly basis	• Recipient survey

(continued)

Table 4.4   *(continued)*

• Proportion of people who exhibit serious challenging behavior, especially in the areas of aggression toward others or their property	• Provider survey, family survey
Valued cultural participation	
• Proportion of people using various community resources on a weekly basis	• Recipient survey
• Proportion of people engaged in real work at various levels of pay	• Recipient survey
• Proportion of people who are involved in meetings and community activities on a monthly basis	• Recipient survey
Personal autonomy and self-determination	
• Proportion of people participating in self-chosen weekly activities outside their homes	• Recipient survey
• Proportion engaged in self-chosen learning skills that relate directly to activities or social roles	• Recipient survey
• Proportion participating in self-advocacy groups	• Recipient survey
• Proportion of people expressing satisfaction with the major areas of their lives (homes, roommates, jobs or other day activities, personal assistance, social lives, etc.)	• Recipient survey

CONCLUSION

How much priority should be given to tracking the risk factors, service access, and consumer satisfaction of those with developmental disabilities, including mental retardation? The relatively low prevalence of these conditions in the population perhaps argues for a relatively low priority, as do the complexity and cost associated with survey-based data collection, which has been suggested as the most viable source of indicators. On the other hand, much of this disability can be prevented, and many of those with these challenges can, with appropriate assistance, lead relatively independent and self-satisfying lives.

On balance, countervailing incentives such as these suggest that some sort of monitoring system is appropriate, both for prevention and for quality assurance. The latter would emphasize the noninstitutional approaches that are becoming characteristic of the care for adults with developmental disability. Building from this assumption, it is necessary to address the practical question of how to implement the proposed monitoring system in a cost-effective way. Sample frame development is fundamental to this issue; this implies that the delivery system can identify the entire relevant population, and access these names, and field the data collection. Community social service and special education program records appear to be reasonably good sources for identifying persons (including their families) who have conditions defined as developmental disabilities or who are in the target classifications of at-risk subgroups for whom the incidence of developmental disability has a higher probability. Noninstitutionalized adults with developmental disabilities who may not be enrolled in human services programs present a greater challenge. With the exception of large national surveys, such as the 1994–95 Disability Supplement to the NHIS, general population surveys are too expensive to mount on a community-by-community basis. Service recipient–based samples, with their inherent bias toward users, are more accessible, but they too carry high data collection costs if repeated on a community basis, and they are biased in reflecting only those in the service system.

One alternative may be to track service access (e.g., from Medicaid service claims and the relative distribution of clients in institutional and noninstitutional care) among all or a sample of communities as a minimum data set and indicator of prevalence and service access. Risk behaviors, which are often more generic, fall into a middle ground and can be tracked via existing resources, such as the Behavioral Risk Factor Surveillance System (BRFSS), conducted in conjunction with the CDC. Service satisfaction, autonomy, and the other self-actualization outcomes discussed throughout the chapter, although of interest to provider and consumer groups, could perhaps be incorporated into geographically targeted samples. These might be probability selected, selected to reflect specific types of communities (e.g., those with comprehensive service systems vs. those with less comprehensive systems), or selected on some other catchment-area basis. The point here would be to concentrate the resources needed to develop the samples and field the data collection. General trends in service appropriateness and outcomes would be inferred from such efforts. The policy response to these results would affect the general approaches to care, not specific communities. In short, on the premise that monitoring care for those with developmental disabilities is desirable, viable and feasible indicators can be obtained. Left to other venues is resolution of the geographic breadth of this endeavor.

Notes

1. See appendix A for a detailed list of NCHS data sets.

2. Studies of noninstitutionalized adolescents (Abramowicz & Richardson, 1975; Stein & Susser, 1975) show that persons with this level of impairment constitute approximately 0.4 percent of the population. Adjustments to include

institutionalized persons would make 0.5 percent a reasonable estimate of the percentage of the total population with moderate to profound retardation.

3. Despite clear evidence of the importance of nutrition to child development, 48 percent of eligible families with preschool children did not participate in WIC, and the proportion of eligible families participating has declined by about 14 percent over the last decade. In 1980, only about 50 percent of those eligible actually participated in the School Lunch and Breakfast programs, and the program received a 25 percent cut in federal dollars for meals between 1980 and 1988 (Select Committee on Children, Youth and Families, 1989).

4. The 1987 National Medical Expenditure Survey (NMES) estimated that 14 percent of residents of places with fifteen or fewer residents had profound mental retardation as opposed to 47 percent of residents of all larger facilities (Lakin et al., 1989). A national study (Hill et al., 1989) of persons living in small (six or fewer people) residential facilities estimated that 20 percent of the residents of small Intermediate Care Facilities for Persons with Mental Retardation (ICFs-MR) had profound retardation, as did about 9 percent of the foster home residents and 13 percent of the non-ICF-MR group home residents.

5. Nationally, only about twenty-eight thousand people received either supported or semi-independent living services in 1992 (the latter being settings in which less than 24-hour-a-day supervision and training is provided in the residential unit) (Prouty & Lakin, 1996).

6. A recent statewide assessment of Minnesota's Home and Community-Based Services (HCBS) waiver program showed recipients to be actively engaged in recreation and leisure activities, but only about 5 percent participated in these activities with people other than family members, people in their residential or day programs, or paid staff members (Lakin et al., 1991).

7. A 1990 survey of state MR/DD agencies indicated that of 281,339 service recipients with known day activities, only 4 percent were in competitive employment or in time-limited training programs directed at competitive employment. Another 8 percent were in supported employment situations (i.e., work environments in which most employees did not have disabilities and in which ongoing support was provided to train, assist, or monitor the individual with mental retardation). In contrast, over 88 percent spent their days in sheltered workshop and day habilitation centers (McGaughey et al., 1991). The numbers differed significantly among states.

8. In 1995, 6,947 residential facilities (total population, 134,384) were certified as ICFs-MR, of which 6 percent were operated by state governments. Although most (89 percent) ICFs-MR are small (fifteen or fewer residents), the great majority of ICF-MR residents still live in large facilities. In 1992, 72 percent of ICF-MR residents lived in facilities with more than sixteen residents (Prouty & Lakin, 1996), and 75 percent of the $8.8 billion spent on ICF-MR services was spent on these large facilities (Braddock et al., 1994). In 1995, only 21 percent of people living in community settings with fifteen or fewer residents and only 13 percent of people living in settings with six or fewer residents lived in ICFs-MR (Prouty & Lakin, 1996).

9. Total ICF-MR expenditures in 1987 were $5.5 billion; in 1989, $6.6 bil-

lion; in 1991, $8.2 billion; in 1993, $9.2 billion; and in 1995, $9.5 billion.

10. Since enactment of the Medicaid HCBS program in 1981, all states have chosen to provide HCBS. The number of program participants grew from 1,381 in 1982 to 62,462 in 1992, in which year states expended approximately $1.6 billion on the HCBS program. By June 1995, the number of participants had grown to 149,185, with states expending approximately $3.7 billion on the HCBS program. The average expenditure of $24,900 per recipient plus an average yearly SSI/SSDI payment of about $5,500 was still less than 50 percent of the average ICF-MR cost of $70,900 per recipient (Prouty & Lakin, 1996).

11. Statistics on 55 percent of HCBS recipients showed that in June 1995 about 25 percent lived with their natural family, 46 percent lived in housing owned or rented by the agency providing services to them, 13 percent in foster home type arrangements, 13 percent in homes that they themselves owned or rented, and 2 percent in other types of arrangements.

12. California, Colorado, Florida, Illinois, Maryland, Michigan, Rhode Island, Wisconsin.

References

Abery, B. 1994. A framework for enhancing self-determination. In M. F. Hayden and B. Abery (eds.), *Challenges for a Service System in Transition* (pp. 345–80). Baltimore: Paul H. Brookes.

Abramowicz, H. K., & Richardson, S. A. 1975. Epidemiology of severe mental retardation in children: Community studies. *American Journal of Mental Deficiency 80*: 18–39.

Accreditation Council on Services for Persons with Disabilities. 1993. *Outcome-Based Performance Measures*. Landover, Md.: Author.

Bellinger, D., Leviton, A., Waternaux, C., Needleman, H., & Rabinowitz, M. 1987. Longitudinal analyses of prenatal and postnatal lead exposure and early cognitive development. *New England Journal of Medicine 316*: 1037–43.

Bercovici, S. 1983. *Barriers to Normalization: The Restrictive Management of Retarded Persons*. Baltimore: University Park Press.

Birch, H. G., Richardson, S. A., Baird, D., Horobin, G., & Illsley, R. 1970. *Mental Abnormality in the Community: A Clinical and Epidemiological Study*. Baltimore: Williams and Wilkins.

Blake, E., Prouty, R., Lakin, K. C., & Mangan, T. 1994. *Reinventing Quality: Improving Community Services for Persons with Mental Retardation and Related Conditions*. Minneapolis: University of Minnesota, Research and Training Center on Community Living.

Braddock, D., Hemp, R., Fujiura, G. T., Bachelder, L., & Mitchell, D. 1994. *The State of the States in Developmental Disabilities*. Washington, D.C.: American Association on Mental Retardation.

Braddock, D., & Mitchell, D. 1992. *Residential Services in the United States*. Washington, D.C.: American Association of Mental Retardation.

Brown, S.S. 1988. *Prenatal Care: Reaching Mothers, Reaching Children*. Washington, D.C.: National Academy Press.

Buescher, P. A., Meis, P. J., Ernest, J. M., Moore, M. L., Michielutte, R., & Sharp, P. 1988. A comparison of women in and out of a prematurity prevention project in a North Carolina perinatal care region. *American Journal of Public Health 78:* 264–67.

Centers for Disease Control. 1991. *The Prevention of Primary and Secondary Conditions: Building Partnerships towards Health—Reducing the Risks for Disability.* Atlanta: Author.

Centers for Disease Control. 1992. Selected behaviors that increase risk for HIV infection, other sexually transmitted diseases, and unintended pregnancy among high school students—United States, 1991. *Morbidity and Mortality Weekly Report 41:* 945–50.

Chavez, G. F., Cordero, J. F., & Becerra, J. E. 1988. Leading major congenital malformations among minority groups in the United States. *Morbidity and Mortality Weekly Report 37:* 17–24.

Committee on Environmental Hazards. 1987. Statement on childhood lead poisoning. *Pediatrics 79:* 457–65.

Consortium for Citizens with Disabilities, Health Task Force. 1991. *Principles for Health Care Reform from a Disability Perspective.* Washington, D.C.: Author, c/o United Cerebral Palsy Association.

Davis, S. 1987. *A National Status Report on Waiting Lists of People with Mental Retardation for Community Services.* Arlington, Tex.: Association for Retarded Citizens of the United States.

Dingman, H. F., & Tarjan, G. 1960. Mental retardation and the normal distribution curve. *American Journal on Mental Deficiency 64:* 991–94.

Farber, B. 1968. *Mental Retardation: Its Social Context and Social Consequences.* Boston: Houghton Mifflin.

Flower, C. D. 1994. Legal guardianship: The implication of law, procedure, and policy for the lives of people with developmental disabilities. In M. F. Hayden and B. Abery (eds.), *Challenges for a Service System in Transition.* Baltimore: Paul H. Brookes.

Gold, L., Kenney, A., & Singh, S. 1987. *Blessed Events and the Bottom Line: The Financing of Maternity Care in the United States.* New York: The Guttmacher Institute.

Gollay, E. 1980. *Operational Definition of Developmental Disabilities.* Columbia, Md.: Morgan Management Systems.

Green, R., & Schleien, S. 1991. Understanding friendship and recreation: A theoretical sampling. *Therapeutic Recreation Journal 25:* 29–40.

Grossman, H. (ed.). 1973. *Manual on Terminology and Classification in Mental Retardation.* Washington, D.C.: American Association of Mental Deficiency.

Hayden, M. F., & DePaepe, P. A. 1993. Medical conditions, level of care needs, and health related outcomes of persons with mental retardation: A review. *Journal of the Association of Persons with Severe Handicaps 16:* 188–206.

Hayden, M. F., Lakin, K. C., Hill, B. K., Bruininks, R. H., & Chen, T. H. 1992. Placement practices in specialized foster homes and small group homes for persons with mental retardation. *Mental Retardation 30:* 53–61.

Hayden, M. F., Lakin, K. C., Hill, B. K., Bruininks, R. H., & Copher, J. I. 1992.

Social and leisure integration of people with mental retardation who reside in foster homes and small group homes. *Education and Training in Mental Retardation* 27: 187–99.

Hayden, M. F., & Shoultz, B. (issue eds.). (1991a). Feature issue on self-advocacy. *IMPACT* 3: 1–20. Minneapolis: University of Minnesota, Institute on Community Integration.

Hayden, M. F., & Shoultz, B. (eds.). (1991b). *Effective Self-Advocacy: Empowering People with Disabilities to Speak for Themselves*. Minneapolis: University of Minnesota, Research and Training Center on Residential Services Community Living/Institute on Community Integration.

Hayden, M. F., Spicer, P., DePaepe, P., & Chelberg, G. 1992. *Waiting for Community Services: Support and Service Needs of Families with Adult Members with Mental Retardation and other Developmental Disabilities*. Policy Research Brief, 4, 1–12. Minneapolis: University of Minnesota Research and Training Center on Residential Services and Community Living/Institute on Community Integration.

Hill, B. K., Lakin, K. C., Bruininks, R. H., Amado, A. N., Anderson, D. J., & Copher, J. I. 1989. *Living in the Community: A Comparative Study of Foster Homes and Small Group Homes for People with Mental Retardation* (Report no. 28). Minneapolis: University of Minnesota Research and Training Center on Residential Services and Community Living/Institute on Community Integration (UAP).

Hirsch, B., & DuBois, D. 1989. The school-nonschool ecology of early adolescent friendships. In D. Belle (ed.), *Social Networks and Social Supports* (pp. 260–74). New York: Wiley.

Infant Health and Development Program. 1990. Enhancing the outcomes of low birthweight, premature infants. *Journal of the American Medical Association* 263: 3035–42.

Institute of Medicine. 1985. *Preventing Low Birthweight*. Washington, D.C.: National Academy Press.

Lakin, K. C., Bruininks, R. H., Hill, B. K., Chen, T. H., & Anderson, D. A. 1993. Personal characteristics and competence of people with mental retardation living in foster homes and small group homes. *American Journal on Mental Retardation* 97: 616–27.

Lakin, K. C., Bruininks, R. H., & Larson, S. 1991. The changing face of residential services. In L. Rowitz (ed.), *Mental Retardation: Year 2000*. New York: Springer-Verlag.

Lakin, K. C., Burwell, B. O., Hayden, M. F., & Jackson, M. E. 1992. *An Independent Assessment of Minnesota's Medicaid Home and Community-Based Serves Waiver Program* (Report no. 37). Minneapolis: University of Minnesota, Research and Training Center for Residential Services and Community Living/Institute on Community Integration.

Lakin, K. C., Hill, B. K., Chen, T. H., & Stephens, S. A. 1989. *Persons with Mental Retardation and Related Conditions in Mental Retardation Facilities: Selected Findings from the 1987 National Medical Expenditure Survey*. Minneapolis: University of Minnesota, Research and Training Center for Residential Services and Community Living/Institute on Community Integration.

Lakin, K. C., & Jones, R. (issue eds.). 1993. Feature issue on the Americans with Disabilities Act and developmental disabilities. *IMPACT 5:* 1–24. Minneapolis: University of Minnesota, Institute on Community Integration.

LaPlante, M. 1988. *Data on Disability from the National Health Interview Survey, 1983–1985.* Washington, D.C.: U.S. Department of Education.

Larson, S. A., Hewitt, A., & Lakin, K. C. 1994. Residential services personnel: Recruitment, training and retention. In M. F. Hayden & B. Abery (eds.), *Challenges for a Service System in Transition.* Baltimore: Paul H. Brookes.

Larson, S. A., & Lakin, K. C. 1989. Deinstitutionalization of persons with mental retardation: Behavioral outcomes. *Journal of the Association for Persons with Severe Handicaps 14:* 324–32.

Larson, S. A., & Lakin, K. C. 1991. Parent attitudes about residential placement before and after deinstitutionalization: A research synthesis. *Journal of the Association for Persons with Severe Handicaps 16:* 25–38.

Lazar, I., Darlington, R., Murray, H., Royce, J., & Snipper, A. 1984. Lasting effects of early education: A report from the Consortium for Longitudinal Studies. *Monographs of the Society for Research in Child Development 47:* 2–3 (Serial no. 195).

Lemkau, P., Tietze, C., & Cooper, M. 1941. Mental hygiene problems in an urban district. *Mental Hygiene 25:* 624–46.

Lemkau, P. Tietze, C., & Cooper, M. 1942. Mental hygiene problems in an urban district. *Mental Hygiene 26:* 100–119, 275–88.

Lutfiyya, Z. M. 1991. Relationships and community: A resource review. *TASH Newsletter 15:* 3.

MacMillan, D. L. 1977. *Mental Retardation in School and Society.* Boston: Little, Brown and Co.

McGaughey, M., Lynch, S., Morganstern, A., Kiernan, W., & Schalock, R. 1991. *National Survey of Day and Employment Programs.* Boston: Boston Children's Hospital, Training and Research Institute for People with Disabilities.

Mercer, J. 1973. *Labeling the Mentally Retarded.* Berkeley: University of California Press.

Meyer, L., & Putnam, J. 1988. Social integration. In V. Van Hasselt, P. Strain, & M. Hersen (eds.), *Handbook of Developmental and Physical Disabilities* (pp. 107–33). New York: Pergamon.

Millman, M. (ed.). 1993. *Access to Health Care in America.* Washington, D.C.: National Academy Press.

Mount, B., & Zwernik, K. 1988. *It's Never Too Early, It's Never Too Late: A Booklet about Personal Future Planning.* St. Paul, Minn.: Metropolitan Council.

National Center for Health Statistics. 1990. Advance report of final natality statistics, 1988. *Monthly Vital Statistics Report 39:* Supplement. Hyattsville, Md.: Public Health Service.

O'Brien, J. 1989. *Against Pain as a Tool in Professional Work on People with Severe Disabilities.* Lithonia, Ga.: Responsive Systems Associates.

O'Brien, J., & O'Brien, C. L. 1991. *More than Just a New Address: Images of*

Organizations for Supported Living. Syracuse: Syracuse University, Center on Human Policy.

O'Brien, J., & O'Brien, C. L. 1993. *Assistance with Integrity: The Search for Accountability in the Lives of People with Developmental Disabilities.* Lithonia, Ga.: Responsive Systems Associates.

Poland, M. L., Ager, J. W., & Olson, J. M. 1987. Barriers to receiving adequate prenatal care. *American Journal of Obstetrics and Gynecology* 157: 297–303.

President's Committee on Mental Retardation. 1970. *The Six-Hour Retarded Child.* Washington, D.C.: U.S. Government Printing Office.

Prouty, R. W., & Lakin, K. C. 1991. *A Summary of State Efforts to Positively Affect the Quality of Medicaid Home and Community-Based Services for Persons with Mental Retardation and Related Conditions.* Minneapolis: University of Minnesota, Research and Training Center on Residential Services and Community Living/Institute on Community Integration.

Prouty, R. W., & Lakin, K. C. (eds.). 1995. *Residential Services for Persons with Developmental Disabilities: Status and Trends through 1994.* Minneapolis: University of Minnesota, Research and Training Center on Community Living/Institute on Community Integration.

Prouty, R. W., & Lakin, K. C. (eds.). 1996. *Residential Services for Persons with Developmental Disabilities: Status and Trends through 1995.* Minneapolis: University of Minnesota, Research and Training Center on Community Living/Institute on Community Integration.

Racino, J. A., Walker, P., O'Connor, S., & Taylor, S. J. 1992. *Housing Support and Community: Choices and Strategies for Adults with Disabilities.* Baltimore: Paul H. Brookes.

Reichle, J., & Light, C. 1992. Positive approaches to managing challenging behavior among persons with developmental disabilities living in the community. *Policy Research Brief 4:* 1–12. Minneapolis: University of Minnesota Research and Training Center on Residential Services and Community Living/Institute on Community Integration.

Reichle, J., York, J., & Sigafoos, J. 1991. *Implementing Augmentative and Alternative Communication: Strategies for People with Severe Disabilities.* Baltimore: Paul H. Brookes.

Rudolph, C., & Lakin, K. C. 1994. *An Evaluation of a Demonstration Behavioral Support and Crisis Response Program.* Minneapolis: University of Minnesota, Center on Community Living/Institute on Community Integration.

Rynders, J., & Schleien, S. 1991. *Together Successfully: Creating Recreational and Educational Programs that Integrate People with and without Disabilities.* Arlington, Tex.: The Arc-U.S.

Schleien, S., Meyer, L., Heyne, L., & Biel, B. 1993. *Lifelong Leisure Skills and Lifestyles for Persons with Developmental Disabilities.* Baltimore: Paul H. Brookes.

Select Committee on Children, Youth and Families. 1989. *U.S. Children and their Families: Current Conditions and Recent Trends.* Washington, D.C.: Government Printing Office.

Skarnulis, E., & Lakin, K. C. (issue eds.). 1990. Feature issue on consumer controlled housing. *IMPACT 3:* 1–20. Minneapolis: University of Minnesota, Institute on Community Integration.

Smull, M., & Harrison, S. 1992. *Supported Living for Persons with Severe Reputations.* Alexandria, Va.: National Association of State Directors of Developmental Disabilities Services.

Stein, E., & Susser, M. 1975. Public health and mental retardation: new power and new problems. In M. J. Begab & S. A. Richardson (eds.), *The Mentally Retarded and Society: A Social Science Perspective.* Baltimore: University Park Press.

Tarjan, G. 1964. The next decade: Expectations from the biological sciences. In *Mental Retardation: A Handbook for the Primary Physician.* Chicago: American Medical Association.

Tarjan, G., Wright, S. W., Eyman, R. K., & Keran, C. V. 1973. National history of mental retardation: Some aspects of epidemiology. *American Journal of Mental Retardation 77:* 369–79.

Taylor, S. J. 1988. Caught in the continuum: A critical analysis of the principle of the least restrictive environment. *Journal of the Association for Persons with Severe Handicaps 13:* 41–53.

Taylor, S. J., & Bogdan, R. 1989. On accepting relationships between people with mental retardation and non-disabled people: towards an understanding of acceptance. *Disability, Handicap and Society 41:* 21–36.

Taylor, S. J., Lakin, K. C., & Hill, B. K. 1989. Permanency planning for children and youth: Out of home placement decisions. *Exceptional Children 55:* 541–49.

U.S. Department of Education. 1981. *Fourth Annual Report to Congress on the Implementation of Public Law 94–142: The Education of All Handicapped Children Act.* Washington, D.C.: Author.

U.S. Department of Education. 1985. *Seventh Annual Report to Congress on the Implementation of the Education of the Handicapped Act.* Washington, D.C.: Author.

U.S. Department of Education. 1992. *Thirteenth Annual Report to Congress on the Implementation of the Individuals with Disabilities Education Act.* Washington, D.C.: Author.

U.S. General Accounting Office. 1990. *A Generation at Risk* (GAO/HRD-90-138). Washington, D.C.: Author.

U.S. General Accounting Office. 1992. *Federal Investments Like WIC Can Produce Savings* (GAO/HRD-92–18). Washington, D.C.: Author.

U.S. Public Health Service. 1988. *The Nature and Extent of Lead Poisoning in Children in the United States: A Report to Congress.* Atlanta: Author.

U.S. Public Health Service. 1990. *Promoting Health/Preventing Disease: Year 2000 Objectives for the Nation.* Washington, D.C.: U.S. Department of Health and Human Services.

Ward, M., & Halloran, W. 1989. Transition to uncertainty: Status of many school leavers with severe disabilities. *Career Development for Exceptional Individual 12:* 26–37.

5/ CARE FOR ADULTS WITH A DISABILITY, NOW AND AS THEY AGE

Bryan J. Kemp

For the first time in history, most people who acquire a permanent disability before middle age can expect to have a near-normal life expectancy. In the years before 1950, few people who had an impairment serious enough to cause significant disability lived past middle age; infections, illnesses, accidents, self-inflicted harm, and iatrogenic factors combined to limit their life expectancy. Today, improvements in rehabilitative and primary medical care, greater understanding of underlying processes of disabling illness, greater advocacy by consumers (people with a disability), and generally increased public health have combined to produce a growing number of people who are living for decades with a disability. People with cerebral palsy, polio, spinal cord injury, rheumatoid arthritis, and other impairments can expect to live into their sixties, seventies, and eighties (Ansello, 1988). Even among the population with severe disability, life expectancy is good. Sasma and colleagues (1993), for example, computed survival curves on fifty-five hundred males with spinal cord injury, one of the most catastrophic impairments, and found that life expectancy was 85 percent of that of the population without disability, with an average life expectancy after injury of approximately forty years. These changes in life expectancy require a revision in how disabling conditions are viewed, one that anticipates the problems that people with a disability can expect to experience over their lifetimes, the services that need to be provided, and the system monitoring that will be needed to ensure a quality life.

A primary purpose of this chapter is to stress the need for such a "longitudinal" view of disability to supplement the traditional "acute" view. Typically, rehabilitation services have concentrated on the person with a newly acquired disability and have been directed toward assisting that person to achieve maximum physical, functional, and socioeconomic independence as soon after onset as feasible. The underlying assumption has been that the person would then stay at that level of ability or would conveniently die of "complications" before old age. However, people with a disability do age, and as they age, new problems emerge. Focusing attention only on people who have an acute disability (i.e., over a relatively short period of time) gives a different picture of service needs and problems than looking at the same people over a lifetime. Their problems change and new ones develop; they lose contact with service providers and "fall between the cracks" of funded services. This chapter examines the care needs of young adults and adults with newly acquired disabilities, as well as the needs of these people as they grow older. Much of the discussion can likely be extended to the changing health needs of persons with mental illness, chronic substance abuse, or even disabling medical conditions or topics addressed elsewhere in this volume.

To promote conceptual clarity and adhere to generally accepted conventions,[1] it is important to differentiate several terms frequently used in the rehabilitation field, which have a bearing on this chapter. These terms are *pathology, impairment, disability,* and *handicap.* Many of the inconsistencies and much of the confusion in rehabilitation practice and research stem from a misunderstanding of these terms. Pathology is defined as dysfunction at the *cellular* level and generally defines whether one has an illness (or injury), as well as which kind. For example, if cells multiply abnormally, a cancer may develop (an illness). If bone cells are destroyed in sufficient number, a fracture is the result.

Impairment refers to dysfunction at the *organ* level. A person is said to have an impairment of an organ when the pathology affects the organ's functioning to a significant degree. The organ's functioning can be assessed physiologically or by simple performance testing. Low vision is an impairment of the eye, which can be caused by many illnesses and injuries, including glaucoma, detached retina, and macular degeneration. An impairment may or may not then cause disability.

Disability refers to dysfunction at the level of *task performance;* a task is usually made up of a complex set of functions combining skill, strength, coordination, timing, endurance, and flexibility. The task may be work performance, instrumental activities of daily living (IADLs: shopping, transportation, chores, etc.), or activities of daily living (ADLs: dressing, grooming, bathing, toileting, etc.). A disability is specific to the task and, because it involves multiple functions, usually has multiple

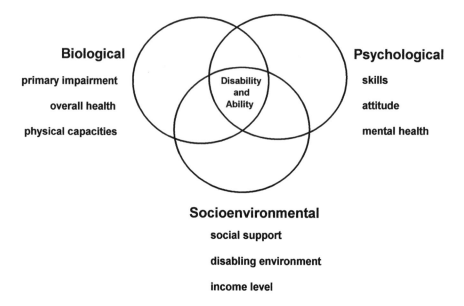

Fig. 5.1.   Biological, Psychological, and Socioenvironmental Factors
in Producing Disability

causes (Brummel-Smith, 1993). Rarely is a disability caused solely by a physical impairment. Psychological, environmental, and social factors also contribute to the degree of the disability. This is an important, fundamental principle in rehabilitation, namely, that disability is a product of "biopsychosocial" influences acting together, changing over time, and varying from person to person. Not all pathology produces impairment, and not all impairment produces disability. Hypertension (an impairment of the cardiovascular system), for example, usually causes no disability, although it is one of the most common chronic diseases in the United States. People simply take antihypertensive medicine and lead normal lives.

Finally, handicap refers to dysfunction at the *social* level. People with disabilities are said to be handicapped when they are precluded, usually by the actions of others, from participating fully in the socioenvironmental world. As Vash (1981) points out, the onus for the handicap belongs to society through neglect or negative attitudes, not to the person. Figure 5.1 illustrates how biological, psychological, and socioenvironmental factors interact to create disability.

ESTIMATES OF IMPAIRMENT AND DISABILITY IN ADULTS

This section considers how many people in the United States aged eighteen to sixty-four have a disability, what degree of disability they have, which impairments underlie these disabilities, and which sociodemographic variables are associated with disability. The ages eighteen to sixty-four are used because they are the primary adult years. Persons aged sixty-five and older are considered separately in chapter 7, while other chapters consider the specific needs of adults who have chronic disease (chapter 6), who have severe mental illness (chapter 8), and who abuse alcohol and drugs (chapter 9).

Federal agencies are the primary sources of information concerning disabilities. These agencies measure and report on the prevalence of disability, using many different definitions of it, including *(a)* activity limitation, *(b)* functional limitation, *(c)* need for personal assistance, and *(d)* work disability. Activity limitations and functional limitations are the most general. Need for assistance with ADLs and IADLs pertains to people with more severe, long-term disabilities.

One of the most commonly cited sources for information about disability prevalence is the National Health Interview Survey (NHIS),[2] published by the National Center for Health Statistics. The NHIS collects data on civilian, noninstitutionalized people through surveys of households; in 1988, approximately forty-seven thousand households were surveyed. Persons aged eighteen to sixty-four are asked about disability related to work or keeping house. Data from the NHIS rely, as do most studies, on self-report and are therefore limited in their validity. This approach can be criticized because it requires respondents to make difficult judgments about their own health. They are asked, for example, to indicate which of their medical problems accounts for a given functional limitation, when, in fact, multiple causes or another cause altogether could be responsible (National Center for Health Statistics, 1989). People are generally recognized as not being able to account for their functional problems (cf. Kane, Ouslander & Abrass, 1989).

The U.S. Bureau of the Census has conducted surveys of disability since 1983 to study the economic well-being of households. In 1984, it included questions about disability in its Survey of Income and Program Participation (SIPP) (U.S. Department of Health and Human Services, 1989).[3] This survey collects self-report information on nine sensory and functional limitations and receipt of Social Security benefits. In 1986, the survey asked whether people needed assistance with these activities. Several studies (reviewed in Ficke, 1992) have specifically used ADL/ IADL measures and the need for assistance with them.

Several agencies also collect administrative data on people with a disability. All states report annually on the number and characteristics of people with a disability who are served by state departments of rehabilitation (DRs). These reports are available through the Rehabilitation Services Administration (RSA) of the U.S. Department of Education. The Social Security Administration keeps records of the number of people receiving disability benefits by age. The Office of Special Education and Rehabilitation maintains records of the number of children in school who have a disability and the underlying physical impairment contributing to it. The major drawback of each of these administrative records is that they underestimate the number of people with a disability, because not everyone is eligible for services, not all eligible people apply, and most programs have age restrictions.

Another approach is typified by sample surveys. In 1985, Louis Harris and Associates (1986) conducted a telephone survey for the International Center for the Disabled and the National Council on the Handicapped. The survey was intended to assess experiences with disability and the impact of disability, especially on social life.

The best data available indicate that the total number of persons in the United States with at least some level of disability (i.e., some degree of limitation in task performance) is about thirty-five million, which includes all ranges of disability and amounts to about 14–15 percent of the population (Pope & Tarlov, 1991). The number of people who have a disability increases linearly with age up to age sixty and then increases exponentially after age sixty-five. The percentage of people with a severe disability does not increase with age until sixty-five. However, the underlying impairments contributing to disability are different for each age group (NCHS, 1989).

Figure 5.2 shows the prevalence of activity limitation caused by chronic conditions by age and severity of disability. These data are from the 1988 NHIS and are based on self-report, using functional limitation criteria for disability. Approximately twenty million people aged eighteen to sixty-four report having a disability, which represents about 57 percent of all persons who have a disability (Fig. 5.3). Men and women have about an equal distribution of disability overall, although men on average have more severe disabilities. The prevalence of disability is higher

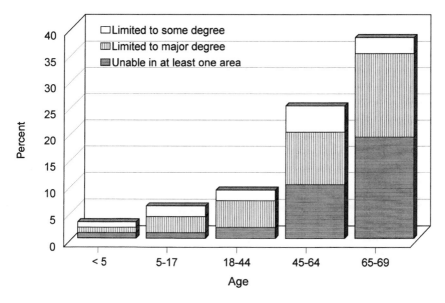

Fig. 5.2. Prevalence of Disability by Age
Source: National Center for Health Statistics, 1989.

among minority groups, including African Americans and Hispanics, by about 10 percent (NCHS, 1989). Bureau of the Census data (SIPP) measuring ADL/IADL disability (a more severe measure) show that nearly four million (2.4 percent) persons aged eighteen to sixty-four need assistance with IADLs and of them, 1.3 million (0.9 percent) also need help with ADLs. These percentages go up with age, particularly over age sixty.

The main physical impairments underlying disabilities in those aged eighteen to sixty-four vary by age (keeping in mind that factors other than physical impairments contribute to disability). In those aged eighteen to thirty years, disability is caused by such conditions as childhood-onset chronic illnesses that are still present when the person reaches age eighteen, such as Down's syndrome, cerebral palsy, polio, deafness, blindness/ low vision, congenital spinal deformities, and several medical illnesses; as well as high rates of spinal cord injury, traumatic brain injury, rheumatoid arthritis, other orthopedic problems (e.g., fractures), and psychiatric conditions that have peak onsets between ages eighteen and thirty. In those aged thirty-one to forty-four, major medical problems, such as cardiovascular disease, respiratory disease, cancer, kidney disease, and diabetic diseases, increase in frequency as do work-related injuries, especially ortho-

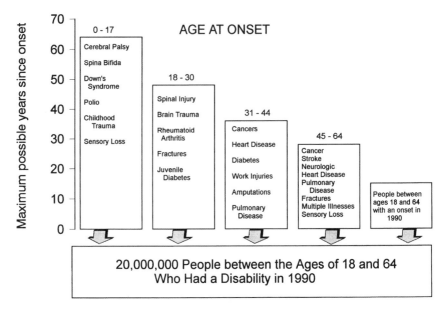

Fig. 5.3. Longitudinal and Cross-Sectional Influences on the
Point Prevalence of Disability

pedic ones involving the back and hand. In addition, this age group contains people who experienced the onset of a disability before age thirty and who now have matured. In those aged forty-five to sixty-four, the previously mentioned major medical illnesses are common, and increases occur in neurological illnesses, such as stroke, Parkinson's disease, and degenerative neurological illness (MS, ALS, etc.); musculoskeletal conditions (see chapter 6); some dementing illnesses (e.g., early-onset Alzheimer's); and sensory impairments of deafness and low vision/blindness.

Two other major factors are related to the degree of disability: socioenvironmental and psychological characteristics. Low socioeconomic status can contribute to disability for two major reasons: *(a)* a person with a disability may lack the resources (financial) to purchase devices to reduce the severity of the disability and make tasks easier (e.g., a van equipped with wheelchair lift, a home computer with a modem, or a reading machine) and *(b)* higher rates of some impairments, such as spinal cord injury, are correlated with socioeconomic status.

Figure 5.4 shows the association of level of income with disability status, indicating that low family income is associated with higher and

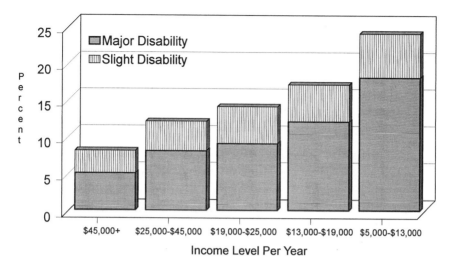

25 —
☐Major Disability
▥Slight Disability

Fig. 5.4. Disability Prevalence as a Function of Socioeconomic Factors.
Source: National Center for Health Statistics, 1989.

more severe disability status, a relationship that may work both ways. People of lower income likely develop more health problems because they lack easy access to health care, and a disability causes changes in work and income status and adds extra expenses, which then lowers income.

Psychological factors, such as discouragement, depression, or low quality of life, can affect disability status, because the person lacks the emotional resources to deal effectively with the adjustments that accompany a disability. Both low life-satisfaction and high depression are associated with more severe disability. The Louis Harris survey (1986) compared ratings of life satisfaction in over 950 persons who had various levels of disability with the responses of a comparison group without disability. While 90 percent of the latter rated their life as "very satisfying" or "somewhat satisfying," 80 percent of persons with slight or moderate disability, 64 percent of people with moderately severe disability, and 50 percent of people with severe disability did so. Of those in the latter two groups, 30 percent and 35 percent, respectively, reported ratings of "somewhat" or "very dissatisfied" with life, compared with 6 percent of the group without disability. Overall, a moderate relationship exists between severity of disability and depression, with more severe disabilities having higher rates of depression. What is more important, given the same level of impairment, depressed individuals have higher levels of disability.

While these data on prevalence and degree of disability are illuminating, they are cross-sectional data and do not reveal the changes, problems, and complications that occur over time as people mature and grow older with a disability. The next section takes up those issues.

CHANGES, PROBLEMS, AND ISSUES AS PEOPLE MATURE AND AGE

The needs and problems of people who have a disability are not as static as cross-sectional prevalence studies and an "acute" orientation indicate. The way things are at any given time is not the way they will always be for the person with a disability, or for his or her family. Planning programs and services that will be effective over the long run, educating professionals and consumers about changes in conditions, designing measures to monitor the quality of services, and resolving bureaucratic jurisdiction dilemmas about who is responsible for care will require knowing not only what has traditionally been understood about rehabilitation but also what recent investigations (within the last ten years) are discovering about the needs and problems of people who have a disability over a long period of time.

As the Institute of Medicine (Pope & Tarlov, 1991) stated, "One of the major goals of disability prevention is to maximize an individual's functioning, well-being, and quality of life *throughout the life course.*" In this age of growing life expectancy, disability policy must be built around a lifelong perspective, anticipating that the person with a disability will have a disability for fifteen to fifty years.

A growing body of research on longitudinal and aging aspects of disability (see Kemp 1992, 1993b for reviews) is summarized below:

- Twenty to twenty-five years after initial onset, most people who have a moderate or severe disability find their physical condition and functional abilities beginning to diminish, often over a relatively short time. People with spinal cord injury, for example, have very high rates of early-onset cardiovascular disease, diabetes, and osteoporosis. People with a history of polio suddenly undergo changes in strength and stamina and develop pain and weakness.
- These changes affect daily functioning, support systems, employment, and quality of life.
- Not only are specialized rehabilitation or health services unavail-

able to help these people maintain their independence and health, but few professionals and service providers have ever heard of later-life changes occurring among people with a previous disability.

- It is becoming clear that later-life changes are the norm for most people with a disability and that rehabilitation services must be designed to assist them.
- The paucity and discontinuity of programs make community-level monitoring of the quality of care over the lifetime of a person with a disability almost impossible at this time.

SERVICE NEEDS OF PEOPLE WITH A DISABILITY

The problems and service needs of people with a disability vary depending upon the age of onset of the disability and the current age of the individual. The needs of a person immediately after the onset of a disability are different from the needs of that individual decades later. Likewise, the needs of a young adult with a recent disability are different from those of an individual who sustains a disability in his or her forties, fifties, or sixties. For all people, however, six basic service needs must be addressed eventually, both at onset and throughout their lives: *(a)* health, *(b)* functional independence, *(c)* education and employment, *(d)* social support, *(e)* economic security, and *(f)* psychological well-being.

Health

The health need is concerned mostly with access to quality primary care (family medicine, internal medicine, pediatrics, and OB/GYN) and secondary care (urology, dermatology, neurology, etc.); rehabilitative medical care is not included here. Diagnostic and treatment services are necessary to maintain health and prevent secondary problems and must be available. For the person with a recent disability, finding a primary care physician can be difficult, because most doctors are intimidated by the supposed and real problems imposed by the disability (ranging from ignorance about diagnosing autonomic dysreflexia in people with spinal cord injury to not having the kind of examining table suitable for a person using a wheelchair). In a white paper publication on the topic, the American Congress of Rehabilitation Medicine (ACRM) concluded that "there is no system of post-rehabilitation primary care, acute care, or long-term care that is responsive to the particular constellation of health care problems commonly experienced by such persons with disabilities" (1993). As people mature with a disability and lose contact with the rehabilitation center where they received rehabilitative care, this problem is further compounded. The person who has had a disability for twenty or twenty-five years often develops joint pain, pressure sores, fractures, osteoporosis, fatigue, sleep problems, infections, and cardiovascular disease (Gellman, Sie, & Waters, 1988; Maynard, 1992; Trieshman, 1987). The high rate of rehospitalization after disability is most often attributed to poor access to primary care, which could have prevented a problem from becoming worse by treating it earlier. So many people with a disability are experiencing health problems not usually found in persons without disability until later in life that many investigators have raised the issue of "premature aging" (e.g., Ohry, Shemash, & Rosin, 1983).

Functional Independence

Rehabilitative care is directed toward improving functioning and includes access to rehabilitation medicine (a secondary or tertiary care specialty), rehabilitation therapies (occupational, physical, and speech therapy), and rehabilitation technology services, such as appropriate assistive devices, job modification, and home enhancement. Almost by definition, people with a relatively new disability need access to inpatient and/or outpatient acute rehabilitation services. These services may occur in a large profit or nonprofit rehabilitation center, such as the Rehabilitation Institute of Chicago or Rancho Los Amigos Medical Center; in a rehabilitation section of a general or community hospital; or in skilled nursing/ rehabilitation facilities. The purpose of these services is to provide an interdisciplinary program that will improve the person's functional abilities to the maximum. Any person in the United States who has a severe enough disability ought to be able to access rehabilitative care. These programs not only help maximize function, but they also educate the person about self-care after discharge and the prevention of secondary complications such as deconditioning, contractures, pressure sores, urinary infections, and new injuries. Health providers have tended to believe that once people with disabilities reach maximum functional ability in rehabilitation, they should remain at that level, and if they do not, it is because they did not look after themselves. One of the major findings in the last ten years is just the opposite: nearly everyone with a major disability will go through functional decline, whether or not they look after themselves well.

About 50–80 percent of all people with major disability can expect substantial changes in their condition and abilities (Kemp, 1992; Lammertse & Yankony, 1991; Trieshman, 1987; Whiteneck et al., 1992). Of the approximately 600,000 people with a history of polio, for example, 90 percent have or will experience significant change or even the more limiting "postpolio syndrome" (Halstead, 1991; Halstead & Weickers, 1987). Other groups have experienced similar changes. People with cerebral palsy have experienced new orthopedic-based functional problems and fatigue (Bleck, 1984). Many people with spinal cord injury have developed weakness, fatigue, disease, pain, and job loss (Garland et al., 1989; Sie et al., 1992; Whiteneck et al., 1992). Persons with Down's syndrome have developed greater cognitive loss, dementia, and declines in functional ability (Ansello, 1988).

Obtaining proper rehabilitation services or even an assessment of these problems is difficult twenty, twenty-five, or thirty years postonset. Few medical rehabilitation centers are knowledgeable about these changes or provide employment assistance or technology-based services. Medical rehabilitative programs are not geared to the returning patient, and because discovery of longitudinal and later-life changes is so recent, many professionals have not yet seen or treated people with late-life complications. Moreover, people with a disability are likely to misinterpret their symptoms and problems as being part of "normal aging"; because they see this aging as normal, even if a little early, they may conclude that nothing can be done about it. To date, however, all the data suggest that this is not normal aging but rather the onset of new conditions attributable to multiple causes.

Technology-based assistive device services are also vital to improving and maintaining function. If a disability is defined as an imbalance between task demands on the one hand and human performance on the other, then changes on either side of this imbalance will improve performance. Attempts can be made to improve the performance of a person with a disability through rehabilitation therapies, surgery, or medicine. Alternatively, task demands can be altered to bring them more in line with the person's abilities. Efforts to change or reduce task demands can range from high technology (computers, electric wheelchairs, robotics) to low technology (reacher sticks, grab bars, walkers). The more appropriate the technology is to the person's needs and preferences, the more it will reduce disability. Most people with a new or recent disability receive much of the assistive equipment they need through rehabilitation centers, DRs, or other government-sponsored agencies. However, as people age with a disability, they develop new functional problems at the same time that they are out of touch with centers that provide technology services. These services include access to an assessment of the need for assistive devices or technology, the equipment itself, funding, repair of existing equipment, and information about new devices. Mann (1992) found that as people age with a disability, they need an average of three to four pieces of assistive equipment to which they do not have access. La Buda (1990) has shown how people with disabilities lose access to information about new technology as well as follow-up services to ensure satisfactory functioning of existing equipment. Without ongoing access to rehabilitation technology services, persons aging with a disability will probably become increasingly incapacitated. Most primary care physicians do not have expertise in prescribing assistive devices or equipment.

Employment and Education

Employment remains one of the most important rehabilitation outcomes, both for economic reasons and for purposes of societal integration of people who have a disability. Each year, thousands of people with a disability return to work. State DRs, the traditional provider of government-sponsored vocational and educational programs for adults with a disability, do a reasonably good job of helping persons with a new or recent disability enter the work force, school, or training programs. However, DRs are less likely to open a new case for services on an older person (fewer than 10 percent of DR clients are over age forty-five) (Government Accounting Office, 1991). Providing services to employed people who have an existing disability but who are experiencing new work problems, while always possible under the DR mandate, has not yet been widely tested for people aging with a disability.

Educational programs are a concern primarily for the person with a disability under the age of eighteen, while vocational programs are a concern for those over eighteen. Community colleges, state colleges, and vocational training centers, often working with state DRs, are the sites of most postsecondary education and training. The major factor preventing more education and employment assistance is limited financing. Given a limited budget, DRs are faced with making policy decisions to help the increasing number of persons with severe disability (who require greater expenditures) or to help more people with less severe disabilities. Over the past decade, the emphasis has shifted to the former.

Support Services

Support services that are vital for people with disabilities to maintain independence can be divided into *formal* and *informal*. The formal support system is provided through government-sponsored programs, which include paid in-home help, housing assistance, transportation, monetary support, and nutrition services. Informal support is provided by family and friends. Informal help from the family is the most common form of everyday support, especially for persons with more severe disability. The family provides approximately 60–75 percent of all assistance to people with a disability; this figure is even higher for the very young and very old populations (Brody, 1986).

Most people who acquire a disability have access to at least some formal support services, such as economic support and health coverage. However, many support needs go unmet or underfunded, such as in-home help, transportation, and housing assistance. The most critical need continues to be adequate personal care assistance (in-home help) for persons with moderate or severe disability. Medicaid will pay for some in-home help, but only if the person is Medicaid eligible (low income); those who are not must fund help themselves. Even when state funding is available, receiving enough in-home help is a problem. Moreover, locating personal care assistance is difficult. There are few training programs for personal assistants, the pay is low, retention is difficult, and reports of neglect or abandonment are not uncommon. The second most needed service for persons with a new disability is transportation (Heuman, 1986). Transportation services are expensive, the purchase of individual vehicles is prohibitively expensive, and organized transportation services for "seniors and handicapped" will not even cross city boundaries because of liability issues. Both of these issues, personal care assistance and transportation, continue to be addressed at barely adequate levels.

Educational and support programs to help families caring for a person with a disability are also an important concern (Kaplan & Mearig, 1977). Most families assist their relatives by serving as de facto personal assistants, but stress, disagreements, and role conflict are common, especially in situations involving severe physical disability, brain impairment, or mental health problems (Eisenberg, Satkin & Jansen, 1984; Moos, 1977). Fortunately, some families can take advantage of educational, support, and counseling programs through rehabilitation centers, disability associations, and schools, but again, these programs are in insufficient supply.

Family problems and dynamics change significantly as the person with a disability matures and ages. First, many people who have a disability from early life marry, and "the family" shifts from the family of origin to the spousal family. This can set the stage for a new set of issues as the person ages and his or her condition changes (Carpenter, 1974). The spouse may not feel prepared to provide more assistance than was necessary when they were first married. The spouse may have a career and resent the need to curtail it to provide more assistance, and the person with the disability may not want to acknowledge the need for more help. If the person with a disability does not marry (as in most cases of severe disability) or if he or she divorces, the responsibility for care over the lifetime may continue to rest with the parents. Thirty or forty years ago most parents expected that they would outlive their children who had a disability, even if the child acquired a disability in his or her twenties. In the last few decades, however, people with severe disabilities have begun to outlive their parents; since the parents are developing illnesses and disabilities themselves, they find it more difficult to provide the same level of care to the child. After one or both parents are deceased, the person with the disability is faced with finding another support system. Early reports indicate that alternatives such as board and care facilities, residential care, and skilled nursing facilities are sometimes considered, but only as a last option. The issue of children with cognitive disability outliving their parents is a growing concern and is thought to affect tens of thousands of individuals with a disability (Ansello, 1988; Nosek, 1990).

Economic Security

A close link exists between disability status and economic hardship, the main one being reduced employment. Unless one has a high-paying job or a two-income family or is financially well off to begin with, a disability causes economic hardship. This results from reduced earning capacity and difficulty in obtaining and maintaining employment, especially for the population with more severe disability. Most people who have a disability must also make enough money to overcome the economic disincentives to employment that exist. These disincentives include loss of adequate medical insurance (provided through Medicare, Medicaid, or workers' compensation for unemployed persons) and the increased costs of maintaining a job, such as higher transportation costs and the necessity to pay for one's personal assistance care out of pocket. Evidence from the National Model Spinal Cord Injury System indicates that people with spinal cord injury have a 60 percent unemployment rate, ten times the rate of the population without disability (National Spinal Cord Injury Statistical Center Annual Report #8, 1990).

Another link between disability and low income, discussed earlier, is that disability rates are higher among lower income persons. Lack of adequate health care and insurance, greater exposure to crime and violence, and employment in jobs with higher accident rates are contributing factors. Coupled with a lower educational level, disability then perpetuates a marginal economic existence.

To combat absolute poverty, two programs for economic security exist, Supplemental Security Income (SSI) or Social Security Disability Insurance (SSDI). The former is a "means tested" benefit based upon having a disability and limited income, which provides a subsistence level of economic benefit. What is more important, it qualifies the person for Medicaid to cover medical expenses and therefore gives access to Medicaid-reimbursed personal assistance services in many states. SSDI is for individuals who have paid enough into Social Security to qualify for early Social Security benefits based upon a disability status. These benefits must be applied for, and the person must have a disability serious enough to preclude employment. SSDI also qualifies a person for Medicare benefits. Both SSI and SSDI are designed to prevent abject poverty and to link with other benefits, such as food stamps, subsidized housing, and cash assistance. They do not guarantee anything close to a comfortable existence.

Psychological Well-Being

Finally, the psychological needs of people who have a disability must be considered. Mental health problems are commonly found in conjunction with major physical health problems. About 25–30 percent of people with a disability will develop a diagnosable mental health problem at some time in their lives (Blazer, 1986; Fuhrer et al., 1993; Kaplan &

Sadock, 1991). The major issues here are *(a)* access to appropriate mental health services to help alleviate the psychological problems and stress that accompany serious illness, chronic disease, and disability and *(b)* more "positive" psychosocial services that promote independence, self-determination, and self-esteem.

Chronic disease and disability present crises to the person, causing profound personal loss, ongoing stress, and multiple social challenges. The most common problems are depressive disorders, anxiety disorders, substance abuse, psychotic disorders, and posttraumatic stress disorders. These problems impact health, functioning, relationships, and quality of life. Fuhrer et al. (1993) found about a 30 percent rate of diagnosable major depression among people with long-term spinal cord injury living in the community, a finding supported by Schultz and Decker (1985) and Trieshman (1987). Exact estimates of the prevalence of substance abuse are unknown, although the National Institute on Disability and Rehabilitation Research (NIDRR) estimates it as close to 13 percent (Corthell & Brown, 1991). People who have a disability have difficulty gaining access to proper mental health care. Mental health problems go unrecognized by health professionals who work with people with a disability, and people with a disability do not avail themselves of mental health services to the extent they should; furthermore, funding for such services is poor (National Institute of Mental Health, 1991).

As people with a disability age and face new crises brought on by functional, physical, and social changes, new psychological stresses occur. People who were not depressed before may become depressed. Kemp (1993a) found about a 20 percent rate of depression among people who developed postpolio syndrome, compared with 3 percent among people with polio without postpolio problems. Depression in turn affects a person's overall physical health and may contribute to the high rate of health problems and low rate of use of health services observed in people with a long-standing disability (cf. Hartke, 1991; Maynard, 1992).

Even though treatment of psychological disorders is necessary, it alone cannot promote the kind of independence and self-control that most people who have a disability want and need. The absence of depression does not guarantee that someone will be happy, productive, and self-directed. A need exists for the kinds of programs and interventions that Vash (1981) terms "psychogogic," meaning they are oriented toward strengthening, coaching, encouraging, guiding, and developing personal potential. These goals are often the focus of Centers for Independent Living, which are peer-directed advocacy-oriented service programs that serve an important function in "empowering" people with a disability to take charge of their own lives. The more independent, assertive, well-adjusted individual will generally cope better with a disability over the life span (Cairns & Baker, 1993); more efforts should be devoted to developing this kind of adaptation. This theme is common to children with chronic conditions and adults with mental retardation, as discussed in chapters 3 and 4.

In summary, the service needs of people who have a disability cut across a number of areas, from medical to support. As people age with a disability, these needs increase. At the same time, a long-term system of care for these persons has failed to materialize, and many hundreds of thousands of people with disabilities are now facing new challenges as they enter their later years.

SERVICE SYSTEM ISSUES

Issues existing at a service system level evolve directly from the needs that people with a disability have both at the time of onset and over the long term. Formal service programs designed to meet the needs of people with a disability fall under four major auspices: health, rehabilitation, aging, and economic support. Health programs provide basic health care and medical rehabilitation care. Rehabilitation care from the formal program viewpoint means services that provide assistance with employment, education, independent living, and assistive equipment. Aging services are designed to assist with support in later life, and economic programs are structured to combat poverty.

The Basic Issues

The core of necessary services exists, at least legislatively and programmatically: over eighty federal programs currently serve the needs of people who have a disability across the life span. However, program eligibility criteria, funding levels, definitions of disability, scope of service, reporting authority, and coordination among programs vary dramatically across these programs. The net result is that the person with a disability typically needs services from different programs, but is often left floundering in a bureaucratic maze. This service system complex does not come with a user's manual.

Jim, for example, sustained a spinal cord injury in an automobile accident when he was twenty-eight years old, which resulted in high-level paraplegia. After emergency intervention for his trauma, he needed acute rehabilitation, most of which was covered by his insurance. Following inpatient rehabilitation, he got help returning to work from the state DR. Jim was fortunate that he already had a two-year college degree. He received a wheelchair through the rehabilitation center, and he has been able to propel himself fairly easily because of his good upper body strength. Over the years, Jim often avoided regular medical care, because he could not find a doctor who understood his spinal cord injury complications. Because he is fairly independent, Jim did not need much help other than what his wife provided. Now fifty-one years old, Jim has worked for twenty-three years after injury. Recently, he developed shoulder pain that makes it difficult for him to propel his chair. He also notices increasing fatigue, and he has gained about thirty pounds over the years. At his last medical examination, he was surprised to learn that he has very high cholesterol levels and borderline diabetes. He is experiencing more difficulty in doing his job and thinks of retiring, but his health insurance benefits are probably better than what he can get if he retires. Besides, he likes his job. He now needs some help at home with certain ADLs, but his wife works nights and is not available. Stress is beginning to build in Jim's life, and he is becoming discouraged. When he calls his old rehabilitation center to make an appointment to discuss his changing situation, he is told that they do not have outpatient social services anymore. When Jim asks the nurse about his recent health problems, she is unable to explain why he has them now.

Jim potentially needs many services: a medical and rehabilitation evaluation, a lighter wheelchair, nighttime help, counseling, health insurance if he retires, and possibly some job modification if he does not. Jim had enough difficulty getting the services he needed when he was originally injured, but at that time he was closely tied to the rehabilitation center that treated him. Now, nearly twenty-five years later, he is not well connected to any programs, the staff he remembers are no longer there, his condition is changing, and he finds that it's not easy to access services. Jim's case is following the common "life course" of disability: a flurry of activity and services at the beginning in the hospital, fewer services out in the community, and a regular puzzle years later.

Programs for People with Disabilities

Rehabilitation, health, aging-related, and economic services have different funding streams, policies, and restrictions. Rehabilitation services were originally established to help injured workers and veterans return to work; later, young adults and children with disabilities were added. The principal laws governing rehabilitation are the Federal Rehabilitation Acts of 1945, 1973, and 1992 and the workers' compensation laws in the states. The 1973 act, particularly as amended in 1978, focused not only on vocational and special educational needs of people with a disability, but also on independent living, supported employment, and technology assistance. Title VII of the 1978 amendments provides a statutory base for independent living centers. The acts provide funding to state DRs to provide these services at the local level. Given limited resources and a policy mandate, DR services usually go to younger persons and those with a new or recent disability, up to age forty (GAO, 1991). Additionally, the American with Disabilities Act provides the most sweeping civil rights legislation for people with disabilities, affecting employment, accessibility, education, and public accommodations. The 1988 Technology-Related Assistance for Individuals with Disabilities Act assists states in providing access to evaluations for assistive devices and services for people who have a disability.

Health services and medical rehabilitation for people who have a disability are covered either through private insurance, Medicaid, or Medicare. People with a disability who have private health insurance encounter the same dilemmas that persons without disability face: the high cost of health insurance and the number of plans converting to a health maintenance organization (HMO). People with a disability who are enrolled in HMOs report difficulties finding a doctor to see consistently, accessing specialists, getting enough appointment time for complex problems, and being examined in ill-equipped offices (ACRM, 1993). Persons with a disability who have Medicaid report having difficulties finding any doctor to see them (because of low reimbursement rates) and having to use emergency rooms for primary care (because they cannot be turned away if it is an emergency). A positive benefit of Medicaid, however, is that it does cover in-home help for low income persons, which is a highly valued benefit. To be eligible for Medicare, one must be eligible for Social Security benefits. People who are Medicare eligible encounter a big disincentive to keeping a job or returning to work, because they lose this health insurance benefit. Medicare coverage (A and B) is important because it covers most costs of hospital care, rehabilitation, physician and therapy services, and mental health care.

Legislation covering older people who have a disability includes not only Social Security and Medicare, but social support programs as well. The Older Americans Act of 1965 provides for a wide range of supportive services (nutrition, transportation, housing, legal services, case management, senior centers, etc.). Even though these support programs could greatly benefit younger people who have a disability, they generally have age-eligibility criteria of sixty or sixty-five. Programs on aging are administered primarily through departments of aging in each state and through them, by area agencies on aging on the local level. The artificial dichotomy between assistance programs for younger and older persons with disabilities reflects the nature of U.S. special-interest politics. Separate programs reflect the interests of separate constituencies, who pushed to develop distinct legislation protecting those interests. Little planning was given to changing needs or to needs of multiple groups that may cut across various entitlement programs. As Jim ages and his needs change, he is out of touch (if not out of luck) with most rehabilitation programs, yet not old enough to qualify for aging services that could greatly benefit him.

Factors Limiting Access to Services

Several factors limit access to services for people who acquire a disability and for those persons as they mature and age:

1. Short-sighted, special-interest policies that cover the needs of a particular segment of society but exclude others by creating artificial or arbitrary eligibility criteria (different programs require different bureaucracies and different measures of success to justify continued funding)
2. Failure to recognize multiple and changing needs of people with a disability, caused in part by short-sighted planning that ignores the fact that people with disabilities will live into late life
3. Underfunding of many programs, although this may be more misfunding than underfunding[4]
4. Lack of coordination among programs (a new application for each type of service needed requires making separate inquiries to different agencies, rather than a single inquiry to a multipurpose center)

Recipient Data (Indicates Extent of Need)

	Health	Function	Employment	Support	Economics	Psychological
	Health					
Provider Data	Function					
(Indicates	Employment		Differences between Need and Utilization			
Supply			Would Reflect Adequacy of Community			
or	Support		Responsiveness to Needs of People with			
Utilization)	Economics		a Disability			
	Psychological					

Fig. 5.5. A Design for Community Indicators

5. Lack of data to monitor the success of health, rehabilitation, and community support systems in providing services to people with disabilities currently and as they age

DATA SOURCES AND INDICATORS OF COMMUNITY ADEQUACY

Two broad, empirical issues face researchers and policymakers interested in assessing how well people with disabilities are being served at the community level: *(a)* what data to collect and *(b)* how to collect them so that they will accurately reflect adequacy of care and quality of life, both cross-sectionally and longitudinally. Besides basic prevalence data, information should be collected on the six basic domains of service needs mentioned earlier: health, functioning, employment/education, economic status, psychological functioning, and social support.

Figure 5.5 illustrates how some of the conditions and service use issues related to tracking community service responsiveness for those with disabilities might be operationalized into an indicator framework. For consistency with other chapters in this volume, the indicators have been grouped under headings that distinguish the incidence of new cases of disability and estimates of disability prevalence. These estimates form a basis of expected demand or need for care against which the performance of the community's delivery system can be compared. In this illustration the initial concern is to assess how well income and care programs have done in identifying the disabled population. This is done by comparing the estimated number of cases with the numbers known to the delivery system. Enumerations of the recipients or those eligible for particular programs will likely not be a perfect match to synthetic and other estimates of need, because of the crudeness of both sets of measures. Nevertheless, these indicators permit an approximation of the fit between demand and those known to the system. Such estimates are useful in comparing among communities or across time as benefit or program eligibility changes, or in setting priorities among conditions or subgroups.

The next level in this model is the process of care. Service use rates calculated relative to the estimated number of disabled persons provide an estimate of the relative use rates for various types and levels of care. This reflects issues in service access. Use rates based on the number of recipients provide an indication of the service efficiency among those gaining access to care. Both sets of rates or indicators can be useful.

Service outcomes are differentiated between those that reflect potential problems in the delivery system and those more specific to individuals. Rates of hospitalization, death, or nursing home placement are suggested as a first-cut indicator of service effectiveness. High rates of hospitalization or mortality at young ages, for example, would suggest potential problems. The measures based on individual cases would be aggregated into community rates (again using either the estimated prevalent population or service recipients as the denominator). The derived rates are especially useful for monitoring change over time, and in planning service capacity and delivery modalities that may be responsive to such changes. Particularly important here is the ability to monitor the relationships among delivery systems. For example, indications of improved health system performance (such as ADL/IADL functioning) or social adjustment should be reflected in such other sectors as employment, income, and mental health.

The data sources and the relative expense of the indicators are varied. The most accessible is Medicare and/or Medicaid claims. These data could be compiled to generate a number of the prevalence, process, and even health status outcome indicators. Such tabulations could be made cross-sectionally, or with panels or cohorts of identified persons who are tracked over time. Claims measures are limited in their generality by the proportion of the disabled population eligible for these programs, but they nevertheless provide a ready resource for fairly comprehensive coverage of the issues discussed. The monitoring of mental health status, access and use of educational and support programs, and living arrangements generally requires some form of survey. These could either be directed to the client or to provider agencies. As discussed elsewhere in this volume, there are good examples of both approaches that might be followed. A beginning basis for any survey is the ability to identify the agencies or clients who would be contacted. Existing lists and inventories of providers and their recipients are the logical starting place. However, as noted earlier, existing rehabilitation systems are not usually oriented to continuing involvement with their clientele. It would be useful to explore the feasibility of developing and maintaining registries of both current and former disabled clients.

The conclusion of this volume presents a strategy for staging indicators and focusing special surveys or more on target issues or populations. The present chapter concludes by examining some of the special issues that would need to be considered if survey data are used as a basis for either indicators or focused studies. Additionally, some of the data sources that might be used to capture information on functional change and employment status are discussed.

A community-based monitoring system for people with a disability

- has to be geographically complete, such as thorough sampling in representative zip codes;
- has to cover the six major service needs (health, function, employment, support, economic, and psychological);
- has to be a longitudinal or cross-sectional design;
- has to collect data from both providers and receivers;
- should not rely solely on a disabled person's self-judgment of conditions;
- should be repeated every three to five years.

Being geographically based is important for maintaining a community focus and assessing change in the population. Data from all six domains should be collected on each person in the sample, and similar data should be collected both from people with disabilities and from health and social service providers. Thus, the health of people with a disability would be assessed by a home-based interview. In this way, a measure of *need* can be estimated from the interview data and a measure of *supply* or use from the provider data (e.g., from records of hospitals, managed care organizations, Medicare). The difference between the two would reflect the adequacy of care at the community level (Table 5.1).

For example, suppose a study involving a representative sample in a

Table 5.1. Prevalence, Process of Care, and Outcomes Indicators

Indicator	Potential Data Source
Incidence	
• By cause or conditions	Hospital discharge abstracts
Prevalence	
• By cause or condition, specific to age, gender, and income level	Synthetic estimate; program eligibility records (e.g., Social Security Disability Insurance, Supplemental Security Income/State Supplemental Payment for Disabled)
Access to care programs	
• Income and health care benefits	Estimated prevalence minus SSDI and/or SSI program recipients
• Rehabilitation care	Incidence minus agency reports from inpatient and outpatient rehabilitation treatment centers; Medicare/Medicaid service claims
• Vocational rehabilitation	Prevalence minus agency reports from state rehabilitation departments
Process of care	
Rehabilitation medicine	
• Occupational, physical, speech therapy	Service claims, perhaps differentiated by newly impaired and prevalent cases; client survey
• Assistive devices	
Medical care	
• Primary care	Service claims, perhaps differentiated by newly impaired and prevalent cases; client survey
• Specialty care	
• Emergency room care	
• Skilled home care	
Empowerment	
• Vocational rehabilitation	Agency reports; client survey
• Other education and training	
• Home modifications	Client survey
• Vehicle modification	
• Attendant aid or similar assistance	Client survey, agency reports
• Support group participation	Client survey, agency reports
Outcomes	
System measures	
• Hospitalization rates	Claims data, client survey
• Mortality	Claims data, program eligibility records
• Nursing home placement	Claims data, client survey
• Employment rates	Client survey, rehabilitation department reports
Individual measures	
• Prevalence of chronic conditions, complications	Claims data, client survey, physician survey
• ADL/IADL capacity	Client or physician survey
• Educational attainment	Client survey, rehabilitation department
• Employment	Client survey, rehabilitation department
• Income	Client survey, rehabilitation department

(continued)

160

Table 5.1.   *(continued)*

• Mental health (e.g., depression, anxiety disorder, substance abuse)	Client survey; claims data; provider survey
• Social adjustment (e.g., support group, peer counseling participation)	Client survey
• Living arrangement (e.g., with family or spouse, alone with or without aide, in specialized housing)	Client survey

four-zip-code area found that 20 percent of the sample with a disability should likely have seen a physician in the last six months because of health problems reported at interview, and another 40 percent needed in-home help. In addition to asking participants about services needed, data from providers would determine how many of these persons were in provider records and what overall percentage of people with a disability was receiving assistance. Providers would need to include disability status as a part of their normal data profile. Data from providers could also supply information not likely to be obtained accurately from participants (e.g., failed appointments, diagnoses, length of visit, hospitalization, prescriptions, supplies, etc.). Social service records could be used to compare the number of people receiving in-home help in a community and the amount of help they received with the numbers derived from the participant sample. In the beginning, quality of service could be limited to satisfaction measures from participants. Prevalence and demographic data (including number of years with a disability) could be collected from participants. Repeated sampling of the same geographic area would estimate changes in the population and allow monitoring of services over time to assess change.

Data from people with disabilities could be collected in a combination of telephone and in-person assessments. Questionnaires could cover all six domains of interest and still be reasonably short. Some data not based solely on self-report should be gathered (e.g., specific medications, cognitive ability, some ADL measures, functional impairment, blood pressure, reasons for changes in function, etc.). These measures would be best assessed by suitable screening instruments and by direct observation that could still be done in a home interview.

The population studied should be a complete or highly representative sampling by small geographic area rather than by large-area random sampling, to focus on community-level monitoring and longitudinal tracking of the same people. A suitable approach would be to interview door-to-door or every x doors to identify people with disability. Accurate contact and follow-up data would have to be preserved to assess this sample again for longitudinal purposes. A cross-sectional design that initially assessed people who had different ages of onset of disability would help to gauge aging effects versus duration of disability effects.

Gathering data from providers is difficult for a number of reasons. In the area of health care, data must come from several sources, including trauma care, primary care, and secondary care; however, there is no single source for these data. Good reporting on people who sustain a major disability through trauma is available through trauma centers and emergency rooms. Data from primary and secondary care physicians relevant to the needs of people with a disability—both those with a recent disability and those aging longitudinally—are more problematic. Most physicians would not take time to comb their files. Protecting confidentially would also be a major concern. As the United States moves toward a system of managed care, systems of routine data collection that protect privacy could be established to capture these data.

Data on medical rehabilitation and other rehabilitation services can be gathered through several separate means; again, however, the difficulty lies in collecting longitudinal data that reflect changing needs. One of the better reporting systems on acute rehabilitation is the National Information System on Rehabilitation Outcomes, currently being used by many rehabilitation centers in the country. This system reports data on changing functioning during rehabilitation using the Functional Independence Measure (FIM) developed by Hamilton and Granger (1990). The FIM assesses daily functioning in thirteen areas and is being used by several centers to assess level of disability and gauge change in functioning. The FIM is weak, however, in assessing community functioning skill; it focuses instead on functioning likely to improve in acute rehabilitation. Nevertheless, it is a good system of measurement and should be universally adapted; it is currently being used by the National Model Spinal Cord Injury System program (Thomas, 1992) and the Traumatic Brain Injury Centers System program (McLaughlin, Davis, & Reswik, 1992), both funded by NIDRR. FIM data could be used to assess changes in functioning longitudinally. One benefit of this approach would be to compare how functioning is maintained or lost in different kinds of communities where people live after rehabilitation (urban vs. rural, midcity vs. suburb). The Model Systems projects are already beginning to gather longitudinal information on people aging with these conditions. An additional method for tracking rehabilitation services, and one that might be very useful for longitudinal purposes, could be based upon work being done through the Technology Assistance Act, which in many states funds technology and assistive device services to people who have a disability. Age of onset and duration of disability could be assessed to gauge the percentage of aging individuals with a disability who use this service.

Employment data are fairly well reported, at least for those who use state DR services, by the RSA, which publishes yearly data on the provision of services and the characteristics of the people served. Data by zip code could be derived from its database to make comparisons in the level of need and between communities. Workers' compensation systems could be another source of cross-sectional data, at least on people who are evaluated for return to work through those means. Both these approaches would still miss information on people who become employed on their own as well as longitudinal information on what happens to people in employment as they age. The National Model Spinal Cord Injury System project (Thomas, 1992) shows that employment of people with paraplegia peaks at a rate of 40 percent and rapidly declines after twelve to fifteen years of employment. A more in-depth study of the causes and consequences of unemployment would be of great benefit. For example, how many people with disability continue working but could use assistance to do so? Since there are not model systems for all disability categories, supplemental national studies of the type proposed here, or carried out through the NHIS or by NIDRR-funded Rehabilitation Research and Training Centers, will be needed to provide estimates or indicators of employment.

People who have a disability most likely do not make much use of the public mental health system in each state, so few accurate data can be gained from those administrative databases. An approach based on community surveys would be helpful to gather both accurate data and life-long prevalence rates. Kemp and colleagues (1987) used a similar methodology to assess levels of depression in a large Hispanic sample and determine how many individuals should be taking antidepressant medications. They compared that number with the number who were taking such medications and concluded that community-level care was poor. Another approach would be to include disability status, including duration of disability, in future Epidemiologic Catchment Area (ECA) studies conducted by the National Institute of Mental Health (Robins, Helzer, & Weissman, 1984).

Measures of formal and informal support, both economic and personal, can be estimated in a variety of ways. Again, simply determining who is receiving formal benefits, be it through records from Medicare, SSI, IHSS, etc., will not answer the question of whether those who need it are getting it, whether they are getting enough, and whether changing needs are being met. Likewise, administrative records cannot assess the impact on the family and their needs. These records, however, when compared with data collected at the community level from people who have a disability, would give a fairly good estimate of the number of people receiving help versus the number who need it. In summary, to get representative data that reflect a community focus, small-area, intensely studied group designs must be conducted, and improved data sources from providers must be developed.

SUMMARY AND RECOMMENDATIONS

Approximately 35 million people in the United States have a disability serious enough to interfere with some aspect of daily functioning, and more than half of them are between eighteen and sixty-four years of age. Moreover, most of these people, along with younger persons with a disability, will live decades longer; most will reach their sixties, seventies, or eighties. As they do, most of them will experience changes in their physical and functional status, employment status, psychosocial functioning, and social support systems. Evidence shows increasingly that the number of problems a person with a disability will experience over his or her lifetime is great, and that current resources do not address these needs. At present, no adequate way exists at the community level to determine the quantity and quality of services that people with a disability receive, either soon after onset or over the long term.

To determine adequacy of services, one must know what the needs are and what the provision of services is. This will require that data be gathered from both people with disability and service providers, since data only from people with a disability is not always reliable, and data from providers alone does not indicate who *should* be receiving services.

It is recommended that accurate data on people with a disability be gathered using census-type approaches, perhaps at the zip code level, to best gauge the status of the population at the community level. The same groups can then be restudied to discover longitudinal changes in the sample and in the community. Gathering data from providers is difficult because there are many providers within various funding systems, and there are no requirements for a central database. Therefore, various estimates of service provision adequacy will be needed to estimate overall community responsiveness. Such data are critically needed to further integrate people with a disability into everyday society, and repeated studies are needed to gauge progress toward that goal.

Acknowledgments—Supported in part by a grant (H133B3004–94) from the National Institute of Disability and Rehabilitation Research, U.S. Department of Education.

Notes

1. This chapter follows the framework of the International Classification of Impairments Disabilities and Handicaps proposed by the World Health Organization, with the exception that what the ICIDH calls disease will be called pathology, in keeping with recent debates on the issue (e.g., Pope & Tarlov, 1991).

2. See appendix A for listing of NCHS data sets referred to in this chapter.

3. See appendix C for listing of all governmental and nongovernmental data sets referred to in this chapter.

4. Torres-Gil and Wray (1993) reported that 79% of state DR agency personnel surveyed said that state and federal funding was grossly inadequate for the job. One surprising finding was that DR staffs felt positive about wanting to extend services to older persons with a disability and confident that they could do so if given the financial resources.

References

American Congress of Rehabilitative Medicine Committee on Social, Ethical and Environmental Aspects of Rehabilitation. 1993. Addressing the post-rehabilitation health care needs of persons with disabilities. *Archives of Physical Medicine and Rehabilitation 79:* S-8–13.

Ansello, E. F. 1988. The intersecting of aging and disabilities. *Educational Gerontology 14:* 351–64.

Blazer, D. 1982. *Depression in Late Life.* St. Louis: C. V. Mosby.

Bleck, E. E. 1984. Where have all the CP children gone? The needs of adults. *Developmental Medicine & Child Neurology 26:* 669–76.

Brody, E. 1986. Informal support systems in the rehabilitation of the aging. In S. J. Brody & G. E. Ruff (eds.), *Aging and Rehabilitation.* New York: Springer.

Brummel-Smith, K. (ed.) 1993. Geriatric rehabilitation. *Clinics in Geriatric Medicine.* Philadelphia: W. B. Saunders.

Cairns, D., & Baker, J. 1993. Adjustment to spinal cord injury: a review of coping styles contributing to the process. *Journal of Rehabilitation 37:* 31–36.

Carpenter, J. O. 1974. Changing roles and disagreements in families with disabled husbands. *Archives of Pharmaceutical Medicine and Rehabilitation 55:* 272–76.

Corthell, D. W., & Brown, J. 1991. *Substance Abuse as a Coexisting Disability.* Research and Training Center. Menomonie, Wis.: University of Wisconsin-Stout.

Eisenberg, M., Satkin, L., & Jansen, M. (eds.). 1984. *Chronic Illness and Disability through the Life Span.* New York: Springer.

Ficke, R. 1992. *Digest of Data on Persons with Disabilities.* Washington, D.C.: National Institute on Disability and Rehabilitation Research.

Fuhrer, M. J., Rintala, D. H., Hart, K. A., Clearman, R., & Young, M. E. 1993. Depressive symptomatology in persons with spinal cord injury who reside in the community. *Archives of Physical Medicine and Rehabilitation 74:* 255–61.

Garland, D. E., Rosen, S. D., Stewart, C. A., Adkins, R., & Huang, G. 1989. Bone and mineral distribution five years or more after spinal cord injury. *Journal of Nuclear Medicine 30:* 857–61.

Gellman, H., Sie, I., & Waters, R. 1988. Late complications of the weight-bearing upper extremity in paraplegic patients. *Clinical Orthopedics 223:* 132–35.

Government Accounting Office. 1991. *Vocational Rehabilitation Program: Client Characteristics, Services Received, and Elective Outcomes.* GAO/T-PEMD 92–3. Washington, D.C.: U.S. Printing Office.

Halstead, L. S. 1991. Assessment and differential diagnosis for post-polio syndrome. *Orthopedics 14:* 1209–17.

Halstead, L. S., & Weikers, D. O. (eds.). 1987. *Research and Clinical Aspects of the Late Effects of Poliomyelitis.* White Plains, N.Y.: March of Dimes.

Hamilton, B., & Granger, C. 1990. *The Functional Independence Measure (FIM).*

Hartke, R. J. (ed.). 1991. *Psychological Aspects of Geriatric Rehabilitation.* Gaithersburg, Md.: Aspen Publishing.

Heuman, J. 1986. *Application for a Rehabilitation Research and Training Center on Independent Living.* San Francisco: World Institute on Disability.

Kane, R. L., Ouslander, J. G., & Abrass, I. B. 1989. *Essentials of Clinical Geriatrics.* New York: McGraw-Hill.

Kaplan, H. I., & Sadock, B. J. (eds.). 1991. *Textbook of Psychiatry.* Baltimore: Williams and Wilkins.

Kaplan, D., & Mearig, J. S. 1977. A community support system for a family coping with chronic illness. *Rehabilitation Literature 38:* 79–83.

Kemp, B. J. 1992. *Rehabilitation Research and Training Center on Aging with a Disability.* Downey, Calif.: Rancho Los Amigos Medical Center.

Kemp, B. J. (1993a). *Rehabilitation Research and Training Center on Aging with Spinal Cord Injury.* Downey, Calif.: Rancho Los Amigos Medical Center.

Kemp, B. J. (1993b). *Final Report on the Rehabilitation Research and Training Center on Aging.* Downey, Calif.: Rancho Los Amigos Medical Center.

Kemp, B. J., Staples, F., & Lopez, W. 1987. Epidemiology of depression and dysphoria in an elderly Hispanic population: Prevalence and correlates. *Journal of the American Geriatric Society 35*: 90–97.

La Buda, D. 1990. The impact of technology on geriatric rehabilitation. In B. J. Kemp, K. Brummel-Smith, & J. Ramsdell (eds.), *Geriatric Rehabilitation*. San Diego, Calif.: Pro-Ed Publishers.

Lammertse, D., & Yankony, G. 1991. Rehabilitation in spinal cord disorders 4. Outcomes and issues of aging after spinal cord injury. *Archives of Physical Medicine and Rehabilitation 72*: 309–11.

Louis Harris & Associates, Inc. 1986. *The ICD Survey of Disabled Americans: Bringing Disabled Americans into the Mainstream*. New York: International Center for the Disabled.

Mann, W. 1992. *Annual Report of the Rehabilitation Engineering Center on Aging*. Buffalo, N.Y.: State University of New York.

Maynard, F. M. 1992. Changing care needs. In G. G. Whiteneck et al. (eds.), *Aging with Spinal Cord Injury*. New York: Demos Publishing.

McLaughlin, W. E., Davis, M., & Reswick, J. 1992. *NIDRR Program Directory*. Washington, D.C.: Office of Special Education and Rehabilitation Services.

Moos, R. H. (ed.). 1977. *Coping with Physical Illness*. New York: Plenum Press.

National Center for Health Statistics. 1989. Current estimates from the National Health Interview Survey, 1988. *Vital and Health Statistics*, series 10, no. 173. DHHS Publ. no.(PHS) 89–1501. Washington, D.C.: U.S. Government Printing Office.

National Institute of Mental Health. 1991. *Consensus Conference on Depression*. Bethesda, Md.

National Spinal Cord Injury Statistical Center Annual Report 8. 1990. University of Alabama at Birmingham.

Nosek, M. A. 1990. Personal assistance—key to maintaining ability of persons with physical disabilities. *Applied Rehabilitation Counseling 21*: 3–8.

Ohry, A., Shemash, Y., & Rosin, R. 1983. Are chronic spinal cord injured patients (CSCIP) subject to premature aging? *Medical Hypotheses 11*: 605–13.

Pope, A. M., & Tarlov, A. R. (eds.). 1991. *Disability in America: Toward a National Agenda for Prevention*. Institute of Medicine. Washington, D.C.: National Academy Press.

Staying fully alive: Can people with disabilities find high quality primary care in the U.S.? 1991. *Rehabilitation Briefs 13*: 9. Washington, D.C.: National Institute on Disability and Rehabilitation Research.

Robins, L., Helzer, J. E., & Weissman, M. M. 1984. Lifetime prevalence of specific psychiatric disorders in three sites. *Archives of General Psychiatry 41*: 949–56.

Sasma, G. P., Patrick, C. H., & Feusser, J. R. 1993. Long-term survival of veterans with traumatic spinal cord injury. *Archives of Neurology 50*: 909–14.

Shultz, R., & Decker, S. 1985. Long-term adjustment to physical disability: The role of social support, control and self blame. *Journal of Personal and Social Psychology 5*: 1162–72.

Sie, I., Waters, R., Adkins, R., & Gellman, H. 1992. Upper extremity pain in the post-rehabilitation spinal cord injured patient. *Archives of Physical Medicine and Rehabilitation 73:* 44–48.

Technology-Related Assistance for Individuals with Disabilities Act. 1988. U.S. Congress, PL 100–147.

Thomas, J. P. 1992. *The National Model Spinal Cord Injury System.* National Institute on Disability and Rehabilitation Research. Washington, D.C.: U.S. Dept. of Education.

Torres-Gil, F. M., & Wray, L. A. 1993. Funding and policies affecting geriatric rehabilitation. *Clinics in Geriatric Medicine 9:* 831–40.

Trieshman, R. B. 1987. *Aging with a Disability.* New York: Demos Publications.

U.S. Department of Health and Human Services. 1989. Task I: Population Profile on Disability. Prepared by Mathematica Policy Research, Washington, D.C.

Vash, C. L. 1981. *The Psychology of Disability.* New York: Springer.

Whiteneck, G., Chanlifue, M., Frankel, M., Fraser, M. H., Gardner, B. S., Gerhart, K. A., Krishman, K. R., Menter, R., Nuseibeth, I., Short, D. J., & Silver, J. R. 1992. Mortality, morbidity and psychosocial outcomes of persons spinal cord injured more than 20 years ago. *Paraplegia 30:* 617–30.

6/ ADULTS WITH CHRONIC DISEASE
Musculoskeletal Conditions As an Exemplar

Carol L. Such, Edward H. Yelin, and Lindsey A. Criswell

Most chronic medical conditions prevalent among adults share numerous attributes. The precise course through the "health care service career" of a person with a chronic disease is uncertain, although it is likely to be characterized by recurring episodes of exacerbation and remission in the shorter term and progressive descent over the longer term. Individuals diagnosed with the same chronic condition may experience dramatically different levels of disease severity, rates of progression, and likelihood of disability. Moreover, access to health care, social services, and peer support, all of which affect one's ability to cope with a chronic medical condition, can vary tremendously among persons with the same diagnosis. Access to these services typically depends upon the individual's geographic location and proximity to family and friends, as well as socioeconomic status. The longevity of chronic medical conditions, the need for increasing health care and social services as the conditions progress, and the incredible variation among persons with the same condition all contribute to the potential usefulness of a community-based indicator system for tracking the resources needed by persons experiencing these conditions.

The purpose of this chapter is to develop a framework for monitoring the progression of adults with chronic medical conditions through the stages of their health care service career. This terminology, which health care planners have drawn from the stages of vocational development, relates to changes in the health care and social service needs of persons with chronic medical conditions as their disease and functional disability grow progressively more severe. Examples of indicators that might be used to monitor changes in the needs of community residents include demographic data to be used as risk factors in estimating the prevalence

169

of a particular chronic medical condition, and assessments of the number of primary care and specialist physicians per capita in a specific locale. The ultimate goal of this work is to allow a local community to anticipate and provide appropriate health care and social services for its residents with chronic medical conditions.

To focus attention on an indicator system rather than on the details of a myriad of chronic medical conditions, this chapter uses musculoskeletal conditions as an exemplar for all adult chronic diseases.[1] A person with a musculoskeletal disease, like those with most chronic medical conditions, generally follows a varied short- and long-term disease course. The degree of pain, morning stiffness, and anxiety about the disease may change markedly throughout the day, and the severity of the condition can progress from something barely noticeable when first diagnosed to a debilitating condition several years later. Variation among people with the same musculoskeletal condition can range from slight discomfort to total disability. Some chronic medical conditions, however, such as hypertension and type II diabetes, do have qualities that set them apart from musculoskeletal conditions, the most important of which may be the usefulness of screening for the presence of the disease. Thus, in using musculoskeletal conditions as an exemplar, these differences must be taken into account.

MUSCULOSKELETAL CONDITIONS AND THEIR TREATMENT

Diseases of the musculoskeletal system are among the most prevalent chronic medical conditions reported in the United States (LaPlante, 1988). Specific diseases within the broad category of musculoskeletal conditions include those as familiar as osteoarthritis and rheumatoid arthritis, as well as less common conditions such as gout, ankylosing spondylitis, and systemic lupus erythematosus. Most people with musculoskeletal conditions have relatively mild forms of disease, while a minority endure much more debilitating and even life-threatening chronic illnesses.

The physical and psychological impacts of musculoskeletal conditions, even the mild forms of disease, can be imposing. Pain is the most often cited reason that persons with arthritis seek medical intervention (Buckelew & Parker, 1989; Davis, Cortez, & Rubin, 1990); fatigue is also commonly reported, particularly among those with rheumatoid arthritis (Tack, 1990). Physical disability strikes many people affected by musculoskeletal conditions. More than 50 percent of people with arthritis in the National Health Interview Survey (NHIS)[2] report some activity limitation resulting from the disease; among working-age adults with arthritis, labor force participation is reduced by 20 percent and 25 percent for men and women, respectively (Felts & Yelin, 1989). Depression is common among people with arthritis, both those who are newly diagnosed and those who have had the disease for years. Persons with newly diagnosed chronic medical conditions tend to be depressed about prospects for the future, while people with longer-term disease are more affected by the inability to engage in activities that require more than limited physical endurance (Fifield & Reisine, 1992).

Despite the high prevalence of musculoskeletal conditions, therapies prescribed for persons with these conditions vary dramatically, and agents used to treat conditions such as rheumatoid arthritis differ markedly in efficacy, toxicity, and cost. Differences in individual practice styles of rheumatologists have been shown to explain much more of the variation in use of medications than do differences in patient characteristics (Criswell & Redfearn, 1994). The optimal set of pharmaceuticals to be prescribed and the appropriate timing of their administration are subject to intense debate among practicing clinicians and warrant further rigorous study. Use of ancillary services, such as physical and occupational rehabilitation and psychological counseling, also varies greatly.

Given the preponderance of mild forms of musculoskeletal conditions and the lack of consensus regarding optimal treatment for specific musculoskeletal diseases, a low-technology approach to therapy is probably appropriate for most people. Those with severe forms of the diseases might benefit from more potent pharmaceuticals, rehabilitative services, and in some cases, surgical procedures. However, screening to identify potentially severe cases of musculoskeletal conditions is unlikely to prove cost effective, because the pain and discomfort that characterize severe forms of these diseases will most likely provide ample incentive to seek medical assistance. As one recent study demonstrated, slightly more than 86 percent of those with a musculoskeletal condition, identified in a random sample of adults living in a California community, reported seeing a physician for their conditions, with the percentage increasing for people with more severe disease (Yelin, Bernhard, & Pflugrad, 1995).

PREVALENCE OF MUSCULOSKELETAL CONDITIONS

Statistics compiled from the 1983–1985 NHIS show arthritis to be one of the most prevalent chronic medical conditions (second only to

Table 6.1.   Number of Musculoskeletal Conditions per 1,000 Community-Dwelling Civilians in the United States by Age and Gender *(Three-Year Average, 1983 through 1985)*

		Age (years)			
Condition	All Ages	Under 45	45–69	70–84	85+
Males and Females					
Rheumatoid arthritis	5.6	1.8	14.3	12.5	17.1*
Osteoarthritis/other arthropathies	125.4	31.1	294.1	478.9	491.2
Males					
Rheumatoid arthritis	3.0	1.4	7.1	6.0*	—
Osteoarthritis/other arthropathies	92.3	23.7	230.4	391.4	377.1
Females					
Rheumatoid arthritis	8.0	2.2	20.8	16.9	25.1*
Osteoarthritis/other arthropathies	156.3	38.4	350.5	537.1	544.7

Source: Data from LaPlante, 1988.
Note: Dash indicates that there were zero respondents among the survey population.
*Figure has low statistical reliability or precision (relative standard error exceeds 30%).

sinusitis) among civilian community-dwelling residents of the United States (LaPlante, 1988). Table 6.1 displays estimated prevalence rates, broken down by age and gender, for persons with rheumatoid arthritis, osteoarthritis, and other arthropathies.[3] Among U.S. residents of all ages, more than thirty million (131 persons per 1000 population) report experience with at least one of these conditions. Nearly 60 percent of the people with rheumatoid arthritis and 55 percent of those reporting osteoarthritis or other arthropathies are in the age range forty-five to sixty-nine. Women of all ages have rheumatoid arthritis or osteoarthritis arthritis more often than men (2.7 and 1.7 times, respectively). African Americans and native Chinese and Japanese people tend to have lower prevalence rates of rheumatoid arthritis than do Caucasians, while several Native American tribes have particularly high prevalence rates for these conditions (Schumacher, 1988). The prevalence of osteoarthritis is also higher among whites than among either Asian or African Americans (Hoaglund et al., 1985; Solomon, Breighton, & Lawrence, 1975).

The NHIS uses three different measures of disability resulting from chronic disease or impairment. All survey respondents are asked whether they are limited in any way from normative activities appropriate for their age group: play for children under age five, school attendance for persons aged five to seventeen, work or housekeeping for those aged eighteen to sixty-nine, and self-care for persons older than sixty-nine. Respondents in the eighteen to sixty-nine age group are asked about work limitations. Survey respondents aged five to sixty-nine who reported any activity limitations and all respondents over age sixty-nine are asked about limitation in activities of daily living (ADLs) (bathing, dressing, eating, mobility within the home) and limitation in instrumental activities of daily living (IADLs) (household chores, household business, shopping, mobility outside the home) (Verbrugge, Lepkowski, & Imanaka, 1990).

Arthritis is the leading cause of activity limitation among community-dwelling civilian residents, affecting four million people (12.3 percent of all persons reporting such limitation). In comparison, heart disease is the second most common cause of activity limitation among people of both genders and all ages, accounting for 11.5 percent of all persons reporting activity limitation (LaPlante, 1988). Table 6.2 shows prevalence rates of activity limitation attributable to rheumatoid arthritis or osteoarthritis and other arthropathies, as well as percentages of all persons with arthritis reporting activity limitation. Largely because of the higher prevalence rate of rheumatoid arthritis among women, 2.8 times as many women as men report activity limitation attributable to rheumatoid arthritis. Women are 2.2 times as likely as men to incur activity limitation from osteoarthritis and other arthropathies, a rate that somewhat exceeds their relative rate of experience with the condition. Prevalence of activity limitation from rheumatoid arthritis among men and women stabilizes, albeit at a high level of disability, after age forty-five, but increases quite dramatically for people with osteoarthritis and other arthropathies as they age.

Of 17.4 million community-dwelling civilian adults reporting limitation in work activities, defined as restrictions in amount or kind of work as well as inability to work, just over two million attribute those limitations to arthritis. As with activity limitation, arthritis is the leading cause of work limitation among all chronic medical conditions, accounting for 11.6 percent of all adults reporting work limitation. Table 6.3 shows prevalence rates of work limitation, broken down by age and gender, and percentages of persons with arthritis reporting work limitation. The higher rate of work limitation attributable to rheumatoid arthritis or osteoarthritis and arthropathies reported by women with either condition is in proportion to the higher prevalence of that condition among women. The prevalence of work limitation attributable to either rheumatoid arthritis or osteoarthritis increases significantly with age for both male and female working-age adults (LaPlante, 1988).

Among people aged five to sixty-nine with some activity limitation

Table 6.2.   Activity Limitation Associated with Specific Arthropathies among Community-Dwelling Civilians in the United States by Age and Gender *(Three-Year Average, 1983 through 1985)*

		Age (years)			
Condition	*All Ages*	*Under 45*	*45–69*	*70–84*	*85+*
Males and Females					
Rheumatoid arthritis					
Rate per 1,000 persons	2.3	0.7	5.8	5.9	3.6*
% of all RA cases	40.9%	0.0%	40.4%	47.2%	21.2%*
Osteoarthritis/other arthropathies					
Rate per 1,000 persons	15.0	2.2	35.6	65.3	105.7
% of all OA cases	12.0%	7.2%	12.1%	13.6%	21.5%
Males					
Rheumatoid arthritis					
Rate per 1,000 persons	1.2	0.4	3.3	3.6	—
% of all RA cases	1.4%	28.7%	46.1%	59.5%	NA
Osteoarthritis/other arthropathies					
Rate per 1,000 persons	9.2	1.9	23.7	37.9	65.2
% of all OA cases	9.9%	8.2%	10.3%	9.7%	17.3%
Females					
Rheumatoid arthritis					
Rate per 1,000 persons	3.3	1.1	8.0	7.4	5.4*
% of all RA cases	40.7%	47.5%	38.8%	43.6%	21.1%*
Osteoarthritis/other arthropathies					
Rate per 1,000 persons	20.5	2.5	46.2	83.7	123.9
% of all OA cases	13.1%	6.6%	13.2%	15.6%	22.8%

Source: Data from LaPlante, 1988.
Note: Dash indicates that there were zero respondents among the survey population. NA means that a denominator was not available.
*Figure has low statistical reliability or precision (relative standard error exceeds 30%).

and all people over sixty-nine years, 7.6 million need assistance with IADLs, ADLs, or both. Arthritis is the most frequently cited cause of this type of limitation, accounting for 14.9 percent of the total group, or just under one million persons. Table 6.4 contains rates of need for assistance with either IADLs or ADLs caused by rheumatoid arthritis or osteoarthritis and other arthropathies. Women with either rheumatoid arthritis or osteoarthritis and other arthropathies are four times more likely than men to need assistance with IADLs or ADLs. This can be explained by noting that the need for such assistance increases with age even faster than the prevalence of the conditions themselves, coupled with the fact that women tend to live to older ages than men (LaPlante, 1988).

The NHIS reports prevalence of chronic conditions and disability at-

Table 6.3. Work Limitation Associated with Specific Arthropathies among Community-Dwelling Civilians in the United States by Age and Gender *(Three-Year Average, 1983 through 1985)*

Condition	Age (years)		
	18–69	18–44	45–69
Males and Females			
Rheumatoid arthritis			
Rate per 1,000 persons	1.4	0.8	4.6
% of all RA cases	30.5%	26.1%	32.2%
Osteoarthritis/other arthropathies			
Rate per 1,000 persons	7.3	2.3	27.5
% of OA cases	8.2%	4.5%	9.3%
Males			
Rheumatoid arthritis			
Rate per 1,000 persons	0.8	0.5	2.8
% of all RA cases	32.1%	21.7%	38.8%
Osteoarthritis/other arthropathies			
Rate per 1,000 persons	5.2	2.0	19.2
% of all OA cases	7.5%	5.0%	8.3%
Females			
Rheumatoid arthritis			
Rate per 1,000 persons	1.9	1.0	6.3
% of all RA cases	30.0%	29.1%	30.3%
Osteoarthritis/other arthropathies			
Rate per 1,000 persons	9.3	2.6	34.8
% of all OA cases	8.6%	4.2%	9.9%

Source: Data from LaPlante, 1988.

tributable to those conditions only for the civilian community-dwelling population. However, 4.6 percent of the U.S. population over age sixty-five lives in nursing homes, and musculoskeletal conditions and connective tissue disorders constitute the fourth most frequent major system or disease category within this group (Lee & Estes, 1990; Praemer, Furner, & Rice, 1992). In 1985, 429,000 nursing home residents reported one or more types of musculoskeletal conditions, with arthritis and rheumatism accounting for 63.4 percent and osteoporosis an additional 11.4 percent (Praemer et al., 1992). In most cases, these musculoskeletal conditions were secondary to other medical conditions or mental status as a cause for placement or continued institutionalization in a long-term care facility (Guccione, Meenan, & Anderson, 1989).

Other musculoskeletal conditions affecting adults, such as gout, ankylosing spondylitis, systemic lupus erythematosus, and osteoporosis, are

Table 6.4. Need for Assistance in IADLs or ADLs Associated with Specific Arthropathies among Community-Dwelling Civilians in the United States by Age and Gender *(Three-Year Average, 1983 through 1985)*

		Age (years)	
Condition	All Ages	5–69	70+
Males and Females			
Rheumatoid arthritis			
Rate per 1,000 persons	0.8	0.5	3.5
% of all RA cases	13.4%	10.6%	27.0%
Osteoarthritis/other arthropathies			
Rate per 1,000 persons	4.1	1.7	34.4
% of all OA cases	3.3%	1.7%	7.2%
Males			
Rheumatoid arthritis			
Rate per 1,000 persons	0.3	0.2	1.6*
% of all RA cases	9.4%	7.2%	29.7%*
Osteoarthritis/other arthropathies			
Rate per 1,000 persons	1.6	0.8	13.3
% of all OA cases	1.7%	1.1%	3.4%
Females			
Rheumatoid arthritis			
Rate per 1,000 persons	1.2	0.8	4.7
% of all RA cases	14.9%	11.9%	26.5%
Osteoarthritis/other arthropathies			
Rate per 1,000 persons	6.5	2.5	47.9
% of all OA cases	4.2%	2.1%	8.9%

Source: Data from LaPlante, 1988.
*Figure has low statistical reliability or precision (relative standard error exceeds 30%).

not reported currently in the sources used for rheumatoid arthritis and osteoarthritis, but their presence should be noted in a national indicator system for tracking adults with chronic medical conditions. The prevalence of these conditions varies considerably depending on factors such as gender, age, ethnicity, and geographic location. One study, for example, found that more than 45 percent of Caucasian women over age fifty have osteoporosis (Melton et al., 1992), while other sources report that prevalence rates are significantly lower for African American women (Kelley et al., 1993).

Resource Use Attributable to Musculoskeletal Conditions

Because of the high prevalence of musculoskeletal conditions, the percentage of health care resources expended on these conditions is correspondingly large, particularly in outpatient settings. According to the National Ambulatory Medical Care Survey of 1985, more office visits were scheduled for treatment of musculoskeletal conditions than for any other anatomic or disease category. Musculoskeletal conditions were cited as the primary reason for 87.5 million office visits, constituting 13.8 percent of all physician office visits for 1985. Musculoskeletal conditions of all types, including fractures, dislocations, and other injuries, accounted for 12.8 percent of all hospitalizations in 1988. Within the category of musculoskeletal conditions, people in the eighteen to sixty-four age group are hospitalized most frequently for musculoskeletal diseases and connective tissue disorders. Fractures account for the largest proportion of hospitalizations for people over age sixty-five, and that proportion continues to increase with age. In 1988, more than three million surgical procedures were performed on musculoskeletal systems, 40 percent of which were reductions of fractures or arthroplasties (Praemer et al., 1992).

Estimates of total direct plus indirect expenditures on musculoskeletal conditions for 1988 amount to nearly $126 billion. Direct costs, including hospital charges, physician visits, pharmaceuticals, nursing home care, and other services, account for just over 48 percent of the total, while indirect costs caused by lost productivity resulting from morbidity and premature mortality make up the rest (Praemer et al., 1992).[4] Arthritis was the cause of 43 percent of total costs for musculoskeletal conditions ($54.6 million) in 1988. Of this amount, indirect costs resulting from lost productivity from morbidity accounted for 75 percent. Charges for nursing home care made up 46 percent of the $12.7 billion spent on direct costs for arthritis care; inpatient hospital care comprised an additional 20 percent of direct costs (Praemer et al., 1992).

TRANSITIONS THROUGH THE SERVICE CAREERS OF ADULTS WITH MUSCULOSKELETAL CONDITIONS

Because of the duration of chronic medical conditions, most persons with chronic disease pass through several stages in their health care service career, requiring different forms and degrees of health care and social services as the severity of the condition worsens. The purpose of a community-level indicator system for chronic disease is to estimate the number of residents and the accessibility of relevant services at each stage of the service career, so that appropriate resources can be made available as they are needed.

1. Adults at Risk	
Locale:	In community
Symptoms:	None
Diagnoses:	None
Disability:	None

2. Adults with Mild Symptoms	
Locale:	In community
Symptoms:	Mild
Diagnoses:	None
Disability:	None

3. Adults with Sustained Symptoms	
Locale:	In community
Symptoms:	Sustained
Diagnoses:	Possible, but not all
Disability:	None to mild

4. Adults with Severe Course of Disease	
Locale:	In community
Symptoms:	Sustained and severe
Diagnoses:	Established
Disability:	Mild to moderate

5. Adults with Severe Course, Significant Disability	
Locale:	In community
Symptoms:	Sustained and severe
Diagnoses:	Established
Disability:	Significant rehabilitation, community services

6. Adults Confined to Home and Bed	
Locale:	In community
Symptoms:	Sustained and severe
Diagnoses:	Established
Disability:	Significant

7. Adults Confined to Institutions	
Locale:	LTC facility
Symptoms:	Sustained and severe
Diagnoses:	Established
Disability:	Significant

Fig. 6.1.   Health Care Service Career For Adults with Chronic Medical Conditions. *Note:* LTC facility is long-term care facility.

Figure 6.1 traces a typical path through the health care service career of an adult with a chronic medical condition. For convenience, this service career has been characterized in seven distinct stages of disease severity and service use. The path begins with adults at risk of developing a particular chronic condition, proceeds to stages characterized by progressive disease symptoms without disability, advances to disease symptoms accompanied by progressive levels of disability, and culminates with such severe disease and disability that the individual is confined to a long-term care facility. For any particular chronic disease, most community residents can be expected to remain in stage 1 throughout their lives, meaning that they are at risk of developing the condition but may never do so. Every person who advances to stage 2 and beyond will have passed through each of the earlier stages; however, individuals will spend varying amounts of time in each stage, stabilizing at any particular level without necessarily passing through subsequent stages. Some people with certain chronic medical conditions may move relatively quickly into the stages involving disability.

In reality, most people probably straddle stages, but for heuristic reasons, the progression will be portrayed as though it proceeds through discrete steps. While most movement through the service career is from lower to higher stages, a significant number of persons also go from higher to lower levels at some points during their lives (Yelin & Katz, 1990). To simplify the presentation, only the forward movement is described below.

In many cases, people with one chronic medical condition have one or more comorbidities, which tend to accumulate with age. Multiple chronic conditions are likely to hasten the pace of transition through the service career described in Figure 6.1, having an impact on physical functioning, depression, and social connectedness. Multiple chronic conditions have an almost exponential impact on functioning and well-being, suggesting that the indicator system should be constructed with particular attention to this population (Berkanovic & Hurwicz, 1990; Verbrugge et al., 1990; Yelin, 1992; Yelin & Katz, 1990). In analyses controlling for comorbid conditions, age was found to have an insignificant impact on the likelihood of disability among persons with chronic disease; that is, the higher prevalence of disability among elderly persons is attributable to the accumulation of chronic medical conditions rather than to the intrinsic effect of aging (Verbrugge et al., 1990). However, female gender and nonwhite race were associated with higher levels of disability, even after controlling for comorbid medical conditions.

Figure 6.2 presents a summary of prevalence rates, useful indicators, and likely therapies for use at each stage of the health care service career of individuals with rheumatoid arthritis, osteoarthritis, or other arthropathies.[5] Each of these stages is described in some detail below and illustrated with a vignette intended to characterize likely life experiences for a person with or at risk of developing arthritis. Disability levels used for the NHIS were not developed with this transition framework in mind, but prevalence rates for activity limitation, work limitation, and limitation in IADLs and ADLs can be construed as roughly comparable to prevalence rates for persons in stages 3 through 5. One caveat, however,

1. Adults at Risk
Prevalence: Most people
Indicators: Risk factors such as age, gender, race
Therapy: None

2. Adults with Mild Symptoms
Prevalence: 131 per 1000 persons
Indicators: Prevalence estimates; financial and transit access to health care; peer support
Therapy: Mild analgesics; self-help course

3. Adults with Sustained Symptoms
Prevalence: 17.3 per 1000 persons
Indicators: Access to health care, social services, and assistive devices; satisfaction with care
Therapy: NSAIDs; palliative measures to relieve pain and joint inflammation

4. Adults with Severe Course of Disease
Prevalence: 8.7 per 1000 persons
Indicators: Extent of disability; depression level; satisfaction with support system; toxicity to medication; exacerbations of disease
Therapy: Palliative measures for relief of pain and joint inflammation; NSAIDs and DMARDs for RA; evaluation of comorbid conditions; social and psychological support

5. Adults with Severe Course, Significant Disability
Prevalence: 4.9 per 1000 persons
Indicators: Secondary health problems; access to and continuity of social services
Therapy: Palliative measures to relieve pain and joint inflammation; NSAIDs; DMARDs; possible joint replacement for RA; treatment of comorbid conditions; social and psychological support

6. Adults Confined to Home and Bed
Prevalence: 0.6 per 1000 persons
Indicators: Complications of disease or disability; adequacy of social support system; emergency and respite care
Therapy: Palliative measures for relief of pain and joint inflammation; treatment of comorbid conditions; social and psychological support; rehabilitation; community services

7. Adults Confined to Institutions
Prevalence: Unknown
Indicators: Comfort level; adequacy of health, psychological, and social services
Therapy: Palliative measures for relief of pain and joint inflammation; treatment of comorbid conditions; social and psychological support; rehabilitation; community services

Fig. 6.2. Prevalence, Indicators, and Therapy for Health Care Service Career of Adults with Rheumatoid Arthritis and Osteoarthritis and Other Arthropathies.
Note: NSAIDs are nonsteroidal antiinflammatory drugs; DMARDs are disease-modifying antirheumatic drugs; RA is rheumatoid arthritis.

is that the NHIS measures work limitation only for people aged eighteen to sixty-nine (LaPlante, 1988); consequently, the estimates offered for the number of people expected to pass through stage 4 are significantly lower than might be appropriate for any given community.

Both rheumatoid arthritis and osteoarthritis can take widely varying courses, so the treatment plan for any one individual must be adapted to the severity of the disease, the goals of that individual, and the environment in which the person resides and works. At all stages of the service career of a person with arthritis, the goals of therapy are to relieve pain and other symptoms, curb or suppress inflammation, delay or prevent joint destruction, avoid undesirable side effects of medications and other therapies, maintain function, and preserve quality of life (Schumacher, 1988). Health care resources are required to pursue these goals, but social services, psychological counseling, and other community services become increasingly necessary as a person passes through the more advanced stages of the service career. Most persons with chronic arthritis have health insurance plans to pay for health care services; payment for additional services is determined by the particular payment plan. Cost shifting between uninsured or publicly insured individuals and those with private health insurance is no more prevalent for arthritis than for other medical conditions.

The size and available resources of a local community are the most significant factors likely to affect the choices made regarding caring for adults with chronic arthritis within the community. Smaller communities may not be able to support the team of physical and occupational therapists and social workers essential to the provision of complete services, much less a rheumatologist or an orthopedic surgeon trained in joint replacement surgery. Physicians in such locales will need to foster alliances with providers in cities large enough to support these specialists, so that local persons with chronic arthritis can be referred to specialists as needed. Other factors likely to influence routine care of a person with arthritis stem more from individual practice patterns of the physician and practice incentives of the health care system than from specific features of the individual's case (Henke & Epstein, 1991).

STAGE 1: Adults at Risk for Some Form of Arthritis

Rita, a typical member of the group at stage 1 of the health care service career, is a healthy, forty-year-old woman, with a husband and two children. She holds a full-time job, plays tennis every Thursday with a friend, organizes active family outings on most weekends, and holds season tickets to the symphony.

All adults who do not acquire any form of arthritis as a child pass through stage 1 of the health care service career. Persons at this stage obviously require no health care resources for treating musculoskeletal conditions, but should have access to primary and preventive care considered standard for all adults. Most screening for arthritis among community adults at risk is unlikely to prove cost effective, because prevalence estimates for severe forms of musculoskeletal conditions are relatively low, and potential screening devices lack specificity.[6] Moreover, people with severe forms of arthritis who do need medical attention will almost certainly seek help because of the excruciating pain involved.

The indicator system at this stage needs to include little more than basic population statistics, which serve as risk factors that provide some estimate of the likelihood of developing certain chronic musculoskeletal conditions. The goal of the system in stage 1 is simply to anticipate likely changes in disease prevalence. The age and gender of the community population serve as appropriate risk factors or indicators to meet this goal, because the incidence of arthritis increases with advancing age, particularly among women. Additionally, persons who have held jobs requiring repetitive stressful movement and older obese women might be monitored for onset of osteoarthritis. Measurements of the accessibility of health care facilities and counts of general practitioners per capita might be used as indicators of access to health care for community residents at this stage.

STAGE 2: Adults with Mild Symptoms

At stage 2, Rita, who is now fifty, engages in many of the same activities as she did ten years ago; however, she needs to slow down occasionally to ease the pain and stiffness in her knees, which she first noticed a few years ago. Most of the time, Rita is not aware of the joint pain, but she takes aspirin and applies heat to ease the pain when it bothers her. She enjoys tennis only intermittently now, and family outings are a thing of the past, which doesn't concern her that much because the children are grown. Currently, Rita engages in volunteer work on weekends to help support the local symphony.

As reflected in Table 6.1, 131 out of 1000 persons in the community can be expected to acquire either rheumatoid arthritis, osteoarthritis, or other arthropathies at some point in their lives, moving from stage 1 into stage 2. Nearly 75 percent are likely to be over age forty-five, and roughly two-thirds will be women (LaPlante, 1988). In many cases, these conditions begin with relatively minor symptoms, requiring no treatment at all; if this is the case, the condition is unlikely to get a discrete diagnosis at this stage. About 15 percent of those with rheumatoid arthritis are likely to remain at this stage for the rest of their lives (Zvaifler, 1989); a much higher proportion of those with osteoarthritis are likely to stabilize at stage 2. Approximately 62 percent of people over age fifty-five with rheumatoid arthritis and 74 percent of people above age fifty-five with osteoarthritis also experience various comorbidities (Yelin, 1992). Therefore, roughly 95 per 1000 community residents face a higher probability of proceeding through subsequent stages and stabilizing at more advanced levels than the remaining 36 of 1000 persons who enter stage 2 with no additional comorbidities.

Beginning in stage 2 and proceeding through all other stages of the service career, most people with arthritis use medications to reduce pain and inflammation of the joints. Almost all persons with arthritis are started on aspirin, and those with rheumatoid arthritis are often prescribed other nonsteroidal antiinflammatory drugs (NSAIDs), such as ibuprofen, to treat symptoms. The choice of drug for a particular person is based on effectiveness, cost, and minimization of adverse reactions, particularly gastrointestinal problems. Simultaneous use of more than one NSAID generally is not recommended, because toxicity is increased while effectiveness is not (Schumacher, 1988). Many of these medications are available on a nonprescription basis, however, and some patients may be unwittingly subjecting themselves to toxic complications from use of multiple NSAIDs.

Other therapies recommended at this stage of arthritis include application of cold or heat, appropriate exercise, rest, and use of particular social services. For example, recent evidence strongly suggests that education about self-management techniques for people with chronic arthritis can result in significant health benefits and reduced health care costs (Lorig, Mazonson, & Halsted, 1993). These results correlated more strongly with an increased sense of self-efficacy in coping with the consequences of chronic arthritis, such as enhanced confidence in talking with the physician, than with use of exercise, application of heat, or other specific behaviors taught in the class. Four years after a self-management course, participants reported a 20 percent decrease in pain and a 40 percent reduction in physician visits, although physical disability resulting from arthritis had increased by 9 percent. Similar changes were not found among a control group of people with arthritis who received no special training.

Goals of the indicator system expand at stage 2 beyond those relevant for stage 1. Prevalence rates pertaining to those with arthritis only, as well as those with arthritis and other comorbidities, are appropriate indicators at this stage. Other indicators pertinent at stage 2 include measurements of financial and transit access to appropriate health care and social service providers, as well as availability of peer support.

STAGE 3: Adults with Sustained Symptoms

By age sixty, Rita has been diagnosed with osteoarthritis, a common condition among women of her age. She takes a mild NSAID regularly for relief of joint pain, which has become almost a daily occurrence. Rita will pass back and forth between stages 2 and 3 for the rest of her life, intermittently seeking counseling and peer support to deal with her depressive symptoms.

People who report activity limitations resulting from arthritis can be expected to pass through stage 3. Most people in stage 3 are likely to have been diagnosed with either rheumatoid arthritis or osteoarthritis. Approximately 17 persons per 1000 in the community are likely to spend time at this stage (Table 6.2), experiencing some activity limitations and requiring at least palliative measures to treat symptoms. Rheumatoid arthritis is a severe form of musculoskeletal condition, resulting in restrictions in many aspects of life. Activity restrictions typically experienced by people with rheumatoid arthritis include difficulties with household chores, shopping and errands, social relations, religious activities, leisure activities, transport, public service, and work. Osteoarthritis generally is a less severe, but more common, form of musculoskeletal condition; prevailing activity restrictions for people with this disease include some difficulties with work, household chores, shopping and errands, and leisure activities (Yelin et al., 1987).

All therapies begun in stage 2 are likely to continue as the person moves into stage 3, but the dosage or frequency of the therapies may be increased. Some people at this stage might find assistive devices helpful in maintaining their level of functioning. Canes or walkers might be used for support, while other aids are available to assist with personal hygiene, dressing, eating, and preparing food. Social and psychological services might become more important for some people at this stage, particularly those with rheumatoid arthritis who are concerned about deformities and other changes in appearance and self-image, as well as what the future might hold for them. Many persons with osteoarthritis do well simply with reassurance that they do not have a more serious form of arthritis (Schumacher, 1988).

Prevalence rates are pertinent indicators to be maintained at stage 3, but they could be enhanced with some record of the level of functioning among people at this stage and predictors of the proportion of people at stage 3 who are likely to advance even further through the service career. For example, instruments such as the Arthritis Impact Measurement Scales (AIMS) or the Stanford Health Assessment Questionnaire (HAQ) might be incorporated into the survey instrument to assess the functional status of persons with arthritis. In addition, joint counts and some version of the McGill Pain Questionnaire might be considered for assessing extent and severity of pain. Also relevant at stage 3 are measurements of appropriate access to health care; use of available social services such as psychotherapy, social work, or case management; activities with peers; access to assistive devices; and satisfaction with care.

STAGE 4: Adults with Severe Disease

Rita's friend, Emily, is in stage 4 of the service career. She is fifty years old and was diagnosed with rheumatoid arthritis six months ago. Disease onset was rapid, moving her abruptly through the first few stages of the service career. Upon diagnosis, Emily received NSAIDs to relieve her painful, swollen wrists and knees, and she has recently begun corticosteroid therapy in an attempt to relieve her joint pain. Recently, depression and concern about her future have been as much an obstacle for Emily as the joint pain itself.

Evidence of work limitation or other age-appropriate activity limitation attributable to arthritis may serve as an indicator that a community resident's arthritis has become sufficiently advanced to force that person to enter stage 4 of the service career. Close to 9 community residents per 1000 with arthritis (aged eighteen to sixty-nine) can anticipate passing through this stage (Table 6.3), necessitating considerably higher levels of health care and social service resources. Including adults over age sixty-nine in the count of persons at stage 4 is likely to increase significantly the ratio of persons per 1000 residents with severe arthritis. Proportionately, more residents with rheumatoid arthritis are likely to proceed as far as stage 4 than those with osteoarthritis or other arthropathies.

People with arthritis who progress to stage 4 are almost certain to have their disease diagnosed. At this point, the primary care physician might be advised to refer the patient to a rheumatologist, at least on a consultative basis, for assistance in determining the most appropriate therapies. This holds true particularly for people with rheumatoid arthritis. Because of the high frequency of comorbid conditions among persons with arthritis, screening for other common chronic conditions might also be included in the treatment strategy. In addition, some experts recommend that persons with rheumatoid arthritis be immunized for influenza and pneumonia at this stage of the service career (Arnold & Hochberg, 1989).

Along with continuation of NSAIDs, second-line therapies, also known as disease-modifying antirheumatic drugs (DMARDs), are likely to be prescribed for people with rheumatoid arthritis who advance to stage 4.[7] Most of these drugs have little immediate effect, but continued use for at least six to eight months may suppress or delay the disease process for most people. Complete suppression of the disease by use of DMARDs has been documented for a minority of people with rheumatoid arthritis (Schumacher, 1988). As with NSAIDs, the choice of the specific DMARD must be tailored to each individual, because of varying effectiveness and toxicity for different users. Use of any DMARD, however, must be closely monitored for potential toxicity. Most people are forced to discontinue use of a DMARD within three years, because of lack of effectiveness or toxicity. When this occurs, therapy with a second DMARD often is begun (Schumacher, 1988; Weinblatt & Maier, 1989).

There is little agreement among internists and rheumatologists about the optimal course of therapy with DMARDs. For example, some controlled, randomized clinical studies of both intramuscular and oral gold have demonstrated the efficacy of these treatments (Weinblatt & Maier, 1989), but results from a longer-term observational study suggested that the use of intramuscular gold therapy had no significant impact on functional status or number of painful joints for adults with rheumatoid arthritis (Pincus & Callahan, 1989). Similarly, while a number of studies report the effectiveness of methotrexate as a treatment for rheumatoid arthritis (Kremer & Lee, 1988; Weinblatt et al., 1988), others suggest that the drug does little to alter the course of the disease over the long term (Wolfe & Cathey, 1991). In sum, further investigation of appropriate medications for rheumatoid arthritis is warranted, both to benefit the individual and to conserve scarce health care resources.

Increased rates of fractures have been reported among women with rheumatoid arthritis who also have osteoporosis from use of prednisone and physical limitation from the effects of their disease (Michel, Bloch, &

Fries, 1991).[8] A bone fracture is likely to cause an individual to proceed from stage 4 to stage 5 (adults with severe course of disease and significant disability), at least on a temporary basis. Women taking 5 mg or more of prednisone for arthritis face a 34 percent probability of experiencing a fracture within a five-year span and may be advised to try to prevent fractures by taking calcium and estrogen and avoiding falls, as well as reducing or stopping the prednisone.

Relatively few community residents with osteoarthritis are likely to reach stage 4 of the service career. However, the high incidence of this condition compared with rheumatoid arthritis suggests that persons with osteoarthritis may comprise the majority of community residents at stage 4. DMARDs generally are not recommended for persons with osteoarthritis; NSAIDs may also be inappropriate, because osteoarthritis does not involve joint inflammation (Bradley et al., 1991). Some physicians, however, do prescribe relatively strong dosages of NSAIDs for persons in advanced stages of osteoarthritis (Schumacher, 1988). Close monitoring for toxic reactions should accompany higher doses of these treatments, particularly since some persons may be simultaneously taking over-the-counter NSAIDs. Application of heat or cold to stiff or painful joints and appropriate levels of exercise are often recommended for people with osteoarthritis who have advanced to this stage.

Assessing the social support system and the psychological status of people at stage 4 may be important to determine whether additional help is needed in these areas. Significant pain and stiffness, coupled with depression, can cause persons at this stage to withdraw rather than pursue contact with peers and friends who might be available to offer assistance and reassurance. Several studies have found prevalence rates of depression of 19–50 percent among persons with rheumatoid arthritis, and the condition tends to persist if not treated. Furthermore, people with similar levels of disease activity can display widely varying levels of physical functioning, suggesting that psychosocial factors play a significant role in influencing the ability to function (Lorish et al., 1991). One study determined that depression plays a more significant role than medical status in understanding a person's psychosocial functioning and adjustment to rheumatoid arthritis (Beckman et al., 1992). Another found that depression affects pain, but a reciprocal relationship was not supported (Parker et al., 1992). A subsequent longitudinal study confirmed that depression among persons with rheumatoid arthritis correlated significantly with earlier or concurrent functional decline and pain (Katz & Yelin, 1995).

Finally, the relationship between satisfaction with the available support system and psychosocial adjustment has been found to grow stronger among people with rheumatoid arthritis as the level of disability grows more severe, suggesting that satisfaction with the support system acts as a buffer for stress and other complications of the disease (Affleck et al., 1988).

The indicator system for people at stage 4 should expand the measurements used in stage 3 to include not only functional status and number of painful and stiff joints, but also extent of disability, depression level, individual satisfaction with the available support system, possible toxicity to medication, serious exacerbation of the disease, and secondary health complications, such as fractures. Instruments currently available for assessing emotional and social health status include the McMaster Health Index Questionnaire (MHIQ) and the Functional Status Questionnaire (FSQ). Indicators of access would be much like those used at stage 3: measurements of access to a primary care physician, a consulting rheumatologist, physical and occupational therapists, and social and psychological counselors, and provision of assistive devices as needed. Continuity of the support available should also be monitored as an indicator, because disruptions of support have been shown to cause significant levels of distress among people with arthritis (Affleck et al., 1988). The Medical Outcomes Study (MOS) Social Support Survey might be used to evaluate this construct (Sherbourne & Stewart, 1991).

STAGE 5: Adults with Severe Disease and Significant Disability

At age sixty-five, Emily has been receiving gold, corticosteroids, and methotrexate, but none of these drugs has prevented the significant disability she now experiences. Moreover, she has needed additional medication to treat the gastrointestinal complications resulting from the NSAIDs she continues to use. Emily's husband assists her with locomotion outside the home, does most of the cooking (because she is not able to handle the pots and pans), and helps her with eating and dressing when her arthritis flares.

People at stage 5 are not only likely to incur limitation in activities and work, but may also require assistance in ADLs and IADLs. Among people aged eighteen to sixty-five who report activity limitation plus all people who are over age sixty-nine, about five persons per thousand are expected to enter stage 5 at some point in their lives (Table 6.4). Slightly more than one-third of residents at stage 5 are likely to be over age sixty-nine.

Joint replacement surgery might be considered at this stage for people with either rheumatoid arthritis or osteoarthritis, principally to ease pain. Although restoration of motion and function may be achieved, these are secondary objectives of the surgery. Optimal results from joint surgery are most likely when surgery is scheduled as the joint becomes destroyed and the patient receives adequate physical therapy to increase strength before surgery. Delay in joint replacement surgery can reduce the chance of restoring near normal movement. People with arthritis who undergo surgery must be monitored closely for possible infections, which need aggressive treatment when discovered (Schumacher, 1988).

Risk factors for disability resulting from arthritis are similar to those arising from other conditions, increasing primarily with the number of comorbid conditions and secondarily from demographic factors, such as advanced age, lack of education, nonwhite race, and never-married status. Obesity is the one risk factor uniquely relevant to disability stemming from arthritis, having a significant impact on difficulty with walking and functional limitation, including the need for assistance with IADLs or ADLs as the disease worsens (Verbrugge, Gates, & Ike, 1991). A two-year follow-up study of people over age sixty-nine found that obese people with arthritis experience disability more frequently and at a faster pace than people whose weight is in the normal range. People with arthritis are more likely to recover the ability to walk and perform ADLs and IADLs, but are less likely to regain the ability to perform physical activities requiring strength, endurance, or dexterity (Verbrugge, 1992). A longitudinal study following people with rheumatoid arthritis for up to 12 years found that the median length of time from diagnosis to moderate disability is 11 years, while the median time to severe disability is 20.8 years. Predictors of the development of disability among people with rheumatoid arthritis include self-reported measures of global assessment, pain, and functioning (Wolfe & Cathey, 1991).

Because of the significant level of disability among persons at stage 5, social support and community services become at least as important on a day-to-day basis as health care services. Therefore, the indicator system for people at this stage should continue to monitor the measurements relevant at stage 4, with somewhat greater emphasis on indicators measuring access to and continuity of social services. Measurements of secondary physical complications resulting from the primary disability should also be added to the list of indicators. Because disability among persons with arthritis tends to flare and then remit, prevalence numbers of people at this stage are likely to be somewhat unstable (Reisine & Fifield, 1992).

STAGE 6: Adults Confined to Home and Bed

Emily, now age seventy, is confined to home almost all the time because of her rheumatoid arthritis. On bad days, she does not get out of bed. Although she is grateful for the care and assistance her husband gives her, she is lonely and depressed because she cannot get out and socialize as she did in the past. She feels as if all she can do is watch TV and read books and magazines.

Few community residents with rheumatoid arthritis and even fewer (if any) with osteoarthritis are likely to proceed as far through the service career as stage 6; however, the resource needs of these people are formidable (Badley & Tennant, 1993; Locker, 1983). Approximately 10 percent of persons diagnosed with rheumatoid arthritis will become so severely ill that confinement because of disability is inevitable (Zvaifler, 1989). Applying this percentage to the figures in Table 6.1, fewer than one person per thousand community residents is likely to be confined to home or an institution because of rheumatoid arthritis. No similar estimates are available for people with osteoarthritis or other arthropathies.

Early mortality has been associated with rheumatoid arthritis that has advanced to severe physical disability (Leigh & Fries, 1991); estimates of loss of life because of rheumatoid arthritis range from three to eighteen years (Symmons, 1988). Use of prednisone and never-married status were also found to predict early mortality. These results, however, should not be interpreted to mean that prednisone causes early death; rather, the relationship could mean that prednisone is prescribed primarily to persons with extremely severe disease. Nevertheless, further investigation of possible toxic effects resulting from prednisone therapy is warranted. Mobility and general health perception were also significant predictors of early mortality, even controlling for physical function (Kazis, Anderson, & Meenan, 1990). Bacterial infection and renal disease, often resulting from immunosuppression induced by drugs used to treat rheumatoid arthritis, were common causes of death in this population.

Persons with such severe disability from arthritis that they are confined to home or bed for lengthy periods of time tend to have unrelenting disease, so the prevalence numbers at stage 6 are unlikely to fluctuate much. The indicator system at this point in the service career should be modified to concentrate more significantly on exercise and physical and occupational therapy to reduce stress caused by disability. In addition, it should monitor the availability of transportation to social and community services, including adult day care centers. The possibility of rehabilitation also needs to be investigated for people at stage 6. Again, indicators should include prevalence of increasing difficulty with mobility and physical activity, psychological measures such as anxiety and depression, and social complications restricting interactions with family and friends, which are attributable to the disability or to the disease itself. Access measurements should be developed to assess the adequacy of social supports and respite and emergency resources for assisting the person with arthritis with routine functioning, as well as for offering support to their primary caregivers.

STAGE 7: Adults Confined to Long-Term Care Institutions

Within six months of her husband's death, Emily decides that she must resign herself to living in a nursing home, because she does not have much money and cannot expect her children to care for her for the rest of her life. She understands that Medicaid will help with the nursing home expenses, and her daughter lives close enough to the nursing home to visit fairly often. The arthritis pain is a constant companion, but she would gladly endure twice the pain if she could maintain herself in her own home.

Differences in the adequacy of one's social support system and socioeconomic status are probably the primary factors distinguishing persons with arthritis at stage 7 of the service career from those at stage 6 (Zedlewske & McBride, 1992). However, deterioration in physical functioning and ability to perform self-care also contribute significantly to nursing home placement (Vladek, 1989).

No estimates are available for the expected prevalence of institutionalization due to arthritis within a community. Using the 1985 National Nursing Home Survey, which represents approximately 300,000 nursing home residents in the United States, one study found that over 23 percent of nursing home residents experienced some form of arthritis (Guccione et al., 1989). Most of those surveyed, however, did not consider arthritis to be the major determinant of their need to be institutionalized. Although arthritis was not among the major contributors to placement in a long-term care institution, it was a major cause of institutionalization for 15 percent of all residents without dementia. Nursing home residents with arthritis tended to be older than those without the condition; controlling for age, they also tended to experience more pain, require more assistance in functioning, and use a wheelchair on a regular basis. Furthermore, few, if any, were considered likely to be reintegrated into the community.

Because most people at stage 7 will probably live out their lives in a long-term care institution, the indicator system should concentrate on assessing the comfort of the individual. Participation in social interactions and limited exercise should be emphasized. The possibility of rehabilitation, including total joint replacement, is appropriate for those with some prospect of reentering the community. Indicators of access should measure the adequacy of health, psychological, and social care in ways that are sensitive to the needs of the person with this extreme level of disability.

DEVELOPING A MONITORING SYSTEM

Given the importance of chronic medical conditions within the population and the amount of health care resources expended on treating them, development of a longitudinal indicator system regarding the status of persons affected by chronic medical conditions is warranted. The ultimate goal of this endeavor is to provide a means by which all levels of government, as well as public and private payers, can assess needs for improving the delivery of health care services to community residents at various stages of their service careers. Such a system will be particularly useful for national policy purposes.

Although the appropriate unit of analysis of an indicator system for chronic medical conditions is the local medical market, development of such a system is practical only on a national basis. Medical and technical expertise at the national level is required to build a useful needs assessment instrument for persons with different chronic conditions, to be maintained on an integrated, flexible database. The primary role of the local market will be to determine whether health care and social service resources are available to meet the needs of its residents. Development of a national system that can be stratified by basic demographic characteristics will allow most local communities to perform their own needs assessment by extrapolating national results to the demographics of their own locale at relatively low incremental cost. Local telephone directories and chambers of commerce can supply adequate information about the health care resources of the community.

The nature of chronic medical conditions requires longitudinal data to assess appropriately the impact of the disease and the effectiveness of pharmaceutical and rehabilitative therapies. Pincus & Callahan (1989) documented widely varying conclusions regarding therapy for rheumatoid arthritis, depending on the length of the analysis. For example, results from clinical trials, which rarely run for more than two years, tend to support the efficacy of NSAIDs and DMARDs for the treatment of rheumatoid arthritis, while longer-term analyses often call these results into question. This suggests that erroneous conclusions regarding potential therapy for chronic medical conditions might be reached if longitudinal results are extrapolated from cross-sectional databases. Another recent study relates the differences in conclusions regarding therapy for rheumatoid arthritis to the methodology used in the analysis (Edworthy et al., 1993). The authors argue that longitudinal pretreatment data are needed to understand the trend and pace of disease progression before the impact of a particular therapy can be assessed. Disease progress has been shown to mask up to one-third of a therapy's effect. Moreover, information regarding backward movement through the stages of the health care service career, or improvements in condition, would never have been discovered without the aid of longitudinal data collection and analyses.

Previously, very little was done to develop indicator systems focused on providing information relevant to adults with chronic medical conditions. Currently, cross-sectional data collected at the national level permit estimation of the prevalence of a number of chronic conditions and the levels of disability attributable to these conditions. The NHIS collects self-reported data on chronic medical conditions from community-based adults. The Longitudinal Study on Aging (LSOA), initiated in 1984 as a supplement to the NHIS, includes those over age fifty-five who reported some activity limitation, as well as all NHIS respondents over age seventy. These respondents have been surveyed every two years, and the data are integrated with Medicaid, Medicare, and vital statistics records. The National Health and Nutrition Examination Survey (NHANES) uses face-to-face interviews with respondents and includes medical examinations and x-rays, providing a useful complement to the NHIS because of the greater detail about medical conditions.

Other data collection efforts have focused on people with a particular chronic condition, following them periodically for a number of years, but these efforts typically are staged within fairly narrow geographic boundaries.[9] However, no satisfactory model exists currently that would permit a local community to assess easily the needs of its residents with chronic medical conditions and to monitor developments in the delivery of services over time.

One model that would permit estimation of relevant parameters through the health care service careers of persons with chronic disease calls for following every tenth cohort of the NHIS longitudinally for at least ten years. An appropriate survey instrument would first screen each respondent to determine which chronic medical conditions, if any, are present, and which stage of the service career is applicable; it would then proceed with a set of questions specific to the appropriate condition and stage. Finally, a panel of national experts for each chronic medical condition could be established to provide guidance in identifying types of health care and social services likely to be needed at each stage of the service career. Pursuing this endeavor as a supplement to the current cross-sectional NHIS would streamline the logistics of developing the survey instrument and the database.

In order to use an indicator system for chronic disease to perform a needs assessment at the local level, the national database must be constructed to allow for stratification based on basic demographic characteristics, such as age, gender, and race. These demographic features are already being collected in many communities, so little additional expense would be involved in extrapolating the national survey findings to fit these locales. A community with demographics that differ markedly from national averages might choose to expend more resources to extend the national system by placing greater emphasis on particular conditions affecting its residents. Retirement communities, for example, might want to enhance the survey instrument to concentrate more on conditions prevalent among the elderly, such as Alzheimer's disease, and the health care resources available to deal with these conditions. Communities with a particularly high prevalence of HIV infection might want to modify the national survey instrument to focus on this condition.

To ensure that community residents with chronic medical conditions have access to the care they need, local communities will have to evaluate the availability and accessibility of health care and social services within their area and the assistance in coordinating services needed by their residents. A comparison can then be made between the resources that already exist within a community and the resources determined at the national level to be required for adequate care. If local resources are insufficient, a community must decide whether those services can be made available locally or whether referrals must be made to specialists located in larger metropolitan areas.

Given the expense of developing and maintaining a comprehensive indicator system for adults with chronic medical conditions, a smaller-scale pilot study is warranted. Such a study might be developed in one large demonstration community, with the accuracy of data extrapolations tested later in one other large city and one smaller community. Using a large test city will determine whether the extrapolations are useful in a location that is likely to have all necessary resources available locally; using a smaller community permits an evaluation of the usefulness of the indicator system to a community that may have to refer some residents to experts outside the immediate area.

Extensive data collection would be required in the test communities to assess directly the needs of residents, to determine the availability of health care and social resources, and to ascertain whether residents in need have access to those resources. Results from the data collected directly could then be compared with results extrapolated from the demonstration community to determine appropriate additions or modifications that might be incorporated into the national indicator system. The pilot study might also be used to determine the data-collection interval that would provide sufficient sensitivity to changes in needs and health care resources without expending more money than necessary on the indicator system.

SUMMARY AND CONCLUSIONS

Chronic medical conditions are a growing phenomenon in the United States as the population ages, requiring a growing proportion of the health care budget. An indicator system of transitions in the stages of chronic disease and service supply could prove to be an effective tool for resource planning pertaining to health care services at both the national and local levels.

Use of health care and social support resources increases significantly as community residents with chronic arthritis progress to more advanced stages of their health care service careers. For any given chronic medical condition, most people will remain at risk or with mild disease symptoms (stages 1 or 2) for their entire lives. The principal health care resources needed by this group are encompassed within an adequate primary health care delivery system.

Residents progressing to stages 3 and 4 of the health care service career are likely to need the services of a primary care physician and a consulting specialist. From time to time, they might also require the services of physical or occupational therapists and psychological counselors. Residents in smaller communities may need to be referred to specialists in larger metropolitan areas to fulfill these needs. Medications used to treat a chronic condition at these stages often are quite potent and may require close monitoring for effectiveness and potential toxic reactions. This again raises the question of how to coordinate the roles of primary care and specialty care most effectively—a theme common among the other chronic conditions discussed in this book.

When the chronic medical condition causes significant disability (stages 5 and 6), rehabilitation services and assistance with personal care are likely to be needed, in addition to services provided in stages 3 and 4. Nursing home facilities may be needed for residents at stage 7 who lack access to necessary home care.

Development of a well-constructed national indicator system and database for chronic medical conditions is key to enhancing the ability of local communities to plan for adequate and efficient provision of health care services to the growing number of residents affected by these conditions. Local community involvement is required for extrapolating the national findings to the local level, as well as for assessing the adequacy of local resources for providing necessary health care services. Shared responsibility for development at the national level and use at the local level can enhance the feasibility of such a system. More important is that such a system might improve both the quality of care and the efficiency of health care services delivery to a significant proportion of the population.

Notes

1. Some sources use the term "musculoskeletal conditions" to refer to rheumatoid arthritis, osteoarthritis, and other arthropathies; others use the same term to include conditions such as gout, ankylosing spondylitis, and systemic lupus erythematosus, as well as rheumatoid arthritis and osteoarthritis. The latter definition is used in this chapter.

2. See appendix A for additional information on all NCHS data sets referred to in this chapter.

3. Prevalence rates for these conditions obtained from other sources may differ, depending on the criteria used to identify each condition.

4. These figures were computed by the human capital approach, meaning that

output and household services are valued at market rates, using 1988 dollars and a 4 percent discount rate. Because musculoskeletal conditions are most prominent among women and the elderly, many of whom may not have worked outside the home, these estimates of indirect costs are likely to be quite conservative.

5. Prevalence rates in Figure 6.2 were calculated by summing the rates for rheumatoid arthritis and osteoarthritis and other arthropathies presented in Tables 6.1 through 6.4.

6. For example, the presence of rheumatoid factor (RF) in the blood is an ineffective predictor of rheumatoid arthritis because 1–5 percent of all persons without rheumatoid arthritis are RF positive, while approximately 25 percent of those with confirmed cases of rheumatoid arthritis are RF negative (Schumacher, 1988; MacGregor & Silman, 1991).

7. DMARDs include antimalarial agents, methotrexate, gold compounds, sulfasalazine, penicillamine, azathioprine, cyclosporin A, and alkylating agents.

8. Prednisone is the most frequently prescribed corticosteroid for rheumatoid arthritis.

9. The panel database for rheumatoid arthritis at the University of California, San Francisco, provides an example of this type of data collection effort.

References

Affleck, G., Pfeiffer, C., Tennen, H., & Fifield, J. 1988. Social support and psychosocial adjustment to rheumatoid arthritis. *Arthritis Care and Research 1:* 71–77.

Arnold, C. M., & Hochberg, M. C. 1989. Development and implementation of an immunization program for patients with rheumatoid arthritis. *Arthritis Care and Research 2:* 162–64.

Badley, E. M., & Tennant, A. 1993. Impact of disablement due to rheumatic disorders in a British population: Estimates of severity and prevalence from the Calderdale Rheumatic Disablement Survey. *Annals of the Rheumatic Diseases 52:* 6–13.

Beckman, J. C., D'Amico, C. J., Rice, J. R., Jordan, J. S., & Divine, G. W. 1992. Depression and level of functioning in patients with rheumatoid arthritis. *Canadian Journal of Psychiatry 17:* 539–43.

Berkanovic E., & Hurwicz, M. 1990. Rheumatoid arthritis and comorbidity. *The Journal of Rheumatology 17:* 888–92.

Bradley, J. D., Brundt, K. D., Katz, B. P., Kalasinski, L. A., & Ryan, S. I. 1991. Comparison of an anti-inflammatory dose of ibuprofen, an analgesic dose of ibuprofen, and acetaminophen in the treatment of patients with osteoarthritis of the knees. *New England Journal of Medicine 325:* 87–91.

Buckelew, S. P., & Parker, J. C. 1989. Coping with arthritis pain. *Arthritis Care and Research 2:* 136–45.

Criswell, L. A., & Redfearn, W. J. 1994. Variation across rheumatologists in the use of prednisone and second-line agents for the treatment of rheumatoid arthritis. *Arthritis and Rheumatism 37:* 476–80.

Davis, G. C., Cortez, C., & Rubin, B. R. 1990. Pain management in the older adult with rheumatoid arthritis or osteoarthritis. *Arthritis Care and Research* 3: 127–31.

Edworthy, S. M., Bloch, D. A., Brant, R. F., & Fries, J. F. 1993. Detecting treatment effects in patients with rheumatoid arthritis: The advantage of longitudinal data. *Journal of Rheumatology* 20: 40–44.

Felts, W., & Yelin, E. 1989. The economic impact of the rheumatic diseases in the United States. *The Journal of Rheumatology* 16: 867–84.

Fifield, J., & Reisine, S. 1992. Characterizing the meaning of psychological distress in rheumatoid arthritis. *Arthritis Care and Research* 5: 184–91.

Guccione, A. A., Meenan, R. F., & Anderson, J. J. 1989. Arthritis in nursing home residents: A validation of its prevalence and examination of its impact on institutionalization and functional status. *Arthritis and Rheumatism* 32: 1546–53.

Henke, C. J., & Epstein, W. V. 1991. Practice variation in rheumatologists' encounters with their patients who have rheumatoid arthritis. *Medical Care* 29: 799–812.

Hoaglund, F. T., Shiba, R., Newberg, A. H., & Leung, K. Y. 1985. Diseases of the hip: A comparative study of Japanese, Oriental, and American white patients. *Journal of Bone and Joint Surgery* 67-A: 1380–83.

Katz, P. P., & Yelin, E. H. 1995. The development of depressive symptoms among women with rheumatoid arthritis. The role of function. *Arthritis and Rheumatism* 38: 49–56.

Kazis, L. E., Anderson, J. J., & Meenan, R. F. 1990. Health status as a predictor of mortality in rheumatoid arthritis: A five-year study. *Journal of Rheumatology* 17: 609–13.

Kelley, W. N., Harris, E. D., Jr., Ruddy, S., & Sledge, C. B. 1993. *Textbook of Rheumatology* (4th ed.). Vol. 2. Philadelphia, Pa.: W. B. Saunders.

Kremer, J. M., & Lee, J. K. 1988. A long-term prospective study of the use of methotrexate in rheumatoid arthritis: Update after a mean of 53 months. *Arthritis and Rheumatism* 31: 577–84.

LaPlante, M. P. 1988. *Data on Disability from the National Health Interview Survey, 1983–85,* an InfoUse Report. Washington, D.C.: U.S. National Institute on Disability and Rehabilitation.

Lee, P. R., & Estes, C. L. (eds.). 1990. *The Nation's Health* (3rd ed.). Boston: Jones and Bartlett Publishers.

Leigh, J. P., & Fries, J. F. 1991. Mortality predictors among 263 patients with rheumatoid arthritis. *Journal of Rheumatology* 18: 1307–12.

Locker, D. 1983. *Disability and Disadvantage: The Consequences of Chronic Illness.* New York: Tavistock Publications.

Lorig, K. R., Mazonson, P. D., & Halsted, R.H. 1993. Evidence suggesting that health education for self-management in patients with chronic arthritis has sustained health benefits while reducing health care costs. *Arthritis and Rheumatism* 16: 439–46.

Lorish, C. D., Abraham, N., Austin, J., Bradley, L. A., & Alarcon, G.S. 1991. Disease and psychosocial factors related to physical functioning in rheumatoid arthritis. *The Journal of Rheumatology* 18: 1150–57.

MacGregor, A. J., & Silman, A. J. 1991. Rheumatoid factors as predictors of rheumatoid arthritis. *The Journal of Rheumatology 18*: 1280–81.

Melton, L. J., III, Chrischilles, E. A., Cooper, C., Lane, A. W., & Riggs, B. L. 1992. Perspective: How many women have osteoporosis? *Journal of Bone and Mineral Research 7*: 1005–10.

Michel, B. A., Bloch, D. A., & Fries, J. F. 1991. Predictors of fractures in early rheumatoid arthritis. *The Journal of Rheumatology 18*: 804–8.

Parker, J. C., Smarr, K. L., Angelone, E. O., Mothersead, P. K., Lee, B. S., Walker, S. E., Bridges, A. J., & Caldwell, C. W. 1992. Psychological factors, immunologic activation, and disease activity in rheumatoid arthritis. *Arthritis Care and Research 5*: 196–201.

Pincus, T., & Callahan, L. F. 1989. Reassessment of twelve traditional paradigms concerning the diagnosis, prevalence, morbidity and mortality of rheumatoid arthritis. *Scandinavian Journal of Rheumatology*, suppl. 79: 67–95.

Praemer, A., Furner, S., & Rice, D. P. 1992. *Musculoskeletal Conditions in the United States*. Park Ridge, Ill.: American Academy of Orthopaedic Surgeons.

Reisine, S., & Fifield, J. 1992. Expanding the definition of disability: Implications for planning, policy, and research. *The Milbank Quarterly 70*: 491–508.

Schumacher, H. R., Jr. (ed.). 1988. *Primer on the Rheumatic Diseases* (9th ed.). Atlanta, Ga.: Arthritis Foundation.

Sherbourne, D. C., & Stewart, A. L. 1991. The MOS Social Support Survey. *Social Science and Medicine 32*: 705–14.

Solomon, L., Breighton, P., & Lawrence, J. S. 1975. Rheumatic disorders in the South African Negro. II: Osteoarthritis. *South African Medical Journal 49*: 1737–40.

Symmons, D. P. M. 1988. Mortality in rheumatoid arthritis. *British Journal of Rheumatology 27 (Suppl I)*: 44–54.

Tack, B. B. 1990. Fatigue in rheumatoid arthritis. *Arthritis Care and Research 3*: 65–70.

Verbrugge, L. M. 1992. Disability transitions for older persons with arthritis. *Journal of Aging and Health 4*: 212–43.

Verbrugge, L. M., Gates, D. M., & Ike, R. W. 1991. Risk factors for disability among U.S. adults with arthritis. *Journal of Clinical Epidemiology 44*: 167–82.

Verbrugge, L. M, Lepkowski, J. M., & Imanaka, Y. 1990. Comorbidity and its impact on disability. *The Milbank Quarterly 67*: 450–84.

Vladek, B. 1989. Long-term care for the elderly: The future of nursing homes. *The Western Journal of Medicine 150*: 215–20.

Weinblatt, M. E., & Maier, A. L. 1989. Treatment of rheumatoid arthritis. *Arthritis Care and Research 2*: S23–S32.

Weinblatt, M. E., Trentham, D. E., Fraser, P. A., Holdsworth, D. E., Falchuk, K. R., Weissman, B. N., & Coblyn, J. S. 1988. Long-term prospective trial of low-dose methotrexate in rheumatoid arthritis. *Arthritis and Rheumatism 31*: 167–75.

Wolfe, F., & Cathey, M. A. 1991. Analysis of methotrexate treatment effect in a longitudinal observational study: Utility of cluster analysis. *The Journal of Rheumatology 18:* 672–77.

Yelin, E. 1992. Arthritis: The cumulative impact of a common chronic condition. *Arthritis and Rheumatism 15:* 489–97.

Yelin, E., Bernhard, G., & Pflugrad, D. 1995. Access to medical care among persons with musculoskeletal conditions. A study using a random sample of households in San Mateo County, California. *Arthritis and Rheumatism 38:* 1128–33.

Yelin, E. H., & Katz, P. P. 1990. Transitions in health status among community-dwelling elderly people with arthritis. *Arthritis and Rheumatism 33:* 1205–15.

Yelin, E., Lubeck, D., Holman, H., & Epstein, W. 1987. The impact of rheumatoid arthritis and osteoarthritis: The activities of patients with rheumatoid arthritis and osteoarthritis compared to controls. *The Journal of Rheumatology 14:* 710–17.

Zedlewske, S. R., & McBride, T. D. 1992. The changing profile of the elderly: Effects on future long-term care needs and financing. *The Milbank Quarterly 70:* 247–75.

Zvaifler, N. J. 1989. An introduction to rheumatoid arthritis. *Arthritis Care and Research 2:* S17–S22.

7/ CHRONIC ILLNESS AMONG ELDERLY PEOPLE

Jay S. Luxenberg and Robert J. Newcomer

The characterization of health status among older adults and the subsequent tracking of this status into programs of prevention, treatment, and rehabilitation are complex. Part of the complexity occurs because the frequency of degenerative diseases affecting health status increases with age. Physiological and anatomic changes related to aging (e.g., increased susceptibility to heat and cold exposure, decreased immune responses to infection, falls, toxicity from medications) also place older adults at increased risk of worsening health and premature death (Minaker & Rowe, 1985). As of 1991, eight of the ten leading causes of death among persons aged sixty-five and older were related to chronic diseases, including diseases of the heart, malignant neoplasm, cerebrovascular disease, arteriosclerosis, diabetes, emphysema, and nephritis (National Center for Health Statistics, 1993). Paralleling the importance of chronic illness in mortality is its general prevalence as a cause of morbidity. Approximately 80 percent of persons aged sixty-five and older have at least one chronic disease. Chronic disease prevalence increases with age. Among people aged eighty and older, 70 percent of the women and 53 percent of the men have two or more chronic conditions. Comorbidity, or the concurrent presence of more than one chronic condition, adds to the complexity of consequences arising from chronic illness. In one recent U.S. national study, 49 percent of noninstitutionalized people aged sixty and older had two or more of nine chronic conditions surveyed, 23 percent had three or more, and 8 percent had four or more (Guralnik et al., 1989). Table 7.1 shows the most prevalent chronic conditions and how their rates vary by age and gender and by age and race.

Chronic conditions often result in the development of similar forms of disability. For example, 38.8 percent of community-dwelling people aged

Table 7.1. Top Ten Chronic Conditions, United States, 1992 *(Number of Chronic Conditions per 1,000 Persons)*

A. By Age and Gender

Condition	All Elderly	Male		Female	
		Age 65–74	Age 75+	Age 65–74	Age 75+
Arthritis	481.9	364.8	417.2	508.7	611.2
High blood pressure	357.6	341.4	314.7	377.7	374.3
Heart disease	324.6	334.7	408.5	220.6	401.2
Hearing impairment	320.4	322.3	452.7	204.3	392.9
Deformity/ortho impairment	185.7	154.9	185.8	167.1	243.0
Cataracts	166.0	112.5	193.2	137.1	245.2
Chronic sinusitis	158.7	123.9	120.2	185.4	183.6
Diabetes	110.4	119.6	—	109.2	110.2
Tinnitus	89.4	95.5	113.7	—	—
Visual impairment	87.0	96.6	131.9	—	99.4
Hay fever/allergic rhinitis	—	—	—	103.0	—
Cerebrovascular disease	—	—	97.7	—	—
Varicose veins, lower extremities	—	—	—	84.4	101.0
Chronic bronchitis	—	—	—	—	—

B. By Age and Race

Condition	All Elderly	White		Black	
		Age 65–74	Age 75+	Age 65–74	Age 75+
Arthritis	481.9	447.8	544.4	431.9	519.4
High blood pressure	357.6	343.8	351.7	572.4	351.7
Heart disease	324.6	276.9	423.0	271.9	252.6
Hearing impairment	320.4	271.8	423.5	152.7	377.3
Deformity/ortho impairment	185.7	165.7	214.7	141.7	236.2
Cataracts	166.0	131.8	219.0	95.5*	254.6
Chronic sinusitis	158.7	161.1	167.3	149.0	—
Diabetes	110.4	104.4	99.2	223.2	158.5*
Tinnitus	89.4	90.4	100.0	—	—
Visual impairment	87.0	—	111.4	—	—
Hay fever/allergic rhinitis	—	83.9	—	91.2*	—
Cerebrovascular disease	—	—	—	112.5	132.9*
Frequent constipation	—	—	—	—	141.1*
Glaucoma	—	—	—	—	106.3*

Source: Data from Benson & Marano, 1994, Tables 57–59, pp. 83–88.
Note: Dash indicates that condition was not among the top ten chronic conditions.
*Estimates for which the numerator has a relative standard error of more than 30%.

sixty-five and over report limitations in their activities because of various chronic conditions, and 10.6 percent are unable to perform a major activity (NCHS, 1994); 16 percent report difficulty walking, with the percentage increasing from 13 percent of those aged sixty-five to seventy-four to 32 percent of those aged seventy-five and older (Havlik, Liu, & Kovar, 1987).

Functional disability rather than specific chronic conditions is commonly used to identify those aged persons assumed to be at high risk for long-term care services. This perspective, however, is essentially reactive and custodial in its approach to quantifying the population in need of services and ignores the potential benefits of preventive intervention with the conditions that produce disability. Kane and Boult (1997), modifying an Institute of Medicine (1991) model of disability, provide a more expansive progression from pathology to service demand. A similar perspective is used in this chapter as a framework for monitoring community responses to the needs of the older population.

Pathological $\rightarrow$ Organ $\rightarrow$ Functional $\rightarrow$ Disability $\rightarrow$ Need $\rightarrow$ Demand
  Lesion   Impairment   Limitation

SELECTED CHRONIC DISEASES AND THEIR TREATMENT

For purposes of this chapter, conditions with differing natural histories and service requirements were selected for discussion. In essence, these conditions are markers for how well the delivery system is operating in the screening, identification, treatment, and management of high-risk conditions. Conditions considered for selection as markers come from those with a combination of high prevalence and high risk of either mortality or activity restriction.

As seen from Table 7.2, heart (or cardiovascular) diseases are the most common cause of death in persons over age sixty-five. Most of these deaths are due to coronary artery disease, congestive heart failure, or stroke. Hypertension, although not a major direct cause of death, is a major risk factor for the outcomes of congestive heart failure and stroke. These outcome conditions have well-defined natural histories and established treatment and are relatively easy to monitor in terms of hospitalization rates, mortality, and functional impairment (Schocken et al., 1992). Hypertension is typically asymptomatic, which raises issues of screening and outreach. The performance of the delivery system in identifying and managing hypertension is thus a useful "indicator of system

Table 7.2. Ten Leading Causes of Death by Age, Gender, and Race, United States, 1991 *(Rates per 100,000 Persons)*

Condition	All Elderly	Male Age 65+	Female Age 65+	White Age 65+	Black Age 65+
Heart disease	4,924.0	2,131.3	1,712.0	1,884.2	2,068.2
Cancer	1,117.3	1,469.3	879.7	1,106.5	1,350.7
Cerebrovascular diseases	394.1	366.6	412.7	388.2	484.6
Chronic obstructive pulmonary diseases	240.6	334.7	177.2	251.4	150.8
Pneumonia/influenza	217.2	240.1	201.7	220.2	196.9
Diabetes	115.0	114.1	115.7	106.8	213.7
Accidents	83.3	102.9	70.0	82.9	92.5
Nephritis	56.6	65.7	50.4	52.6	105.5
Atherosclerosis	52.2	47.5	55.3	53.5	—
Septicemia	50. 0	50.4	49.8	46.8	91.2
Hypertension	—	—	—	—	59.7

Source: Data from National Center for Health Statistics, 1993, Table 6, pp. 22–26.
Note: Dash indicates that condition was not among the ten leading causes of death.

functioning" for all cardiovascular diseases. Another advantage of hypertension as a marker condition for the elderly patient is that the benefit of treatment, even for persons in their eighties, has been confirmed repeatedly by large and well-designed clinical trials (Reeves et al., 1993).

Stroke, one of the potential secondary consequences of uncontrolled hypertension, frequently results in permanent functional impairment and concurrent need for higher levels of care. Poststroke cases yield a useful population for tracking the performance of the health care system throughout a continuum of care needs, including rehabilitation, nursing home placement, home health care, and hospital discharge without further treatment. In many cases, functional outcomes can be improved with appropriate rehabilitation service.

Diabetes, a third condition selected as a marker, also begins frequently with an asymptomatic state—again raising concern about screening. It too has a well-defined natural history with a high frequency of marker adverse end-points: blindness, amputation, renal failure, neuropathy, and accelerated coronary artery disease. Screening techniques and medical treatment options for diabetes are relatively well accepted and standardized.

The final marker condition to be discussed is cognitive impairment due to dementing illness. This condition differs from the preceding ones in that it is not a major cause of death, is not currently recognized as having an asymptomatic state, and has only limited and relatively weak options available for treatment. The clinical course of dementia is much more predictable and steadily progressive than the above conditions. Issues of screening revolve around service needs rather than treatment of an asymptomatic state. Currently, the needs of dementia patients are primarily social rather than medical, and therefore reflect a set of systems different from those of the aforementioned medical conditions.

Hypertension

The standards of defining hypertension and of its treatment and management are regularly updated by the Joint National Committee on the Detection, Evaluation, and Treatment of High Blood Pressure (JNCV) (1993). Although there are many drug therapy and nonpharmacologic options for treating hypertension (Harper & Forker, 1992), national treatment standards are sufficiently accepted to allow fairly easy monitoring of treatment adequacy. Blood pressure is a quantitative measurement well suited for surveillance of screening efficiency and treatment efficacy. The effective and well-tolerated pharmacological agents for hypertension potentially allow treatment to be monitored by drug prescriptions (Applegate & Rutan, 1992).

The availability and efficacy of screening programs for elderly persons can be quantified and monitored by comparing incidence figures for a community with normative rates for hypertension matched for age, race, and gender. The end-points of stroke incidence and other complications of hypertension allow a measure of hypertension control in a population (MacMahon, Cutler, & Stamler, 1989). In a multicenter cooperative project, the WHO-WHL Hypertension Management Audit Project assessed the quality of hypertension control in eighteen European population groups (Strasser & Wilhelmsen, 1992; Wilhelmsen & Strasser, 1993). Five approaches were taken: epidemiological survey, clinical evaluation of samples of patient records, assessment of patient satisfaction, exploration of physicians' attitudes and knowledge, and drug use studies.

Hypertension incidence and prevalence in the United States are well documented on a national basis, most accessibly in the fifth report of the JNCV (1993). Analysis of hypertension by race is found in the Hispanic Health and Nutrition Examination Survey and the National Health and Nutrition Examination Surveys (NHANES)[1] (Espino, Burge, & Moreno, 1991; Espino & Maldonado, 1990; Geronimus, Neidert, & Bound, 1990). The NHANES also allows analysis by education and income. Al-

Table 7.3. Hypertension by Age, Gender, and Race, United States, 1992 *(Number per 1,000 Persons)*

Age	Male	Female	White	Black
65–74 years	341.4	377.7	343.8	572.4
75 + years	314.7	374.3	351.7	351.7

Source: Data from Benson & Marano, 1994, Tables 58 and 59, pp. 85–88.

Table 7.4. Cerebrovascular Disease by Age, Gender, and Race, United States, 1992 *(Number per 1,000 Persons)*

Age	All Elderly	Male	Female	White	Black
65–74 years	65.4	84.6	49.7	61.9	112.5
75 + years	88.0	97.7	82.2	85.5	132.9*

Source: Data from Benson & Marano, 1994, Tables 57, 58, and 59, pp. 83–88.
*Estimate for which the numerator has a relative standard error of more than 30%.

though underreporting and lower detection of hypertension have been described in rural populations, compared with urban and suburban populations, this is less important for elderly persons than for those who are younger (Doyle, et al., 1991). Table 7.3 shows prevalence rates of hypertension by age and gender and by age and race.

Area, health plan, or provider differences may exist between the *ideal* treatment program for hypertension and the *typical* treatment of hypertension in the elderly. Given the excellent treatment data from controlled trials that included very elderly or frail patients, the percentage of elderly hypertensives with justifiable reasons to deviate from standard treatment is very small. The most common contraindications for aggressive treatment of asymptomatic hypertension are side effects that impair quality of life. This is particularly likely in the case of the frail elderly patient with a limited predicted remaining life span. In such situations, the physician may elect a course of limited or no treatment.

Stroke

Stroke mortality rates can be calculated using data from the NCHS and the Bureau of the Census[2] (Casper et al., 1992). Such data are stratified by race, gender, age, metropolitan status, and region of the country. Recent national data on stroke mortality were published in the *Morbidity and Mortality Weekly Report (MMWR)* (1992). Table 7.4 shows preva-

Table 7.5. Diabetes by Age, Gender, and Race, United States, 1992 *(Number per 1,000 Persons)*

Age	Male	Female	White	Black
65–74 years	199.6	109.2	104.4	223.2
75+ years	96.8	110.2	99.2	158.5*

Source: Data from Benson & Marano, 1994, Tables 58 and 59, pp. 85–88.
*Estimate for which the numerator has a relative standard error of more than 30%.

lence rates for cerebrovascular disease (of which the major portion is stroke) by age, gender, and race. Racial differences in stroke mortality have been shown to be moderated by the occupational structure of the community (Casper, Wing, & Strogatz, 1991). Other possible data sources for hospitalizations and Medicare-reimbursed service use related to stoke are discussed below.

Diabetes

Diabetes incidence and complications have been investigated in many studies (e.g., Harris, 1990; Young, Roos, & Hammerstrand, 1991), including a population-based sample of elderly persons (Cohen et al., 1991; Klein & Klein, 1990). U.S. national data with racial and gender stratification are published regularly (Centers for Disease Control, 1990). These data sources provide one basis for needs estimations. A potentially more precise estimate can be derived from the diabetes surveillance system, which uses data from vital records, the National Health Interview Survey, the National Hospital Discharge Survey, and the U.S. Health Care Financing Administration's (HCFA) records.[3] These data provide trend information about the prevalence and incidence of diabetes, diabetes mortality, hospitalizations, and diabetic complications (Wetterhall et al., 1992). Table 7.5 shows diabetes prevalence by race, age, and gender stratification.

One approach to monitoring diabetes in elderly diabetics is through serum or blood glucose control over a period of weeks to months. Serum fructosamine and glycohemoglobin are readily available and reasonably priced markers of glucose control, which allow quantitative comparative measurements between populations over time. Another potentially useful feature of diabetes monitoring is that (point-in-time) glucose measurements can be made by nursing staff or the patients themselves either in the home or in institutions, again allowing quantification of diabetic control.

Age-related changes in the body's glucose handling complicate the definition of diabetes. Thus, while diabetes standards are relatively well accepted for persons in their sixties and seventies, there is less consensus about the very elderly (Froom, 1990). Many persons in the community are unaware of their diabetes, as are their physicians.

Changes in medical knowledge and practice strongly influence the "management" and intensity of monitoring of care. The recent trend toward aggressive management of serum glucose in elderly patients is influenced by scientific studies showing benefit from "tight" control of blood sugar. The frequency of monitoring serum glucose and other markers of long-term control (such as glycosylated hemoglobin) is a function of how tightly the physician is attempting to control the blood sugars. The aggressiveness of management is also affected by the patient's general health and the physician's estimation of the patient's life expectancy. Clinical practice guidelines for treatment of diabetes mellitus have been published by the Expert Committee of the Canadian Diabetes Advisory Board (1992) and the American Diabetes Association (1992). A National Institutes of Health (NIH) consensus conference offers guidelines for dietary and exercise treatment of diabetes (1987). Prescribing practices can be monitored through physician surveys or chart reviews, and patient compliance can be monitored through household surveys.

After screening or initial detection of elevated blood sugar, a common trajectory begins with an evaluation for reversible causes of diabetes, such as hypercortisolism. Following the diagnostic evaluation, patients require education and training to allow them to manage their chronic illness. Patients are often taught to monitor their own blood sugar at home, although this proves impractical for many frail elderly patients. Diabetes is often managed initially with a program of weight loss and exercise. If pharmacological therapy is needed, the physician can choose oral hypoglycemic agents or insulin therapy. Several factors influence this important choice, and patient characteristics are a major one. Some patients are absolutely deficient in insulin production and can only be successfully managed with insulin therapy.

Ideally, the diabetic's clinical trajectory would be one of excellent blood sugar control, consistently approximating normal blood sugar levels. Patients would monitor their blood sugar frequently, and physicians and other health care providers would monitor for any signs of end-organ damage, such as retinopathy, accelerated atherosclerosis, peripheral vascular disease, or kidney disease. Patients would receive regular ophthalmological and podiatric care. No adverse consequences would occur. The patient would remain at home and would have no functional impairment attributable to the diabetes and no excess mortality associated with the disease.

In practice, not all patients follow this ideal trajectory. Some will have periods of poor glycemic control, often associated with intercurrent illness such as infections and periods of dangerously low blood sugar. Others will suffer permanent brain damage or seizures from hypoglycemia. Some patients will develop end-organ damage and become blind, have amputations, or require dialysis. Others will no longer be able to manage their diabetes independently, usually because of functional impairments such as blindness and dementia. Such patients may be able to stay at home with the help of home attendants, visiting nurses, and family caregivers. Others will require elements of the full spectrum of assisted living, and some will have so much impairment that they will require nursing homes. More diabetics will die of myocardial infarctions and strokes than will nondiabetics. Tabulations of the incidence of these outcomes, adjusted for the number of persons "at risk," would be a direct means of assessing treatment effectiveness.

Dementia

Dementia incidence and prevalence estimation depend on the screening techniques used, which is especially true in efforts to distinguish mild dementia from age-associated cognitive changes. Severe, and therefore more functionally impairing, dementia is much less affected by measurement error and interpretational ambiguity. Determining the etiology of the dementia further complicates incidence and prevalence rates for specific causes such as Alzheimer's disease or multiinfarctions. Many studies suggest that patients with multiinfarction dementia do not survive as long as those with Alzheimer's disease; therefore, the proportion of Alzheimer's disease should be higher in prevalence data.

No national estimates exist for dementia, unlike the other conditions discussed. Instead, incidence and prevalence have been estimated from community- or catchment-level population studies. These estimates vary widely. On the low end are prevalence estimates of about 9 persons per 1000 among those aged sixty-five to sixty-nine and 164 among those above age eighty-five (Kokmen, et al. 1989; Letenneur et al., 1993). High-end estimates can be much higher. For example, prevalence of all-cause dementia for an eight-year follow-up in the Bronx, New York, was 228 per 1000 persons aged seventy-five and older (239 among those above eighty-five) (Aronson et al., 1991). A prevalence estimate for Alzheimer's disease in the U.S. population shows even higher rates: 113 per 1000 persons aged sixty-five and over, 476 per 1000 persons over age eighty-five (Evans et al., 1990). Data on prevalence exist for several other well-defined communities (Bachman et al., 1993; EURODEM Incidence Conferences, 1992; Fratiglioni et al., 1991). Table 7.6 shows a sampling of prevalence and incidence estimates, some of which are stratified by age and gender.

At this time, no early medical treatment is likely to alter the long-term outcome of the common dementing illnesses; therefore, issues of screening become less important as a preventive strategy (Canadian Task Force on the Periodic Health Examination, 1991). Case finding for dementia patients essentially means identifying persons in the community or in institutions who could benefit from social services. The natural history of Alzheimer's disease, by far the most common dementia, is one of inexorable progression, requiring increasing levels of supportive care for patients and caregivers. A common care trajectory involves an initial diagnosis, with a diagnostic evaluation to rule out alternative, potentially treatable causes of dementia; referral into supportive care systems; and continuation of routine primary care for other medical conditions. Although there is no uniform agreement on the criteria used in selecting patients for evaluation and the extent of such a workup (e.g., the need for neuroimaging), the basic components of care are fairly standardized and well accepted (Arnold & Kumar, 1993).

Usual care of the dementia patient involves patient and family counseling and education concerning the financial, social, and prognostic implications of the diagnosis of dementia. Ideally, this is followed up with regular monitoring of the patient's needs concerning personal assistance, attendant care, supervision, and alternative living situations. As the disease progresses, the average patient will need supervision of activities by family members or an attendant. Adult day health care and scheduled respite care are options appropriate for some patients. Financial oversight also becomes necessary.[4] The disease may progress to require full-time (twenty-four-hour) supervision, at which point a variety of factors, including finances and availability of caregivers, will determine whether this can be provided in the home. Alternatively, the family may elect an option from the full spectrum of assisted living, from residential care to

Table 7.6. Prevalence and Incidence Estimates for Dementia and Alzheimer's Disease

A. Five-Year Kaplan-Meier Incidence Rates of Dementia and Alzheimer's Disease by Age and Gender, The Framingham Study (Rates per 1,000)

Age Group	Total	Men	Women
Total All Forms of Dementia			
65–69	7.0	9.5	5.6
70–74	26.6	28.2	25.8
75–79	51.6	56.8	49.0
80–84	80.9	57.9	92.7
85–89	118.0	175.0	100.3
Alzheimer's Disease Only			
65–69	3.5	5.0	2.7
70–74	15.7	14.1	16.8
75–79	30.0	21.8	34.0
80–84	53.5	40.9	59.9
85–89	72.8	83.3	69.3

B. Estimates of Alzheimer's Disease Prevalence for the U.S. Population in 1980 Established Population for Epidemiologic Studies of the Elderly (EPESE) Study

Age	Absolute No. (in Millions)	Rate per 1,000
65+ years	2.88	113.0
65–74 years	0.61	39.0
75–84 years	1.25	164.0
85+ years	1.02	475.5

Source: Data for part A are from Bachman et al., 1993, pp. 515–519. Data for part B are from Evans et al., 1990, pp. 267–289.

custodial care to skilled nursing homes (Campbell et al., 1983). Special Alzheimer's disease or dementia units are an option in many communities (Berg et al., 1991).

In dementia, an additional service spectrum is needed, support for caregivers, who provide most personal care to dementia patients (Eisdorfer, 1991). Unrelieved caregiver stress may accelerate the need for placing the patient out of the home and can even lead to abuse of the dementia patient.

As the dementia progresses, the natural history of the disease includes impairment in eating ability, with need for feeding assistance. "Tube" feeding is necessary if the impairment becomes severe enough. The advent of eating impairment is associated with the risk of progressive weight loss and malnutrition, which in turn increase the risk of pressure sores, contractures, immune system impairment, infection, and death. Terminal care can be provided in the home environment, if sufficient help is available, or in nursing homes. Use of all aspects of this complicated disease trajectory can be monitored by prevalence rates within various service system sectors and by the incidence of secondary conditions resulting in hospitalization or use of skilled home health care.

FACTORS AFFECTING USE OF SERVICES

Regardless of the specific cause for disability or acute care risk, frail elderly patients usually need a variety of ancillary services, such as transportation, financial supervision and management, housing and home modification, chore work (e.g., home maintenance, heavy cleaning), adult day care, in-home and other forms of respite care, and case management services. The availability of ancillary assistance influences the trajectory of care for chronic illness and can often help determine whether a frail patient can remain in the home. The availability of these services differs from state to state and even from community to community.

During episodes of acute illness, severely ill patients can be cared for in the home if enough skilled care (such as home health nursing, physical therapy, occupational therapy, and even physician visits) is available. This is also true among persons living in residential care and nursing homes. For example, a nursing home patient who has a stroke or myocardial infarction may not require transfer to an acute care hospital, depending on the availability of medical visits, ECGs, and x-rays in the nursing home.

The choices and preferences of patients and their families can also influence the type and site of care. Younger patients, those with spouses, and those with higher incomes are more likely to receive care in their homes than in long-term care institutions (Braun, Rose, & Finch, 1991). The frequency of physician use and voluntary use of hospital services is directly related to income (and/or insurance coverage) (Branch et al., 1981), even controlling for health status. While financial ability is a critical element in ensuring choice, access can also be affected by travel distance (or time), waiting times for appointments, and the priorities given to those with greater needs. Particular problems in providing adequate home and attendant care are experienced in rural areas, because of travel distance and the associated costs.

Racial and cultural differences can also be seen in the use of health care and long-term institutional services. With other factors constant, minorities tend to use fewer services. This may be a result of multiple factors, including cultural preferences, financial ability, the availability of nearby children (particularly daughters), and discrimination.

Pharmacotherapy is a particularly important aspect of the treatment and management of the marker conditions given focus in this paper. For conditions such as hypertension, the recommendations of national committees (e.g., JNCV, 1993) can influence the choice of drugs. Such standardization suggests that drug therapy is one indicator of the appropriateness of care. However, many factors influence the choice of pharmacotherapy. Cost, convenience, side effects, and the presence of relative contraindications (such as coexistent disease) are among the most obvious factors. More subtly, the availability of supervision may influence whether a once-a-day drug is used instead of a less expensive three-times-a-day drug, or cultural factors may influence the willingness to use alternative administration vehicles, such as patches or inhalers. Physician experience with a particular drug or category of drugs is another important influence, but experience may be affected by marketing. Lastly, closed drug formularies within health plans, Medicaid, and other insurance programs may limit the choice of drugs available.

Health care choices are also affected by how well patient and family are informed about the disease and the range of treatment options available to them. Such educational services are especially important for diabetic patients. Unlike patients with hypertension, for whom dietary and drug therapy compliance is fairly straightforward, patients with diabetes face complicated choices (e.g., insulin vs. oral hypoglycemic agents, tight control vs. less stringent control, self-monitoring vs. laboratory monitoring). Diabetes education has been shown to influence which choices are made and how well the patient's diabetes is controlled (Brown, 1992).

SERVICE FINANCING, REGULATION, AND UTILIZATION CONTROL

To describe the current regulatory and utilization control structures affecting them, the services discussed in the preceding section can be grouped into three categories: Medicare reimbursed, Medicaid reimbursed, and reimbursed out of pocket. Services reimbursed under Medicare (and private supplemental insurance) include hospital, skilled nurs-

Table 7.7. Persons Aged 65 and Older with a Disability by Race and Health Insurance Coverage Status, 1991–92 (Numbers in Thousands)

			With a Disability		With Severe Disability	
	Total Number	Total %	Number	%	Number	%
Total 65 + years	30,688	100.0	16,541	53.9	10,417	34.0
Race						
White, not of Hispanic origin	26,449	86.2	13,980	52.9	8,586	32.5
Black	2,737	8.9	1,727	63.1	1,260	46.0
All others	1,502	4.9	834	55.5	571	38.0
Health insurance coverage						
Covered by private insurance	23,893	77.9	11,964	72.3	7,050	67.7
Covered by Medicaid	2,137	7.0	1,746	10.6	1,418	13.6
Not covered by private insurance or Medicaid	4,659	15.2	2,831	17.1	1,950	18.7
Covered by Medicare	29,893	97.4	16,155	97.7	10,141	97.4

Source: Data from McNeil, 1993, Table 13, p. 40.

ing, skilled home health care, rehabilitative services (e.g., occupational, speech, physical therapy), and inpatient and outpatient procedures and laboratory tests. Table 7.7 shows the number of persons above age sixty-five by race and disability level and by disability level and health insurance coverage. As the level of disability rises, the proportion of persons with private insurance declines. This loss of private insurance is reflected in the doubling of the number of persons covered by Medicaid; however, almost 20 percent of those with a disability have neither private insurance nor Medicaid coverage.

Access to the skilled care benefits reimbursed under either Medicare or private insurance is largely controlled by physicians (i.e., they must order or prescribe this care). Increasingly, however, these decisions are subjected to review and even prior authorization by the payer or the health plan. The review may consider the appropriateness, amount, and duration of the treatment. Clinics and HMOs often have protocols that restrict the authority to order certain tests or procedures; they also have procedures that affect selection of and access to specialty care.

These points of control are intended to reduce "unnecessary" tests, procedures, and other treatments and in so doing, control utilization and expenditures. HCFA and the fiscal intermediaries who administer payments within the Medicare program (and for private insurance) have developed extensive price lists, case-mix adjustment algorithms, relative value scales, and other norms by which to compare the billings of hospitals, physicians, and other providers. Through peer (professional) review organizations (PROs) and claims records, they can also profile individual physicians in terms of the type and amount of services prescribed to their patients.

The stringency of these review and management procedures is a potentially important variable in their effectiveness and in utilization and expenditure outcomes. Another important variable is the practices used by physicians, patients, and others to circumvent these controls. The exclusion of activities associated with nursing home visits is one illustration of restrictions on physician billing. Coming simply to "pronounce" someone dead is not reimbursed; therefore, other reasons for this visit will be reported to obtain reimbursement. In other words, while utilization controls may influence practice and patient outcomes, they may also influence reporting and record systems.[5]

Another important factor influencing the reporting of care is the differential reimbursement from Medicare for psychiatric and nonpsychiatric diagnoses. Because of this, when a patient is visited in a nursing home, Alzheimer's disease or dementia is unlikely to be reported. An arbitrary physical complaint will be used, even though the dementia might be the sole factor precipitating the visit. Comorbidity of physical and psychiatric illness is often treated by the primary care physician, yet rarely does this show up in reported diagnoses. A diabetic patient might have significant anxiety or depression, prompting the need for relatively frequent physician visits. Often these will be coded for the diagnosis diabetes, and the frequent visits might be interpreted as reflecting poorly controlled or complicated diabetes rather than psychotherapeutic need.

Another arbitrary factor is that physicians often report a single diagnosis or limited diagnoses, even though a patient may have multiple diagnoses, which might include one of the chosen marker conditions. For example, an office visit might include discussion and treatment of constipation, a sleep disorder, hypertension, and a skin cancer. Medicare billing forms and other systems often preclude the inclusion of multiple diagnoses. In other cases, the site of service may be incorrectly recorded to reflect physician or patient convenience factors, as in the common situation of a home visit for a frail patient cared for by a relatively healthy spouse. The physician might see the spouse at the same time as the homebound patient and bill for a (cheaper) office visit, because the spouse was seen at home for convenience rather than medical necessity. Conversely, the care of the healthy spouse might be reported as a home visit, implying a greater need than really existed.

Medicaid (and private insurance) payments for physician, hospital, and other Medicare-reimbursed providers generally follow the utilization controls used by Medicare and its fiscal intermediaries. When a beneficiary is eligible for both Medicare and Medicaid, Medicaid (and the private insurance company) is liable only for copayments and deductible charges. Medicare is responsible for most of the claim. To gain more control over spending, state governments have attempted to increase the proportion of Medicaid recipients who are members of managed care plans. The assumptions underlying this policy are that managed care reduces cost by more efficient delivery and increases the ability of the government to negotiate reimbursement rates. Neither of these assumptions has been confirmed unequivocally.

Medicaid reimburses a variety of services relevant for long-term care that are not covered by Medicare.[6] These services are generally available under home- and community-based care waivers (e.g., homemaker, chore, companion, adult day care, case manager) or as optional benefits (e.g., personal care, extended nursing home stays) to Medicaid regulations. Other sources of state-controlled resources may also be used to finance these services (e.g., Social Security Act Title XX social services funds, state and county general revenues, Older Americans Act funds). While physician authorization may be required for some of these services, the pervasive practice is to have home- and community-based care and nursing home placements authorized by a case manager. This process generally involves a uniform standardized assessment and periodic reassessments and includes the type, amount, and duration of benefits. All states have some form of case management system in place, which usually operates at the community level. Great variation exists in the clientele screened in this process. Most typical are Medicaid-eligible patients applying (or who have been referred) for home and community care benefits or nursing home placement.

Patients paying for these home- and community-based care services out of pocket are generally not subjected to assessment by a case manager unless they are viewed as likely to spend down to Medicaid eligibility within sixty to ninety days. Only a few states require all applicants for long-term care services to go through their uniform assessment process.

Medicaid or HMO closed drug formularies can also influence care provision. Odious paperwork or the slow processing of reimbursement for nonformulary drug requests can serve as barriers or impede the use of drugs not on the formularies. If the cost of drug care is weighted heavily toward choosing drugs on the formulary, other factors that influence compliance, such as patient convenience and lack of side effects, can be overwhelmed. Whole categories of drugs that might influence quality of life, but not mortality, can be omitted from formularies (e.g. anxiolytics, antiemetics).

States and communities vary in the range of community-based care available under public reimbursement and in the extensiveness and effectiveness of the prior authorization process. One factor contributing to these variations is the extent of the state's discretionary initiative to pool or to integrate funding for long-term care services. Among the variety of federal and state revenue sources (beyond Medicaid) for social services are Title XX of the Social Security Act (homemaker/chore services), the Older Americans Act (meals programs and transportation services), and general revenues committed by state or local government. If these funding sources are included in an integrated long-term care program, their access and use usually fall under the case manager structures outlined above. Without this integration, usually a case manager or some other authorization will control access to funding for each service.

Ironically, as more state resources are placed at risk, these utilization control processes generally become more stringent, leading to tighter control of home- and community-based care than of much more expensive care, such as hospital care. Currently, Medicare funding mechanisms dictate much of the choice available to elderly persons as well as the care trajectory followed. Long-term care programs and community care benefits are usually accessed after a hospitalization or when nursing home placement is imminent. More rarely, these services are used to enhance the effectiveness of primary care in reducing the risk of a hospitalization (e.g., in the management of congestive heart disease) or as an adjunct to rehabilitation services.

DATA SOURCES AND INDICATORS

The responsiveness of the monitoring system begins with recognizing the potential number of persons within a catchment area and their probabilities of requiring services within a given period. At the most basic level, both the Social Security Administration (SSA) and HCFA provide a periodic count of the number of persons eligible for SSA/Medicare (by age, gender, and disability eligibility) within specific geographic areas (e.g., counties or zip codes). Also available are state- and county-level tabulations of Medicaid recipients (whether aged, blind, disabled, other categorically eligible group, or medically needy).

Within states and localities, going beyond basic demographics into estimates of disease or condition prevalence typically involves synthetic estimates that can assign a weighted probability for age, gender, race, and sometimes even a living arrangement for each disease or condition. The most widely used bases for these estimates, as discussed above (and in other chapters), are the prevalence estimates developed by the NCHS. These surveys also provide instruments and a standard or trend line against which to compare results obtained from geographically targeted studies or data systems.

For the elderly and those with disability, the major source of client or beneficiary-specific information is Medicare claims records.[7] These data include information on a variety of inpatient (e.g., hospital, skilled nursing home) and outpatient services (e.g., physician visits, home health care, durable medical equipment), as well as information on the procedures reimbursed and the diagnoses of persons discharged from hospitals. Claims records are strongest in assessing the patient mix within hospital settings and in tracking outpatient procedures. All physician visits under traditional fee-for-service and many managed care systems require that diagnostic codes accompany the evaluation and management codes. This is used to ensure the appropriate level and intensity of care.

Until recently, the linkage of diagnoses with procedures was generally absent in the outpatient records; other comorbid conditions affecting a patient's health status are often absent in both inpatient and outpatient records. Only in nursing homes is the Skilled Nursing Facility Resident Assessment Minimum Data Set available to report periodically on the functional and cognitive status and diagnostic conditions of patients. Although this is a federally mandated database, states can add supplemental questions. This system, however, is not fully operational.

Utilization

Medicare claims data have been used to compile a vast number of area-level files used for specific time-limited analyses, for example, *Hospital Data by Geographic Area for Aged Medicare Beneficiaries: Selected Procedures*. This file includes information on the use of hospital-based procedures and outcomes of treatment (measured by hospital stays, readmission, length of stay, and mortality) associated with fourteen common procedures including coronary artery bypass graft, hip and knee replacement, and prostatectomy. Similar information is available by eleven diagnostic categories (e.g., heart disease, cancer, stroke). Data can be compiled by county, Standard Metropolitan Statistical Area (SMSA), and state. The database can be used to examine geographic variation in the use of inpatient hospital services, factors associated with high and low rates of hospitalization for certain conditions, and the relationship between hospitalization rates and thirty-day mortality following admission.[8] Similar treatment and outcome data could be compiled for the target conditions given focus in this paper.

Among the problems affecting the use of Medicare claims data is the proportion of the Medicare population for whom such information is available. Claims data are not collected for beneficiaries enrolled in

Medicare risk contract HMOs or under the Medicare Hospice program. Nationally, this is a minor problem, because fewer than 10 percent of beneficiaries are enrolled in these plans; however, this data void can be significant in some communities, where as many as 40–60 percent of all Medicare beneficiaries are enrolled in HMOs. Health plans are adopting records systems that can track individual patient encounters, but these are not yet integrated with Medicare claims systems.

Service Supply

A wide variety of sources can provide relatively current community-level information about service supply. The most comprehensive and inclusive of these is the *Area Resource File* (formerly known as the *National Master Facility Inventory*), a county-level database for each county in the United States (with the exception of Alaska, which has a statewide inventory). It summarizes data from many sources into a single file. Data elements include

- county descriptors (e. g., name, PROs, SMSA, city size, shortage area designation);
- the number of licensed health professionals (e.g., MDs, DOs, DDSs, pharmacists, podiatrists, RNs, LPNs, dental hygienists);
- the number of hospitals and nursing homes (e.g., size, type, utilization, staffing, services);
- population data (e.g., size, composition, employment, housing, morbidity, mortality (by cause, race, gender, age);
- health professions training data (training programs, enrollments, graduates);
- expenditure data (e.g., hospital expenditures, Medicare enrollments and reimbursements, Medicare prevailing charges);
- economic data, (e.g., total, per capita and median income; income distribution, AFDC recipients); and
- environmental data (e.g., land area, elevation, latitude and longitude, climate data).

Not all data are updated annually, but many elements could be if key data sources were accessed directly.[9]

The *Area Resource File* does not systematically include many social services (e.g., nonskilled home care, transportation, meals programs, assisted living facilities) and "recreational" programs (e.g., exercise classes, support groups), which can be important in meeting the broad range of care needed by the chronically ill. While compiling inventories of such services within any one community is relatively inexpensive, it becomes a large undertaking to do so nationally. The infrastructure for doing this in the field of aging is in place in the *National Data Base on Aging*.[10] These data are compiled for the Administration on Aging by a voluntary annual survey of state and area agencies on aging (about one-third of the area agencies are surveyed each year). The service area for area agencies on aging (AAAs) is usually one or more counties. The information collected includes staffing patterns and services supported by these agencies, as well as their funding sources and expenditures. How comprehensive the reports on community-based care resources or uses are varies with the agency's breadth of responsibility.

Effective incorporation of this database into a chronic illness indicator or service monitoring system will likely require establishing a uniform minimum data set. Such a data set would systematically inventory the supply and use of community-based care and the functions of nursing home preadmission screening (and its referral outcomes), as well as chronicle the other forms of long-term care case management systems and their referral outcomes. This effort would extend the information currently being collected by many of the AAAs and their state units on aging.

An inventory of community-level providers of various types has several practical applications in an indicator system. Most immediately, the supply and use rates of these services are a direct measure of responsiveness, particularly to changes in reimbursement, benefit eligibility, and other conditions affecting operational costs. For example, is there growth in adult day care when these services are covered under Medicare or Medicaid? How is the supply of home care attendants affected by changes in reimbursement, service acuity levels, or other higher-paying employment opportunities in the community?

A comprehensive service inventory can also be used as a sample frame in which special surveys could be directed to track specific information. The *National Ambulatory Medical Care Survey* (NAMCS) and the *Survey of Rehabilitation Hospitals and Programs* (SRHP) represent two such surveys. The purpose of the SRHP, for example, is to monitor the number and census of inpatient and outpatient programs, types of services provided, referral sources, source of payment for rehabilitation programs, staffing, and financial performance. The sample is compiled from the hospitals identified in the American Hospital Association's annual survey of hospitals, which has been conducted on a biannual basis. Results are available at city- or community-level aggregation.

Quality of Care/Service Outcomes

The most common forms of outcomes tracking currently in use involve mortality rates, length of stay, rehospitalization rates, and duration of service. These indicators have the virtue of being monitored through administrative claims records or vital statistics. Standard diagnostic codes are available for patients who have received a Medicare-reimbursed service, such as hospitalization, rehabilitation hospitalization, physical therapy, occupational therapy, speech therapy, podiatry, ophthalmology, oxygen therapy, or physician visit. If a sufficiently long time frame is studied, these codes could identify most patients with hypertension, stroke, diabetes, congestive heart failure, and many other conditions. Dementia is somewhat harder to identify, as it is rarely included in the evaluation/management or discharge diagnoses, because of the lower Medicare reimbursement rate for psychiatric diagnoses. This problem can be overcome by using a single incidence of dementia (or a defined small number of occurrences) across multiple time frames to categorize a patient. Once the patient is classified as having dementia, outcome variables such as falls and death can be linked to this condition regardless of whether dementia is listed as a codiagnosis at the time of subsequent physician encounters.

Mortality rates, rehospitalizations, and the level and intensity of care can be connected to diagnosis procedures and to specific providers.[11] For certain conditions that occur at a point in time and are then associated with a chronic course (e.g., stroke), different codes within the Medicare record apply for the acute event and the chronic impairment (e.g., acute stroke = 436, chronic sequelae of stroke = 438). For such conditions, either the acute event or the chronic sequelae would categorize the patient into a condition-specific subgroup. Outcome variables, such as subsequent hospitalizations or institutionalization, could be monitored by keeping track of the sites of subsequent claims for this individual and by linking claims data to death records. For other marker conditions that persist indefinitely after diagnosis, such as hypertension, diabetes, or dementia, the initial use of such a diagnostic code could categorize the patient. Subsequent diagnostic codes for target outcome diagnoses, such as stroke, myocardial infarction, or peripheral vascular disease, would allow some monitoring of the care trajectory for patients with these marker conditions.

Appropriate outcome variables for hypertension include awareness of the diagnosis, blood pressure, drug use, and signs of end-organ damage (e.g., stroke, renal failure, hypertensive retinopathy, left ventricular hypertrophy, congestive heart failure). Criteria for diabetes include awareness of the diagnosis, fasting glucose levels, glycosylated hemoglobin or fructosamine levels as reflections of mean glucose levels, drug use, and signs of end-organ damage (e.g., diabetic retinopathy, cataracts, peripheral neuropathy, atherosclerotic disorders such as myocardial infarction and peripheral vascular insufficiency, diabetic nephropathy). Provision of ophthalmological and podiatric care would also be considered important variables in good care for diabetic patients. For congestive heart failure, awareness of the diagnosis, functional impairment, need for oxygen, and drug use can be measured.

Dementia offers a different set of outcome measures. Awareness of diagnosis is not useful, because self-awareness is compromised by the disease state itself. Although the FDA approval of tacrine does offer a drug therapy, the role of such pharmacotherapy is controversial and not useful for monitoring population health care. Life expectancy after diagnosis is so strongly influenced by diagnostic issues that it is rarely a useful indicator for comparing populations. Use of services for patients and caregivers is therefore one of the most useful parameters for comparing the outcomes of groups. Cognitive and functional measures could also permit comparison of the outcomes of different groups, providing that testing procedures were uniform. The outcome variable most readily available from present data sets is probably site of visit for primary care services, which would separate patients living at home but able to get to physician's offices from those receiving home care, care in board-and-care facilities, and care in nursing homes. Transitions from level to level could be measured as well, if case history files were compiled.

Hospitalization rate, mortality rate, and use of services are appropriate measures of outcome for all the above diagnoses. Satisfaction surveys (e.g., hospital discharge surveys) have been used to further refine measures of outcome or quality of care. Community care services are usually outside the scrutiny of these systems—in part because their number complicates the collection of information, and in part because entry to these services (at least for publicly subsidized cases) often requires prior screening and approval. If sample surveys were used, these service systems could be included.

Complaints and citations are available as a supplement to client-level data. These data could be used as quality of care indicators for nursing homes (and, to a much lesser extent, assisted living) and other licensed community care programs. Such data vary considerably, because of area-level differences in regulatory stringency, enforcement practices, and the legal and administrative processes used to resolve contested citations. The *State Long-Term Care Ombudsman Report* illustrates the types of data systems that might be put into place from complaints and citation systems. State units on aging annually collect data on complaints and conditions in long-term care facilities, as reported from local ombudsman programs. The information compiled includes program staffing and the percentage of complaints investigated, verified, and resolved.

Another approach to "outcomes" measurement is again illustrated by special surveys. Rehabilitation units and programs (or any other targeted service) could be surveyed for the incidence of selected conditions, types of treatment offered, causes, and outcomes. Physicians could be surveyed about the incidence of patients with dementia, hypertension, diabetes (and other conditions), and the treatments provided.

Table 7.8 provides a listing of suggested indicators, which have been organized into separate dimensions of prevalence, access to care, process of care, and outcomes. Service supply, estimates of unmet need based upon expected use rates, and expenditures form the core and minimum data set. Such measures are available from agency reports and often exist in currently available national data systems. The process of care for inpatient and outpatient care represents a refinement over the gross access measures and takes advantage of the data aggregations possible from Medicare claims. These measures can be organized by several alternative aggregations, including age, gender, age by gender, and perhaps Medicare-only compared with those who are eligible for both Medicare and Medicaid. These measures can be further refined by aggregations according to diagnostic or condition classification or by subpopulations receiving particular procedures. This refinement may be especially useful for health plans or other Medicare managed care systems, or for selected PRO monitoring.

The monitoring of social service use cannot take advantage of Medicare claims and, while very important, has a lower priority. This status is affected by two considerations: the substantially lower per capita expen-

Table 7.8. Indicators of Community Responsiveness to the Health and Community Service Needs of the Aged

Prevalence
Synthetic estimate of disease or condition
(Estimation models derived from national data; measured by rates per 1,000 target population)
- Prevalence by age and gender in community settings
- Prevalence by age and gender in institutional settings
- Estimated rates of selected service use

Access to care
Service supply adequacy
(Service supply from *Area Resource File* and other local data, including agency surveys; measured by service units, or units minus estimated need)
- Physician
- Hospital
- Rehabilitation
- Nursing home
- Other therapeutic programs
- Skilled/nonskilled home care
- Specialized living arrangements
- Other social service

Service expenditures
(Expenditures compiled from claims data and agency-reported utilization; measured by expenditures per capita or expenditures per recipient)
- Physician
- Hospital
- Rehabilitation
- Nursing home
- Other therapeutic programs
- Skilled/nonskilled home care
- Specialized living arrangements
- Special education/employment training
- Other social service

Process of care
(Mean units and expenditures by service recipient subgroups; measured by diagnosis/condition, procedure group, age, gender, or categorical group, or any combination of these)
Outpatient health care
(Visits and procedures compiled from Medicare claims data)
- MD visits
- Emergency room visits
- Diagnostic tests and procedures
- Immunizations
- Therapeutic surgical procedures
- Tests/procedures for monitoring treatment/management
- Follow-up care/continuity after inpatient stay
- Specialty referral
- Rehabilitation
- Skilled home care

(continued)

Table 7.8   *(continued)*

Inpatient care
(Visits and procedures compiled from Medicare claims data)
• Hospital
• Nursing home
• Rehabilitation
• Other therapeutic setting
Social services
(Visits and procedures compiled from agency surveys, or client follow-back surveys)
• Other therapeutic programs
• Nonskilled home care
• Specialized living arrangements
• Other social services

Health and other outcomes
(Rates per 1,000 target population; measured by diagnosis/condition, or procedure group,
age, gender, or categorical group, or a combination of these)
Patient or client
(Visits, procedures, complications, and expenditures per episode of care compiled from
Medicare claims; mortality from death registry; physiological measures, functional sta-
tus, psychological status, satisfaction, and expressed unmet need from client follow-
back surveys)
• Mortality rate
• Rehospitalization rate
• Rates of health conditions or complications secondary to primary problem (e.g.,
  stroke, renal failure)
• Average total costs for selected episodes of care
• Condition-specific physiological measures (e.g., frequency of attacks, pulmonary func-
  tion)
• Functional status (e.g., disability, developmental capacity)
• Psychological status
• Satisfaction with care
• Expressed unmet need for care
Family/caregiver outcomes
(Follow-back surveys from selected caregivers, chosen from among the population of ser-
vice recipients)
• Familial support
• Satisfaction with care
• Expressed unmet need for care

---

ditures associated with these services and the proportionately higher cost
of data collection that must rely on either agency or client surveys.

The final set of indicators is organized under the heading of outcomes.
Basic measures such as mortality rates and rehospitalization rates should
likely have a high priority. Measures such as complications and costs per
episode of care can be derived from Medicare claims data and might be
appropriately compiled by health plans or when triggered by adverse
rates in the preceding indicators. As with the process measures, multiple

aggregations (e.g., age, gender, condition) are possible. Physiological measures, functional status, and the other client dimensions are also suggested, but as such data require primary data collection in the form of client surveys, the use of such measures should be highly targeted and not part of a routine reporting system. The nursing home minimum data set is an exception to this and could be reported periodically. Family and caregiver outcomes extend the monitoring system into a tracking of consequences for informal or nonfunded providers. This highly important area is often a focus of program evaluations and political rhetoric. Monitoring of caregiver outcomes is most effective when it is focused on target programs, with targeting based on adverse rates of the preceding indicators (e.g., high rates of institutionalization, potentially inadequate community service supply). Caregiver data will generally have to be obtained from surveys, the most efficient of which are connected either to subsamples of service recipients or to other identified subgroups (such as those with specific conditions or high rates of service).

DISCUSSION AND CONCLUSIONS

A number of national and regional data systems monitor the prevalence of chronic health conditions and service use among the elderly. However, prevalence and use estimates that are specific to communities or counties will sometimes be desirable, given the mix of public and private providers and benefit structures, the diversity of populations, the needs and services involved, the inherent competition for resources, and the importance of community-based care in long-term care. Four chronic diseases—hypertension, stroke, diabetes, and dementia—have been used to illustrate the operation of primary care, prevention, rehabilitation, and custodial care within both medical and social service systems and to demonstrate the feasibility of developing community-level indicator systems. Administrative records (particularly Medicare claims data) and other existing data systems are available for compiling and tracking benefit structures, service eligibility, service supply, case management procedures, service utilization, and outcomes of care for the chronically ill elderly at the community level. Claims-based data systems are likely to expand as part of changes occurring in health care quality assurance, as discussed in chapter 2.

While there is reason to be optimistic about the future and the feasibility of these systems, several important measurement and analytical problems need to be recognized in using administrative data sources as a monitoring system (either statewide or nationally). For example, prevalence estimates based on service use will likely differ from those based on synthetic modeling. Part of this problem stems from a lack of refinement in the synthetic estimates, which may require more sophisticated methods than simply weighting prevalence by the age, gender, and racial mix of the population. Prevalence estimates of specific diagnoses vary according to the sample frame, be it the community, the outpatient ambulatory clinic, the inpatient hospital setting, or the nursing home. One reason for this is that institutionalized or hospitalized patients usually have more severe illness than those with the same diseases living in the community.[12] Rates of comorbidity and disability may also differ in these settings. For example, among nursing home patients aged sixty-five and older, the prevalence of functional dependency is five to forty times higher than it is among noninstitutionalized persons of the same age (NCHS, 1994). There is also a higher likelihood of cognitive impairment in institutionalized persons than in other populations.

When prevalence variations by living arrangement and site of service are used, estimates of the population prevalence of disease and disability may vary among communities (or across time), according to the availability and use of long-term care facilities and home-based care. Disease-specific utilization rates could also be affected. In other words, prevalence and utilization comparisons across communities and across time are affected by the delivery system, as well as by the population profile.

Using administrative records to ascertain disease and make comparisons across time or communities raises the clinical issue of whether all older patients, including those who are frail or who have multiple conditions, are treated with the same diagnostic intensity when presenting with comparable signs or symptoms. For example, the likelihood of hospitalization after a stroke appears to decline with advancing age in some communities, which may be the result of differences in treatment choices or in the selection of alternative diagnoses on the records. Diagnostic and disease ascertainment are also likely related to fiscal and geographic access to health service. Rates may be artificially higher where access to hospital care or other services is more available. Similarly, the regulations related to payment or benefit eligibility may bias data to diagnoses that are covered.

The lack of adjustment for significant cultural and familial factors known to influence the care trajectory of patients with chronic illness may also contribute to the differences between rates (such as diagnosis, health conditions, and utilization) derived from administrative records and survey-based estimates. Simple factors, such as the availability of nearby children (particularly daughters), influence the viability of the home-care option and the corresponding distribution of the population into care alternatives. Self-reporting of health conditions and service use (particularly if proxy respondents are involved) also introduces measurement differences into estimates. The agreement between self-report of disease prevalence for common chronic diseases (e.g., angina, cancer, cataracts, diabetes, fractures, hypertension, myocardial infarction, stroke) and physician diagnosis of disease on a medical record is high, but has a margin of error (e.g., 76–98 percent agreement in persons aged sixty-five and older) (NIH, 1987; Young et al., 1991). Apart from possible memory recall problems, there is another explanation for these differences. Because of the slow, progressive nature of chronic diseases, patients often present to a clinician for evaluation only when they become clearly ill or when the symptoms become intolerable. This is thought to contribute to the disparity between population-based assessments of prevalence and severity and those from clinical settings (Minaker & Rowe, 1985).

Ultimately, the selection of measures and the comprehensiveness of data systems is driven by considerations of cost, desired timeliness, and the nature of the questions being investigated. Epidemiology looks at risk factors (perhaps best obtained through reporting systems), and service planning is interested in use and substitution as affected by supply, cost, and access (risk factors are held constant over the short term). In their current form, administrative records systems are generally more appropriate for service planning and policy analyses, although their timeliness is limited by a two- to three-year time lag between the claim encounter and data availability.

More timely information may require the replication of national surveys using community-level sample frames or, alternatively, using national sample frames for current trends and administrative records for long-term monitoring. If more frequent tracking of "responsiveness" is desired, various ongoing surveys (e.g., the Current Population Survey, New Beneficiary Survey [SSA]) have had supplemental questions for specific information purposes. The delivery system inventories suggested in this chapter could provide a ready sample frame for such surveys.

Notes

1. See appendix A for a listing of all NCHS data sets referred to in this chapter.

2. See appendix C for a listing of all governmental and nongovernmental data sets referred to in this chapter.

3. See Appendix B for a listing of all HCFA data sets referred to in this chapter.

4. The recent advent of FDA-approved pharmacological therapy for dementia (tacrine) may have an influence on the trajectory of care for some of these patients. Theoretically, by improving the cognitive ability of dementia patients, the need for assisted living and attendant care will be delayed. The speed with which physicians adopt new therapies and the success of newer drugs at alleviating the symptoms of cognitive loss will have the potential to affect the trajectory of care of these patients.

5. There are also less direct methods of utilization control. One of these is control over eligibility for Medicaid, which is accomplished through income and resource standards that limit the number of persons who are eligible for coverage. Another approach to utilization control is through the supply and distribution of services. During the 1970s, for example, health systems agencies and state health planning agencies were developed to compile community-level information on service supply and population needs and to use this information as a "rational" basis for the allocation of health care resources. This strategy aimed to limit cost by limiting the supply of hospital and nursing home beds and high-cost equipment. This certificate-of-need approach has since been largely abandoned in favor of more direct controls over supply and use. Among these are DRG-based Medicare payments for hospitals and procedure-based fee incentives for physicians. Increased copayments and deductibles have also provided an incentive for Medicare-eligible persons to join managed care systems. Social and community service supply continues to be controlled by licensing, staffing-level requirements, and reimbursement rates. All these features vary among states (affecting the operational cost and competition for these programs) and contribute to the effect of market forces on supply and demand. Social service program expenditures are also directly limited for public-sector clientele by a governmental ability to fix the budget available for these programs.

6. Home care and nursing home care are also potentially reimbursable under private long-term care insurance, but the number of persons under benefit with active policies is presently negligible in most communities.

7. These data are currently available in several accessible formats from HCFA. Among them are the Medicare Automated Data Retrieval System (MADRS), which is a beneficiary-specific claims file, and various annual report files (e.g., Medicare Annual: Person Summary File, Medicare History Sample, Medicare Part B 5-Percent Sample Bill Summary Records).

8. Another similar use of the Medicare claims file is the Medicare Beneficiary File System. Medicare Inpatient Claims and Summary Inpatient Claims by Current DRG and by Hospital are also available on an ongoing basis from the American Hospital Association (AHA).

9. For example, information on hospital beds and services (including health

promotion programs and rehabilitation programs) can be obtained on a regular basis from the AHA; listings of Medicare- and Medicaid-certified providers (both institutional and noninstitutional) can be obtained from HCFA; physician listings are available from the American Medical Association.

10. Other, perhaps more general, resources for community-level data are state health planning and development agencies, and the National Association of Health Data Organizations (NAHDO). The AHA maintains a list of health planning agencies and an inventory of other community resources.

11. Among the data sources for such information are the Medicare Hospital Mortality Rate File (HCFA), National Mortality Statistics (NCHS), Rehospitalization by Geographic Area for Aged Medicare Beneficiaries: Selected Procedures (HCFA), the Linked Medicare Use and NCHS Mortality Statistics File (HCFA), and the Uniform Clinical Data Set (UCDS), which HCFA has proposed as a national Medicare program database. The UCDS is in a pilot phase, and its utility in monitoring the quality and outcomes of care is being assessed (Audet & Scott, 1993).

12. The likelihood of placement or residence in these various settings changes with age. Over 99.9 percent of adults under age sixty-five dwell in a community setting, and less than 11 percent are likely to be hospitalized in a single year (excluding deliveries) (Hing, 1987). In contrast, among those aged sixty-five to seventy-four, 1.4 percent reside in nursing homes. This rate increases to 6.8 percent for those aged seventy-five to eighty-four and to 21.6 percent for those aged eighty-five and over (Rabin & Stockton, 1987). In addition, the rate of hospitalization (i.e., at least one hospital admission in a given year) increases to about 16 percent for those aged sixty-five to seventy-four and 23 percent for those aged seventy-five and over.

References

American Diabetes Association. 1992. Clinical practice recommendations—1991–1992. *Diabetes Care 2*: 1–80.

Applegate, W. B., & Rutan, G. H. 1992. Advances in management of hypertension in older persons. *Journal of the American Geriatric Society 40*: 1164–74.

Arnold, S. E. & Kumar, A. 1993. Reversible dementias. *Medical Clinics of North America 77*: 215–30.

Aronson, M. K., Ooi, W. L., Geva, D. L., Masur, D., Blau, A., & Frishman, W. 1991. Dementia. Age-dependent incidence, prevalence, and mortality in the old old. *Archives of Internal Medicine 151*: 989–92.

Audet, A., & Scott, H. D. 1993. The Uniform Clinical Data Set: An evaluation of the proposed national database for Medicare's Quality Review Program. *Annals of Internal Medicine 119*: 1209–13.

Bachman, D. L., Wolf, P. A., Linn, R. T., Knoefel, J. E., Cobb, J. L., Belanger, A. J., White, L. R., & D'Agostino, R. B. 1993. Incidence of dementia and probable Alzheimer's disease in a general population: The Framingham Study. *Neurology*, 515–19.

Benson, V. & Marano, M. A. 1994. Current estimates from the National Health Interview Survey. *Vital Health Statistics,* no. 10, National Center for Health Statistics, Public Health Service, Hyattsville, Md.

Berg, L., Buckwalter, K. C., Chafetz, P. K., Gwyther, L. P., Holmes, D., Koepke, K. M., Lawton, M. P., Lindeman, D. A., Magaziner, J., & Maslow, K. 1991. Special care units for persons with dementia. *Journal of the American Geriatric Society 39:* 1229–36.

Branch, L., Jette, A., Evashwick, C., Polansky, M., Rowe, G., & Diehr, P. 1981. Toward understanding elders' health service utilization. *Journal of Community Health 7:* 80–92.

Braun, K. L., Rose, C. L., & Finch, M. D. 1991. Patient characteristics and outcomes in institutional and community long-term care. *Gerontologist 31:* 648–56.

Brown, S. A. 1992. Meta-analysis of diabetes patient education research: Variations in intervention effects across studies. *Research on Nursing and Health 15:* 409–19.

Campbell, A. J., McCosh, L. M., Reinken, J., & Allan, B. C. 1983. Dementia in old age and the need for services. *Age and Ageing 12:* 11–16.

Canadian Task Force on the Periodic Health Examination. 1991. Periodic health examination, 1991 update: 1. Screening for cognitive impairment in the elderly. *Canadian Medical Association Journal 144:* 425–31.

Casper, M., Wing, S., & Strogatz, D. 1991. Variation in the magnitude of black-white differences in stroke mortality by community occupational structure. *Journal of Epidemiology and Community Health 45:* 302–6.

Casper, M., Wing, S., Strogatz, D., Davis, C. E., & Tyroler, H. A. 1992. Antihypertensive treatment and US trends in stroke mortality, 1962 to 1980. *American Journal of Public Health 82:* 1600–1606.

Centers for Disease Control. 1990. Regional variation in diabetes mellitus prevalence—United States, 1988 and 1989. *Journal of the American Medical Association 264:* 3123–24.

Cohen, D. L., Neil, H. A., Thorogood, M., & Mann, J. I. 1991. A population-based study of the incidence of complications associated with type 2 diabetes in the elderly. *Diabetic Medicine 8:* 928–33.

Doyle, D. B., Lauterbach, W., Samargo, P., Robinson, C., & Ludwig, W. 1991. Age- and sex-biased underdetection of hypertension in a rural clinic. *Family Practice Research Journal 11:* 395–404.

Eisdorfer, C. 1991. Caregiving: An emerging risk factor for emotional and physical pathology. *Bulletin of the Menninger Clinic 55:* 238–47.

Espino, D. V., Burge, S. K., & Moreno, C. A. 1991. The prevalence of selected chronic diseases among the Mexican-American elderly: Data from the 1982–1984 Hispanic Health and Nutrition Examination Survey. *Journal of the American Board of Family Practice 4:* 217–22.

Espino, D. V., & Maldonado, D. 1990. Hypertension and acculturation in elderly Mexican Americans: Results from 1982–84 Hispanic Health and Nutrition Examination Survey. *Journal of Gerontology 45:* M209–M213.

EURODEM Incidence Conferences. 1992. European studies on the incidence of dementing diseases: Bordeaux, France, 1989 and Cambridge, UK, 1990. *Neuroepidemiology 1:* 1–122.

Evans, D. A., Scheer, P. P., Cook, N. R., Albert, M. S., Funkenstein, H. H., Smith, L. A., Hebert, L. E., Wetle, T. T., Branch, L. G., Chown, M., Hennekens, C. H., & Taylor, J. O. 1990. Estimated prevalence of Alzheimer's disease in the United States. *The Milbank Quarterly 68:* 267–89.

Expert Committee of the Canadian Diabetes Advisory Board. 1992. Clinical practice guidelines for treatment of diabetes mellitus. *Canadian Medical Association Journal 147:* 697–712.

Fratiglioni, L., Grut, M., Forsell, Y., Viitanen, M., Grafstrom, M., Holmen, K., Ericsson, K., Backman, L., Ahlbom, A., & Winblad, B. 1991. Prevalence of Alzheimer's disease and other dementias in an elderly urban population: Relationship with age, sex, and education. *Neurology 41:* 1886–92.

Froom, J. 1990. Glycemic control in elderly people with diabetes. *Clinical Geriatric Medicine 6:* 933–41.

Geronimus, A. T., Neidert, L. J., & Bound, J. 1990. A note on the measurement of hypertension in HHANES. *American Journal of Public Health 80:* 1437–42.

Guralnik, J. M., LaCroix, A. Z., Everett, D. F., & Kovar, M. G. 1989. Aging in the eighties: The prevalence of comorbidity and association with disability. *Advance Data from Vital and Health Statistics,* no. 170, National Center for Health Statistics, Public Health Service, Hyattsville, Md.

Harper, K. J., & Forker, A. D. 1992. Antihypertensive therapy: Current issues and challenges. *Postgraduate Medicine 91:* 163–66, 171–74, 179–86.

Harris, M. I. 1990. Testing for blood glucose by office-based physicians in the U.S. *Diabetes Care 13:* 419–26.

Havlik, R. J., Liu, B. M., & Kovar, M. G. 1987. Health Statistics on Older Persons, United States, 1986. *Vital and Health Statistics,* series 3, no. 25 DHHS Publ. no. (PHS) 87–1409: National Center for Health Statistics, Public Health Service, Hyattsville, Md.

Hing, E. 1987. Use of nursing homes by the elderly: Preliminary data from the 1985 National Home Survey. *Advance Data from Vital and Health Statistics,* no. 135, DHHS Publ. no. (PHS) 87–1250): National Center for Health Statistics, Public Health Service, Hyattsville, Md.

Institute of Medicine. 1991. *Disability in America: Toward a National Agenda for Prevention.* (ISBN 0–309-040378–6) Washington, D.C.: National Academy Press.

Joint National Committee on Detection, Evaluation, & Treatment of High Blood Pressure (JNCV). 1993. The fifth report of the Joint National Committee on Detection, Evaluation, and Treatment of High Blood Pressure (JNCV). *Archives of Internal Medicine 153:* 154–83.

Kane, R. L., & Boult, C. 1997. Defining the service needs of frail older persons. In V. Mor (ed.), *Living in the Community with Disability.* New York: Springer.

Klein, B. E., & Klein, R. 1990. Ocular problems in older Americans with diabetes. *Clinical Geriatric Medicine 6:* 827–37.

Kokmen, E., Beard, C. M., Offord, K. P., & Kurland, L. T. 1989. Prevalence of medically diagnosed dementia in a defined United States population: Rochester, Minnesota, January 1, 1975. *Neurology 39:* 773–76.

Letenneur, L., Jacqmin, H., Commenges, D., Barberger Gateau, P., Dartigues, J. F., & Salamon, R. 1993. Cerebral and functional aging: First results on prevalence and incidence of the Paquid cohort. *Methods of Information Medicine 32:* 249–51.

MacMahon, S., Cutler, J. A., & Stamler, J. 1989. Antihypertensive drug treatment. Potential, expected, and observed effects on stroke and on coronary heart disease. *Hypertension 13* (5 suppl.): I45–50.

McNeil, J. M. 1993. *Americans with Disabilities: 1991–92.* Washington, D.C.: U.S. Government Printing Office.

Minaker, K. L., & Rowe, J. 1985. Health and disease among the oldest old: A clinical perspective. *Milbank Memorial Fund/Health Society 62:* 324–49.

Morbidity and Mortality Weekly Report. 1992. Cerebrovascular disease mortality and Medicare hospitalization—United States, 1980–1990. *Morbidity Mortality Weekly Report (MMWR) 41:* 477–80.

National Center for Health Statistics. 1993. *Vital Health Statistics of the United States, 1991* (suppl. 42). Public Health Service, Hyattsville, Md.

National Center for Health Statistics. 1994. Current Estimates from the National Health Interview, 1992. *Vital and Health Statistics,* no. 10 (189): Public Health Service, Hyattsville, Md.

National Institutes of Health. 1987. Diet and exercise in noninsulin-dependent diabetes mellitus. *NIH Consensus Statement 6:* 1–21.

Rabin, D. L., & Stockton, P. 1987. *Long Term Care for the Elderly: A Fact Book.* New York: Oxford University Press.

Reeves, R. A., Fodor, J. G., Gryfe, C. I., Patterson, C., & Spence, J. D. 1993. Report of the Canadian Hypertension Society Consensus Conference: 4. Hypertension in the elderly. *Canadian Medical Association Journal 149:* 815–20.

Schocken, D. D., Arrieta, M. I., Leaverton, P. E., & Ross, E. A. 1992. Prevalence and mortality rate of congestive heart failure in the United States. *Journal of the American College of Cardiology 20:* 301–6.

Strasser, T., & Wilhelmsen, L. 1992. Impediments to the control of hypertension. Hypertension Management Audit Group. *Clinical and Experimental Hypertension 14:* 193–212.

Wetterhall, S. F., Olson, D. R., DeStefano, F., Stevenson, J. M., Ford, E. S., German, R. R., Will, J. C., Newman, J. M., Sepe, S. J., & Vinicor, F. 1992. Trends in diabetes and diabetic complications, 1980–1987. *Diabetes Care 15:* 960–67.

Wilhelmsen, L., & Strasser, T. 1993. WHO-WHL Hypertension Management Audit Project. *Journal of Human Hypertension 7:* 257–63.

Young, T. K., Roos, N. P., & Hammerstrand, K. M. 1991. Estimated burden of diabetes mellitus in Manitoba according to health insurance claims: A pilot study. *Canadian Medical Association Journal 144:* 318–24.

8/ CARE FOR INDIVIDUALS WITH SEVERE MENTAL ILLNESS

Donald M. Steinwachs, Judith Kasper, and
Anthony Lehman

A number of early and well-known studies (e.g., Faris & Dunham, 1939; Srole et al., 1962) viewed prevalence of mental illness as a social indicator, that is, a reflection of the well-being of a community. Estimates of the prevalence of severe mental illness, while not interpreted in the same sense today, remain important as a means of identifying the size and scope of the population to whom indicators of adequacy of care should be applied. Efforts have been ongoing at the national level to develop data systems to provide prevalence estimates. Still lacking, however, is a conceptual approach for evaluating adequacy of care, which could lead to the development of empirical indicators. This chapter addresses these issues, taking schizophrenia as a prototype for severe mental illness and drawing on the experience of a study under way to evaluate treatment effectiveness for schizophrenia.

Schizophrenia is a particularly appropriate indicator condition, because persons with this condition have a broad range of needs, which subsume many of the needs of persons with other types of mental disorders. These include treatment for acute illness episodes, maintenance care to prevent relapse, rehabilitative care, and social services. The capacity of a health care delivery system to respond to the needs of persons with schizophrenia is likely to be an excellent indication of the system's capacity to respond to the needs of other patient groups with severe mental illness.

The following discussion is organized into several sections, beginning with a discussion of schizophrenia as a model for developing a community indicator system for severe mental illnesses. To provide a basis for discussing such indicators, the care needs and service patterns of individuals with schizophrenia are described. An understanding of "best" ser-

235

vice patterns and expected outcomes provides an approach to developing indicators of the adequacy of care. Additional factors limit access to "best" care, however, including inadequate financial resources, insufficient availability of services, and lack of consumer acceptance. The feasibility of collecting indicators on key elements of the care process, outcomes, and costs is discussed. The final section provides recommendations for indicator development at local and national levels.

Schizophrenia As a Model for Monitoring Severe Mental Illness Care in the Community

Ideally, an indicator system for severe mental illness would include measures of the process and outcomes of care relevant for the range of severe and persistent psychiatric disorders. Although this is the long-term goal, the proposed starting point in this effort is selection of a single major psychiatric disorder, schizophrenia, which can be used as a model for indicators of mental illness.

Schizophrenia is probably the most common severe and disabling mental disorder, affecting approximately 1 percent of adults. Like those with other severe mental disorders, persons with schizophrenia suffer from psychotic symptoms, as well as a range of disabilities that contribute to deficits in social, work, and independent living skills. The range and severity of disability varies among individuals. Approximately one-third experience a single acute psychotic episode leading to hospitalization and then lead relatively normal lives. The remaining two-thirds, who are more severely ill, suffer recurrent acute psychotic episodes that contribute to long-term disabilities, depriving many of productive and satisfying lives. In the past, many of these individuals had symptoms that did not respond to available drugs; as a result, they experienced long-term institutional care. With newer drugs, the number of such individuals is declining. Advances in drug therapy are now making it possible to provide community-based care for almost all individuals with schizophrenia, reserving inpatient care for the management of short-term acute episodes.

Another perspective on the impact of schizophrenia is the cost of the illness to society. Estimates for 1990 costs totaled $33 billion, which included $18 billion for direct patient care services and $15 billion for indirect costs associated primarily with lost productivity. Schizophrenia accounts for almost half the total costs of all severe mental illnesses, estimated at $73 billion (Rice & Miller, 1996).

NEEDS AND SERVICE PATTERNS OF PERSONS WITH SCHIZOPHRENIA

There is a growing consensus that schizophrenia should be viewed from a vulnerability-stress, or biopsychosocial, perspective (Zubin & Spring, 1977). This view emphasizes the underlying biological vulnerabilities that predispose an individual to the development of schizophrenia, as well as the importance of psychological and social factors in the onset and course of the disorder. Several specific treatments are effective in improving social and independent living skills at the biological and psychological levels. Empirical data have recently confirmed the enhanced efficacy of combining treatments. These integrative approaches form the basis for modern comprehensive treatment of schizophrenia and have set the stage for many exciting therapeutic advances in treatment.

Typically, the course of schizophrenia spans the entire adult years of an individual. Given the heterogeneity of the schizophrenia syndrome (attributable to variability in biological causes and subtypes) (Carpenter & Heinrichs, 1981), the various stages of normal development encompassed by the adult years during which the illness is active (Group for the Advancement of Psychiatry, 1992), and the many variations of social circumstances and personal life history that occur across an individual adult life span, it is not at all surprising that the course of schizophrenia is so varied. Recent investigations have confirmed that manifestations of schizophrenia occur in relatively discrete clusters, with significant independence between clusters. Hallucinations and delusions define a cluster of expressive psychotic symptoms, while restricted emotional responsiveness, low drive, and impoverished mentation define a second cluster (negative symptoms or the deficit syndrome), and attention disturbance and cognitive dysfunction define a third. While the psychosis domain usually precipitates diagnosis and treatment intervention (and occurs most often during adolescence or young adulthood), substantial evidence shows that the other two clusters may precede the onset of psychosis by many years. These latter two domains have not been adequately targeted in treatment intervention studies, although they underlie many aspects of dysfunction that are targeted in rehabilitation approaches. Most treatment has focused on the remarkably disruptive symptom manifestations of psychosis.

The course of schizophrenia can be divided into two main phases, which occur in varying patterns across an individual's life: *(a)* acute symptom episodes and *(b)* periods of persistent disability. Acute symptom episodes are characterized by the emergence of, or a marked increase in, the positive symptoms of the disorder (delusions, hallucinations, bizarre behaviors, thought disorder). As currently defined in the Diagnostic and Statistical Manual of the American Psychiatric Association (DSM-III-R) (American Psychiatric Association, 1987), the diagnosis of schizophrenia requires at least one such episode. Persistent disability is a typical but not inevitable feature of schizophrenia and usually affects multiple areas of functioning: school, work, relationships, and self-care. The natural history of these two phases of the illness has been described in longitudinal studies of schizophrenia (Carpenter & Kirkpatrick, 1988; McGlashan, 1988). The variations range from the relatively benign—one acute episode accompanied by a temporary period of disability with return to essentially full functioning—to the extreme opposite—an insidious onset of functional disability and positive symptoms that persist over many years. Recommendations for the treatment of schizophrenia at the very least must encompass interventions appropriate to each of these phases of the illness.

Clinical Psychiatric Treatments

Typical clinical treatment for persons with chronic mental illnesses combines pharmacotherapy with psychological counseling. Pharmacotherapies that significantly reduce symptoms are available for all the major mental disorders and form the backbone of treatment for these disorders. As a rule of thumb, about two-thirds of patients with a chronic mental disorder will have a favorable initial symptom response to appropriate medication. The symptom response rates in the literature for antipsychotic medications, antidepressants, and antimanics (e.g., lithium) are all in the 65–70 percent range (Kaplan & Sadock, 1985).

In recent years, pharmacotherapeutic strategies have been developed for patients who do not respond to these conventional medications. For schizophrenia, new classes of antipsychotic drugs are being developed and are proving useful for treating patients who do not respond to the conventional antipsychotics (e.g., haloperidol [Haldol], fluphenazine [Prolixin], chlorpromazine [Thorazine], and thiothixene [Navane]). Examples of these novel antipsychotic drugs include clozapine, risperidone, and remoxipride. Approximately 30 percent of patients who do not respond to conventional antipsychotic drugs, for example, respond favorably to clozapine (Kane et al., 1988).

Symptom reduction is a major goal of clinical treatment for chronic mental disorders. These illnesses have devastating effects on an individual's self-esteem and morale, which may in part account for the high suicide rates among these patients, as high as 10 percent (Kaplan & Sadock, 1985). Furthermore, this demoralization contributes to poor compliance with treatment, thus creating a downward cycle. The main goals of psychological interventions for patients are to reduce demoralization, enhance the patient's capacity to cope with the illness, and improve self-esteem.

Psychological treatments include both individual and group therapies. Current practice emphasizes a supportive mode of counseling, which encompasses empathic listening, active problem solving around issues of everyday life, and education about the illness and treatment (Wasylenki, 1992). The theory underlying this approach is that chronic mental illness impairs the patient's capacity to relate to others and to recognize and cope with stresses, which may then result in relapse or other problems. The purpose of the therapeutic relationship is to offset these deficits with emotional support, practical advice and training about everyday life, and enduring contact with someone who is objective, yet who knows and cares about the patient. The supportive therapeutic relationship provides certain potential benefits, specifically, a context in which to educate the patient about schizophrenia, the role of medications, and the importance of recognizing early signs of relapse. It also provides a more individualized approach to pharmacotherapy, which in turn may yield better medication compliance and symptom control.

Support and practical advice can also help reduce the distress experienced by these patients in everyday life. Failure to deal effectively with such stresses can lead to symptom relapse. Thoughtful listening and suggestions from the therapist can enhance the patient's sense of hope and competence in the face of these problems. Patient education about the association of symptoms with stress and the importance of managing distress can improve the patient's sense of control and ability to cope.

A more specific and structured type of group treatment, developed in recent years, is "social skills training" (Anthony & Liberman 1986). Social skills training groups target the social disabilities that accompany chronic mental illness; the technique uses structured behavioral techniques, including role-playing, modeling, feedback, rehearsal, behavioral coaching, and rewards to enhance patients' skill levels. The types of skills taught vary widely and include communication skills (listening, processing, and sending), assertiveness skills, problem-solving skills, and skills related to specific activities of daily living (medication management, shopping, use of transportation, money management, leisure time activities, and use of community resources).

Family Interventions

During the past decade, various types of family interventions have been proposed, based upon the premise that families of persons with chronic mental illnesses need support, information, practical advice, and training in how to cope with the challenges posed by this illness (Anderson, Reiss, & Hogarty, 1986; McFarlane, 1983). These programs differ in their approach and characteristics, but share a common focus on educating the family about chronic mental illness and its treatment, and assisting in the resolution of family problems that arise because of the illness.

Rehabilitation

Over the past four decades, the locus of care for persons with chronic mental illness has shifted from the inpatient hospital setting to the community. The response has been an explosive growth of community-based psychosocial rehabilitation and support programs for these patients, including vocational rehabilitation services and psychosocial rehabilitation centers.

Programs to improve the work functioning of persons with mental illness have existed for a long time, dating back to the rural public asylums of the last century, which often included a farm on which patients worked. In more recent times, this concern about work opportunities and performance has translated into various types of vocational rehabilitation programs, which include hospital-based workshop programs, lodge programs with a focus on work, sheltered workshops, vocational counseling programs, job clubs, psychosocial clubhouse programs, and supportive employment. These programs can be subsumed under two general types: "train and place" programs and "place and train" programs.

The traditional "train and place" model, which includes all transitional and sheltered vocational rehabilitation programs, first assesses and trains the patient in general work habits and particular job skills. Individuals are assessed on work aptitudes and preferences, assisted in improving their work habits, and *trained* to do a certain kind of work. Once they have achieved a certain level of competence and consistent performance, they are *placed* at a regular job site. The advantages of this model are that it provides the opportunity to assess and work with people before they are exposed to the rigors of a real job setting. Its major shortcomings are that it may not adequately prepare patients for the transition from a sheltered rehabilitation center to the regular work world. For example, rehabilitation settings typically limit choices about types of work. Training also delays earning a wage.

In response to these problems, a new model of vocational rehabilitation has developed, the "place and train" model. Under this approach, people work with a vocational counselor to identify their vocational goals, the type of job they would prefer, and the fit with their abilities. Individuals are then *placed* at actual job sites and *trained* to do a specific job in a specific setting. Under this model, often known as "supported employment," the individual works with a job coach, who assists the patient in whatever way necessary to learn and keep the job. This approach is highly individualized, avoids the stressful transition from sheltered to unsheltered work settings, and allows a wage to be earned more quickly. Supported employment is costly, however, and it depends on the willingness of employers to participate in this type of on-the-job training for persons with disabilities.[1]

Housing

Housing services are perhaps one of the most important, yet least studied, aspects of psychosocial interventions for persons with chronic mental illness. Considerable variety characterizes the continuum of community residential care settings for persons with chronic mental illness, and the literature is replete with terminology for these settings. One general paradigm is the "linear continuum" of housing, under which patients move through a series of increasingly independent settings, including transitional halfway houses, long-term group residences, cooperative apartments, intensive care community residences, and board-and-care homes.

Because of a variety of problems with this linear continuum paradigm, a second major shift in housing for persons with chronic mental illness is now under way. The "paradigm of supported housing" (Ridgway & Zipple, 1990) emphasizes mainstream housing integrated fully into the community, with support services provided as needed but not on-site. Housing is not viewed as a treatment or service setting. Because this paradigm emphasizes individual choice and normalization of the patient's living environment, it has attracted considerable attention and advocacy throughout the country.

Integrating Services

Because persons with chronic mental illnesses need a complex array of services, considerable attention has been focused on how to best integrate these services. "Case management" now commands wide conceptual acceptance as an approach for organizing effective services for persons with chronic mental illness. A wide variety of possible activities have been subsumed under the term case management, including outreach, patient assessment, case planning, referral to service providers, advocacy for the patient, direct casework, development of natural support systems, reassessment, advocacy for resource development, quality monitoring, public education, and crisis intervention. Case management can be provided by individuals, teams, or systems. Great variability in the characterization and implementation of case management contributes to much of the ambiguity and confusion that exists in the field.

The best known example of an intensive model of clinical case management is assertive community treatment (Stein & Test, 1980). In a fourteen-month randomized study comparing hospital treatment plus standard aftercare with an innovative and assertive outreach- and community-based treatment program, the patients in the experimental program had lower rates of hospitalization, higher levels of functioning, and greater life satisfaction, with no differences in levels of family burden. Costs for the two programs were essentially equivalent. These results have been replicated elsewhere. Studies of other case management models, however, have produced mixed results (Olfson, 1990).

Together, these studies suggest that under the right circumstances, intensive case management can be highly effective in sustaining appropriately targeted patients with chronic mental illness in the community and enhancing their outcomes. However, case management is not an overall panacea. Major questions remain unanswered about which patients require this type of service, at what intensity, and at which stages in their illness.

Locus of Care

In this era of brief hospitalization, psychosocial treatments occur primarily in community-based settings, including clinics, private offices, day treatment programs, psychosocial rehabilitation centers, vocational rehabilitation centers, and residential care settings. Research on alternatives to long-term hospitalization for persons with chronic mental illness has shown no advantages to extended hospital care when community-based care is a feasible alternative (Braun et al., 1981). Even in the community, however, new pressure is growing to shift the locus of care yet again, from centers of treatment to mainstream community contexts, such as mobile treatment teams, home-based family counseling, "place-and-train" vocational services, and supported housing.

COMORBID CONDITIONS AND EFFECTS ON NEEDS AND SERVICE PATTERNS

Many people with schizophrenia and other mental illnesses suffer from other comorbid conditions that affect treatment needs and require additional efforts at service coordination and case management. As with other forms of disability, the impairments that accompany schizophrenia often lead to difficulties in negotiating service systems, including primary medical care.

Persons with schizophrenia suffer from the same range of medical conditions that affect the rest of the population. They may have reduced access to effective treatment, however, because their illness interferes with their ability to communicate and relate effectively to others, including health care providers. Other factors that may delay or inhibit seeking general medical care include resistance to seeking care, inability to pay, and hesitation among some health care providers to serve these individuals because of their behavior or appearance. An effective service system must take into account these barriers to general medical care, if the needs of these patients are to be met successfully.

Substance abuse is a particularly important comorbidity. Although estimates vary according to clinical settings, 25–50 percent of persons with schizophrenia may suffer from a comorbid substance use disorder (Regier et al., 1990). Substance abuse complicates accurate diagnosis, may reduce efficacy of treatments and treatment compliance, and is strongly related to relapse and rehospitalization (Turner & Tsuang, 1990). Two basic models are used for treating persons diagnosed with both schizo-phrenia and substance abuse: "integrated" and "parallel" programs. Integrated programs provide treatment for both the mental and substance use disorder within one agency (typically a mental health program), thus increasing the likelihood that treatments will be coordinated. Under the parallel program model, treatment for schizophrenia is provided in a mental health program, and the mental health treatment team seeks substance abuse treatment from another agency. This model is effective if the mental health treatment team is assertive about ensuring that the patient receives the substance abuse treatment, and if the substance abuse provider is comfortable with serving persons with comorbid severe mental disorders.

FACTORS AFFECTING ACCESS TO OR RECEIPT OF APPROPRIATE CARE

A range of factors can affect access to care and the appropriateness of the care provided. Factors expected to affect access to care include local availability of services, out-of-pocket payment (insurance coverage), perceived need for services, and the ability to navigate the mental health care system (e.g., arranging and keeping appointments). These factors and others, such as characteristics of the mental health provider (specialty, training, and pattern of practice), may affect whether the care received is appropriate.

Availability

The availability of services varies widely. Psychiatrists are poorly distributed geographically, although psychiatric nurses and social workers who provide a great deal of the care are better distributed. No estimates are available of areas that are "underserved" in terms of specialty mental health providers or services.

In a national sample of members of the National Alliance for the Mentally Ill (NAMI), family members reported that many types of services were not available. For example, one-third of those who tried to find a program to assist with training in daily living skills were unable to find one. About one-fifth of those seeking a structured day program and half of those seeking a structured weekend program were unsuccessful in locating a program in their area (NAMI Family Survey, unpublished data,

1990; Steinwachs, Kasper, & Skinner, 1992).[2] Because NAMI members are often active advocates for services for their relatives with mental illness, the experience of the NAMI population may represent a "best case" in services for severe mental illness.

Financial Barriers

Even when services are available, financial barriers may restrict access to care. Private insurance usually provides coverage for clinical care, but it may place restrictive limits on number of services and total expenditures per year or impose higher copayments or deductibles on the user of mental health services. Even if clinical care is fully covered, rehabilitative services, case management, housing assistance, and family support services may not be. Thus, private insurance rarely provides sufficiently broad coverage to ensure access to the full range of services needed by those who are disabled by mental illness.

Medicare coverage for mental illness is not substantially better than private insurance, although it has been improved over time to provide better coverage for medical management of psychiatric disorders. Individuals disabled by mental illness who qualify for Medicare through Social Security Disability Insurance (SSDI) eligibility (after a two-year waiting period) are still not adequately covered for the range of services needed.

Possibly the most comprehensive coverage for mental health services is provided by Medicaid. During the 1980s, legislation was passed allowing states to expand Medicaid coverage to cover home and community-based services and to pay for case management. The result has been an expansion of covered services in many states to include psychosocial rehabilitation, case management, crisis care, and personal care services. Not all states have exercised the available waivers and options, however, and even in states with expanded coverage, service availability may be limited by rates of reimbursement, availability of providers, and program eligibility.

In summary, financial barriers caused by inadequate insurance coverage are key factors in restricting access to needed services. For those who lack coverage and who cannot afford to pay out-of-pocket, the only source of care is the public sector, including services funded by state and county revenues and by the Department of Veterans' Affairs, for those eligible.

Public Sector Services

Publicly supported services are likely to be the only source of psychosocial rehabilitation, job training, housing assistance, and case management services for those who are uninsured or inadequately insured, excluding persons with Medicaid coverage. States and communities show wide variability in the levels of support for public services and in the scope of services available through public systems. In 1988, estimates of per capita expenditures for state and county mental hospitals ranged from $7 per capita in Arkansas to $89 in New York State; and for freestanding psychiatric outpatient clinics, from $.11 in North Carolina and Colorado to $9 in Wyoming and $10 in Alaska. Total state mental health spending per capita ranged from a high of $174 in Massachusetts and $173 in New York to a low of $45 in Idaho and $49 in Mississippi (Center for Mental Health Services and National Institute of Mental Health, 1992). The best-funded public systems are generally well integrated, provide a wide range of services, and have high participation rates by those who have severe mental illnesses. A well-integrated system of care ideally has

- a "single point of entry";
- a comprehensive array of services under one administrative roof (those enumerated in the preceding section on Needs and Service Patterns);
- a commitment to addressing all the patient's needs (rather than "carving out" a narrow range of service responsibilities);
- a long-term commitment to serving the patient;
- an emphasis on individualized care that addresses needs identified by the patient and the patient's family as well as the treatment team;
- flexibility in the delivery of services, in particular, the capacity to bring services to the patients when needed; and
- a "team approach" that permits sharing of service burden by an interdisciplinary team.

In practice, few service systems achieve all of these goals, but the better ones *(a)* have at least a single point of ongoing responsibility for the patient within the system, *(b)* provide continuity of care across service system components, and *(c)* offer flexible services designed to address individual needs.

Acceptance by Consumers

Considerable anecdotal experience supports the observation that services designed to meet specific needs are not acceptable to all individuals who could benefit from them. In the NAMI survey, families reported that one reason services were not sought or received was that the family member with mental illness (the "consumer") refused the services. For example, about 30 percent of the respondents identified the consumer's anticipated refusal as the reason they did not look for a structured day program. Similarly, family members reported that 20 percent of the consumers who needed assistance or supervision in taking medications refused help. This issue appears to be increasingly important, and it affects the capability of the service system, whether public or private, to achieve a high level of participation and maintain continuity of care.

Disability Policies

Many people with severe mental illness qualify for disability income and health insurance benefits under SSDI or Supplemental Security Income (SSI), and some qualify under both. SSDI is for persons who have become disabled and who meet work history criteria based on Social Security contributions, while SSI covers low-income persons with a disability. Together, they are the major federal programs providing income assistance to persons with disability. Patients with cognitive impairments, including severe mental illness, typically need assistance to complete the application processes for these entitlements. In addition, many who meet the disability criteria are unable to meet the work history requirement for SSDI.

Disability coverage is reviewed and renewed every three years and can be lost if the individual is no longer totally disabled. As a result, job training and job skills may be viewed as a threat to secure sources of disability income and health insurance. Many individuals with mental illness may avoid "productive activities" rather than incur the risk of losing disability coverage. In the NAMI survey, about 40 percent had SSDI coverage, 38 percent qualified under SSI, and 15 percent were covered under both programs because of a brief work history and low SSDI income payments. Coverage reported in this survey is thought to be higher than the national average, reflecting the advocacy of NAMI families for their relatives with mental illness. Whether lack of work force participation and other productive activities is influenced primarily by the absence of appropriate services or by the disincentives of disability program eligibility criteria is difficult to discern and is an issue that deserves more attention.

Patterns of Practice

There are wide variations in patterns of care for individuals with severe mental illness, such as schizophrenia. How much of the variation relates to the availability of services, to single-specialty orientation, to insurance coverage, or to other factors is not known. The Schizophrenia Patient Outcomes Research Team (PORT), funded by the Agency for Health Care Policy and Research (AHCPR) and the National Institute of Mental Health (NIMH), is expected to provide new information about the relationship of these practice patterns to variations in outcomes.[3] The PORT is moving through four stages over a five-year period: *(a)* a comprehensive literature review of treatment approaches; *(b)* an analysis of Medicaid and Medicare claims data to examine practice variations; *(c)* interviews with a two-state sample of persons with a diagnosis of schizophrenia to provide data for analysis of patient outcomes; and *(d)* development of treatment recommendations and dissemination to service providers.

Attributes of System Failure

When service systems fail for persons with schizophrenia, a wide variety of adverse outcomes may ensue. Failure to address needs or serious fragmentation of service can damage the treatment alliance with patients and their families, leading to an undue sense of burden and alienation. Such stresses, often combined with the system's failure to deliver critical treatments or noncompliance with treatment, can result in relapse and unnecessary emergency room visits and hospitalizations. Even worse, extreme system failures too often lead to homelessness, incarceration for minor crimes related to psychosis, and suicide (about 10 percent of persons with schizophrenia commit suicide).

The ideal point of entry to the system for persons with schizophrenia is a mental health clinic. In reality, however, these individuals are often only, or primarily, in contact with the police, an emergency room, or a homeless shelter. Contacts with health, social, and legal institutions should lead to treatment in appropriate clinical settings in the community and not to inappropriate alternatives, such as jail or wandering the streets.

Because of the multiplicity of service needs for individuals with severe mental illness, funding sources and service agencies are fragmented, which leads to numerous possibilities for system failure. Even for those receiving treatment, systems of care meet some needs very well and others minimally or not at all. In the NAMI survey, family members reported high levels of assistance with crisis care and keeping appointments with mental health professionals, services that fall principally into the clinical treatment area. Services that addressed needs for assistance with community living skills were less adequate, and services to assist with managing relationships or engaging in productive activity were not meeting the substantial needs reported in these areas. The composite is a very uneven level of system performance.

DATA SOURCES AND INDICATORS

Indicators of adequacy of care for people with severe mental illness should address three major concerns.

- Are those who need care receiving care?
- What is the process of care for those receiving care?
- How does the process of care relate to outcomes?

The first task is to identify key indicators of system performance in the areas of *(a)* access to care, *(b)* process of care, and *(c)* outcomes of care for persons with severe mental illness. These should be selected for their usefulness to policymakers, program administrators, clinicians, and consumers in tracking the performance of community care systems. Once indicators have been selected, their development and feasibility will depend on the availability of appropriate data sources.

For each of the three areas of performance, Table 8.1 provides the population of interest, key indicators, and sources of information needed to develop and monitor these indicators. The overall purpose of these indicators would be to reflect the success of the population with severe mental illness in gaining access to care, as well as in receiving appropriate and effective treatment. The discussion that follows is organized around development of the indicators in Table 8.1.

Table 8.1. Indicators of the Adequacy of Care for Severe Mental Illness *(Schizophrenia)*

Access to care

Indicators	% of individuals with a severe mental illness currently receiving care from a mental health specialty provider
	% of individuals with a severe mental illness identifying a usual source of care
Population	All persons with severe mental illness (e.g., schizophrenia)
Source of information	Individuals identified as cases based on provider records or claims data or through a population survey (alternatively family members of these individuals)

Process of care

Indicators	Mix and type of services received (e.g., medications, counseling, case management, psychosocial rehabilitaion, special housing, vocational training)
	Rates of use of inpatient and emergency services
	Continuity of care over time
Population	Persons in treatment
Source of information	Claims data from programs such as Medicaid or provider records (this information could also be obtained from patients/family members)

Outcomes of care

Indicators of treatment outcomes	Unmet needs for care and assistance
	Clinical symptoms
	Satisfaction with care
	Daily functioning
	Quality of life
	Violence (violent acts, victim of violent acts)
	Suicide (threats/attempts)
	Arrests
	Homelessness
Population	Persons in treatment
Source of information	Patient/family
Indicators of system failure	Suicide
	Arrests of people with severe mental illness
	Rehospitalizations (adverse outcome)
	Tenure in the community (brief tenure is adverse outcome)
Population	All persons with severe mental illness
Source of information	Multiple including claims/records or patient/family

Indicators of Access to Care

A major indicator of access to care is the proportion of persons with severe mental illness who are receiving specialty mental health services. Access to outpatient or community-based care is of most interest because it has the potential for maintaining people in the community. A second indicator that could be expected to reflect access to and patterns of use of psychiatric care is whether persons with severe mental illness report a usual source of outpatient psychiatric care.

Developing access indicators presents difficulties primarily because a prevalence estimate of severe mental illness in the population at large is needed. Users of services can often be identified through provider or payment record systems, but determining what proportion they represent of those who need services (the denominator population) is much more difficult. Some prevalence estimates of severe mental illness overall and by specific diagnoses have been developed from national data (Barker et al., 1992; Regier et al., 1984), and they provide a rough guide that could be used at the community level to estimate the size of the population in need (e.g., rates per 100,000 population of persons with schizophrenia or other severe mental illness). Basic demographic data, such as age and race or ethnic group, which are available from national data, could also be used to develop more-targeted estimates of expected prevalence within subgroups, against which users' rates could be evaluated. In many instances, estimates based on national data will not accurately reflect the specific characteristics of communities, such as rural/urban or socioeconomic mix, making the applicability of prevalence estimates developed from national data problematic. Nonetheless, large differences between synthetic prevalence estimates and the population under treatment could serve as an indicator of poor access to service.

Substantial progress has been made in developing reliable and valid indicators of severe mental illness for use in sample surveys, but identifying psychiatric disorders through lay interviewing techniques, as opposed to clinical evaluation, remains problematic. Recent promising efforts to develop approaches for identifying people with severe mental illness in community populations include the use of a combination of self-reported functional status measures and psychiatric diagnoses in a supplement to the National Health Interview Survey[4] (NHIS) (Barker et al., 1992) and diagnostic instruments developed for community epidemiological studies (Regier et al., 1984; Robins et al., 1981; Robins et al.,

1988). These types of approaches are clearly needed to identify the population for whom to develop indicators of adequacy of care; however, they are not inexpensive or simple to administer. An additional obstacle is the low prevalence of severe mental illness, which requires screening large numbers of people to find cases and establish prevalence rates. The cost and difficulty of undertaking detailed prevalence studies may make them impractical for many communities.

Characteristics of access, including having a usual source of outpatient mental health care, are best obtained through the direct report of consumers or close family members or friends. Developing data of this type, particularly systematic, routinely collected data, presents challenges at the community level because of the resources required to collect the information. One approach may be to focus on persons identified through contact with the service system, recognizing that this provides information on the characteristics of access arrangements for individuals who have been able to obtain some services.

Indicators of Process of Care

Over the years, the national reporting program for mental health statistics (Redick et al., 1986) has been a major source of statistics on mental health services provided in the United States. Indicators of types of services received (primarily inpatient stays and outpatient volume), rates of service use, and expenditures for services, at the state and national level, are available in *Mental Health United States* and other publications (Center for Mental Health Services and National Institute of Mental Health, 1992). These data are obtained through providers of mental health services, and they reflect provider characteristics (e.g., staffing, services provided) and patient information that is available at the provider level, including volume of use by site of care (Annual Census of Patient Characteristics),[5] and person-level clinical and service information (Longitudinal Client Sample Survey of Outpatient Programs). Because these data are national in scope, they are a good source of process indicators of care to those with severe mental illness; and because they have been collected on a continuing basis, they enable observation of trends. Numbers of psychiatric inpatient stays, for example, can be tracked over the past thirty years. In addition, these data are available at the state level, and some states can provide data for small areas within the state.

The major limitation of the national reporting system is that it provides only partial coverage of the mental health service system. Inpatient care from both public and private sector providers is included, resulting in almost complete coverage of inpatient services in the United States. On the outpatient side, however, only public-sector providers participate in reporting data on services provided. Also missing from the national reporting system are services provided in settings that do not specialize in mental illness treatment, as well as nontraditional community care settings, such as group homes or clubhouses.

Process indicators reflect the experience of persons in treatment, and many can be developed from facility records or claims data. For important segments of the population with severe mental illness, such as those with Medicaid coverage, indicators of the mix and type of services used (including specific services such as inpatient or emergency care) can be constructed from claims data. Inpatient and emergency care are high-cost care and could be viewed as indicators of system failure (e.g., emergency room care for crisis management). States are becoming increasingly adept at using Medicaid claims to evaluate Medicaid program performance, and the Health Care Financing Administration (HCFA) is now developing a national capacity for analyzing Medicaid experience. However, Medicaid claims and national reporting system data largely reflect experience with care in the public sector. Assessing processes of care for consumers in the private sector is more difficult at both the community and national levels, because private insurance claims and private provider records are generally less accessible for evaluation.

More-sophisticated process indicators, such as continuity of care, present a different challenge. Continuity-of-care indicators require a data system in which users can be tracked over time so that gaps in treatment or patterns of inappropriate care can be identified. This may be beyond the capabilities of many communities, although state information systems, including Medicaid, can be developed for this purpose.

Outcomes of Care

While process indicators are useful, particularly in raising questions about variability in service use, they are inadequate for evaluating adequacy of care unless they are linked to outcomes. Several outcomes are proposed in Table 8.1 for inclusion in a community-based system of indicators of adequacy of care. Clinical outcomes include symptom control and avoidance of hospitalization for acute psychiatric crises. Employment status and daily functioning, including performance of tasks needed for independent living, are indicators of the success of the service system in helping people engage in routine activities appropriate to their age and interests. Quality-of-life measurement represents an effort to reflect, in a systematic way, whether services and treatment for mental illness meet the expectations and preferences of consumers. Indicators of system failure can be assessed through rates of suicide, violence, and homelessness. These would probably prove difficult to tie to specific treatment approaches and are certain to be influenced by factors outside the mental health service system; nevertheless, they are likely to be useful indicators of overall adequacy of response to the needs of people with severe mental illness.

Indicators of outcomes of care will usually require information that comes from direct report of consumers and/or family members. Other sources of information may be available for indicators of system failure and perhaps employment status, but assessments of quality of life and daily functioning, as outcomes of specialty mental health treatment, require the consumer's perspective.

RECOMMENDATIONS AND CONCLUSIONS

The complexity involved in developing sensitive and specific indicators of the adequacy of care to individuals with severe mental illness is apparent. Community-based data on people with severe mental illness are critical to efforts to develop indicators of adequacy of care. Not only is existing information limited, but past efforts to assess the adequacy of community care have generally excluded important population subgroups, such as children, homeless people, and prison populations. Gaining access to the homeless and prison populations is difficult, and these individuals are either not identifiable or absent from many routinely used sources of data (e.g., national household surveys, Medicaid claims). Case identification and definitions of mental health services (e.g., school-based counseling) have proven problematic with regard to children, and both are important objectives of the effort under way to conduct an Epidemiology Catchment Area (ECA) study among children.

Even though the challenge is formidable, using a range of data sources to develop fundamental access and process-of-care indicators is feasible. Routine data sources, including claims and administrative data, can provide indicators of access and process for important segments of the population with severe mental illness, but not for all. Medicaid data, for example, provide the opportunity to develop both national and state-specific indicators for individuals with this coverage, although only for those currently in treatment.

The primary problems in relying on existing data sources are that they do not include all segments of the population with severe mental illness and that they lack sensitive indicators of patient outcomes, including quality of life. This information can only be obtained through patient/family interviews.

Strategies are beginning to be tested for developing improved indicators. Steinwachs and Lehman are currently sampling individuals with severe mental illness (using Maryland Medicaid data) and conducting interviews with these individuals in the community. The project will test *(a)* the ability to identify persons with severe mental illness by use of Medicaid enrollment and claims data; *(b)* the utility of Medicaid data for describing the pattern of treatment the individual is receiving; and *(c)* the relationship between pattern of treatment documented in Medicaid claims and patient-reported outcomes, including quality of life, satisfaction, symptom status, and overall health status. This may lead to a model that provides indicators on a significant group of individuals with severe mental illnesses.

The survey of family members conducted in collaboration with NAMI represents another model for tracking indicators. The population has greater breadth than the Medicaid population, but membership in a voluntary organization suggests a select group. The sample includes persons with severe mental illness living with family members who are interested in participating in an advocacy group. NAMI chapters at the state and community level could serve as a sampling frame, as could provider-specific patient populations. To serve as the basis for indicator development, surveys of patients and family members would need to be undertaken on an ongoing basis, probably annually. Decisions would need to be made as well about the information value and costs of cross-sectional versus longitudinal surveys.

The ongoing refinement of health care purchasing practices through either public or private payers suggests that the use of claims/administrative data for practice monitoring and quality assurance will increase. A "report card" for severe mental illness can be envisioned, one that combines measures of access, treatment, and patient-reported outcomes. It is not yet clear, however, which specific access, process, and outcome measures should be obtained routinely to evaluate the effectiveness and efficiency of services and systems caring for persons with severe mental illness.

Even if the nation were to move toward universal health care coverage (or less ambitiously, expanded eligibility for Medicaid), some components of the care of persons with severe mental illnesses would likely lie outside what is usually defined as a health insurance benefit. These include housing services, job training, and some of the long-term care services needed by individuals with a disability living in the community. Furthermore, mental health benefits are expected to be capped, at least initially, which will result in services needed by those with the most severe mental illness being covered for only part of each year. This will pose additional problems in assessing the adequacy of care and patient outcomes for persons with severe mental illness.

The health care reform debate of the 1990s demonstrated the role of information in health policy formulation. At the same time, unfortunately, it has revealed how little is known about access, treatment, patient outcomes, and the overall effectiveness of the health care system. This experience should lead to a new understanding of the need for a dynamic and synergistic process in which health policy provides a framework for defining information needs. As new information is developed from research and evaluation efforts, it can be used by policymakers to refine and/or modify health policy. The objective is to provide accessible, high quality, and efficient systems of care to meet the health needs of all Americans.

Notes

1. At least four organized models of psychosocial rehabilitation can be identified: the Fountain House Clubhouse model, the Fairweather Lodge, the Boston University model, and the UCLA Social Skills Training model (Anthony & Liberman, 1986). Founded in 1948 in New York City, Fountain House, one of oldest and best known psychosocial rehabilitation programs in the United States, seeks to enhance patients' sense of hope and competence. The Fairweather Lodge model began during the 1960s as a response to the problem of recidivism among patients discharged from the hospital. Small groups of patients in the hospital are taught daily living, coping, and work skills and are encouraged to function as semiautonomous groups, fostering mutual responsibility and learning the skills necessary to live in the community. When ready, the group moves together into a community lodge with a homelike setting, where they function essentially as a family. The latter two programs emphasize behavioral and social learning theories to teach patients social and community-living skills.

2. The NAMI survey interviewed a nationally representative sample of individuals belonging to the advocacy organization, which claims a national membership of about fifty-nine thousand people. An 81% response rate was achieved, providing information from 1,401 family members about the characteristics, needs, and unmet needs for assistance of their family member with mental illness. A more detailed description of the study is provided in Steinwachs, Kasper, and Skinner, 1992. The study was conducted by the Center on the Organization and Financing of Care for the Severely Mentally Ill with funding through a grant from the John D. and Catherine T. MacArthur Foundation to NAMI.

3. The Schizophrenia PORT is a joint undertaking of the University of Maryland School of Medicine and the Johns Hopkins University School of Hygiene and Public Health (principal investigator is A. F. Lehman, M.D., at the University of Maryland).

4. See appendix A for a listing of all NCHS data sets referred to in this chapter.

5. See appendix C for a listing of all governmental and nongovernmental data sets referred to in this chapter.

References

American Psychiatric Association. 1987. *DSM-III-R: Diagnostic and Statistical Manual of Mental Disorders.* Washington, D.C.: American Psychiatric Association.

Anderson, C. M., Reiss, D. J., & Hogarty, G. E. 1986. *Chronic Mental Illness and the Family.* New York: Guilford Press.

Anthony, W. A., & Liberman, R. P. 1986. The practice of psychiatric rehabilitation: historical, conceptual, and research base. *Chronic Mental Illness Bulletin* 12: 542–59.

Barker, P. R., Manderscheid, R. W., Hendershot, G. E., Jack, S. S., Schoenborn, C. A., & Goldstrom, I. 1992. *Serious Mental Illness and Disability in the Adult Household Population: United States, 1989.* Advance Data from Vital and Health Statistics: no. 218. Hyattsville, Md.: National Center for Health Statistics.

Braun, P., Kochansky, G., Shapiro, R., Greenberg, S., Gudeman, J. E., Johnson, S., & Shor, M. F. 1981. Overview: Deinstitutionalization of psychiatric patients, a critical review of outcome studies. *American Journal of Psychiatry* 138: 736–49.

Carpenter, W. T., & Heinrichs, D. W. 1981. Treatment relevant subtypes of schizophrenia. *Journal of Nervous and Mental Disease 169:* 113–19.

Carpenter, W. T., & Kirkpatrick, B. 1988. The heterogeneity of the long-term course of schizophrenia. *Schizophrenia Bulletin 14:* 645–52.

Center for Mental Health Services and National Institute of Mental Health. 1992. *Mental Health United States* (DHHS Publ. no. SMA 92–1942). Washington, D.C.: U.S. Government Printing Office.

Faris, R. E. L., & Dunham, H. W. 1939. *Mental Disorders in Urban Areas.* Chicago: University of Chicago Press.

Group for the Advancement of Psychiatry. 1992. *Beyond Symptom Suppression:*

Improving Long-Term Outcomes of Schizophrenia. Washington, D.C.: American Psychiatric Press.

Kane, J., Honigfeld, G., Singer, J., McItzer, H., and the Clozaril Collaborative Study Group. 1988. Clozapine for the treatment-resistant schizophrenic. *Archives of General Psychiatry 45:* 789–96.

Kaplan, H. I., & Sadock, B. J. 1985. *Comprehensive Textbook of Psychiatry/IV.* Baltimore: Williams and Wilkins.

McFarlane, W. R. (ed.). 1983. *Family Therapy in Chronic Mental Illness.* New York: Guilford.

McGlashan, T. H. 1988. A selective review of recent North American long-term follow-up studies of schizophrenia. *Schizophrenia Bulletin 14:* 515–42.

Olfson, M. 1990. Assertive community treatment: An evaluation of the experimental evidence. *Hospital and Community Psychiatry 41:* 634–41.

Redick, R. W., Manderscheid, R. W., Witkin, M. J., & Rosenstein, M. J. 1986. *A History of the U.S. National Reporting Program for Mental Health Statistics 1840–1983* (DHHS Publ. no. ADM 86–1296). Washington, D.C.: U.S. Government Printing Office.

Regier, D. A., Myers, J. K., Kramer, M., Robins, L. N., Blazer, D. G., Hough, R. L., Eaton, W. W., & Locke, B. Z. 1984. The NIMH Epidemiologic Catchment Area Program. *Archives of General Psychiatry 41:* 934–41.

Regier, D. A., Farmer, M. E., Rae, D. S., Locke, B. Z., Keith, S. J., Judd, L. L., & Goodwin, F. K. 1990. Comorbidity of mental disorders with alcohol and other drug abuse. *Journal of the American Medical Association 264:* 2511–18.

Rice, D. P., & Miller, L. S. 1996. The economic burden of schizophrenia: conceptual and methodological issues, and cost estimates. In M. Moscarelli, A. Rupp, & N. Sartorius (eds.), *Schizophrenia: Handbook of Mental Health Economics and Health Policy.* Vol. 1 (pp. 321–34). New York: John Wiley & Sons.

Ridgway, P., & Zipple, A. M. 1990. The paradigm shift in residential services: From the linear continuum to supported housing approaches. *Psychosocial Rehabilitation Journal 13:* 11–31.

Robins, L. N., Helzer, J. E., Croughan, J., Williams, J. B. W., & Spitzer, R. L. 1981. *NIMH Diagnostic Interview Schedule: Version III.* Rockville, Md.: National Institute of Mental Health.

Robins, L. N., Wing, J., Wittchen, H. U., Helzer, J. E., Babor, T. F., Burke, J., Farmer, A., Jablenski, A., Pickens R., Regier, D. A., et al. 1988. The Composite International Diagnostic Interview: An epidemiological instrument suitable for use in conjunction with different diagnostic systems and in different cultures. *Archives of General Psychiatry 45:* 1069–77.

Srole, L., Langner, T. S., Michale, S. T., Kirkpatrick, P., Opler, M. K., & Rennie, T. A. C. 1962. *Mental Health in the Metropolis.* New York: McGraw-Hill.

Stein, L., & Test, M. A. 1980. An alternative to mental hospital treatment I: Conceptual model, treatment program, and clinical evaluation. *Archives of General Psychiatry 37:* 392–97.

Steinwachs, D. M., Kasper, J. D., & Skinner, E. A. 1992. *Family Perspectives on Meeting the Needs for Care of Severely Mentally Ill Relatives: A National Survey.* Final Report to NAMI.

Turner, W. M., & Tsuang, M. T. 1990. Impact of substance abuse on the course and outcome of schizophrenia. *Schizophrenia Bulletin 16:* 87–95.

Wasylenki, D. A. 1992. Psychotherapy of chronic mental illness revisited. *Hospital and Community Psychiatry 43:* 123–27.

Zubin, J., & Spring, B. 1977. Vulnerability: A new view of chronic mental illness. *Journal of Abnormal Psychology 86:* 103–26.

9/ CHRONIC ALCOHOL AND DRUG ABUSE

Constance Weisner

While the overall prevalence of alcohol and drug use has decreased over the past ten years, the decrease has not been consistent across population subgroups and geographical areas (Harrison, 1992; Midanik & Clark, 1994). Evidence suggests that many who continue to abuse alcohol and drugs are diagnostically complex multiple substance users for whom morbidity and mortality consequences are severe (Hubbard, 1990; Tims, Fletcher, & Hubbard, 1991). Clients in treatment for opiate addiction, for example, have a mortality rate seven times higher than that of a general population sample of comparable age, and heavy alcohol consumption is the strongest predictor of death (Joe & Simpson, 1990). Further, the ninth leading cause of death in the late 1980s was chronic liver disease and cirrhosis (the main chronic health hazard associated with alcohol abuse), which caused more than twenty-six thousand deaths in 1989 (National Center for Health Statistics, 1992).

Thus, the physical and social costs of alcohol and drug problems to society are high. Data synthesized from several studies show that over 25 percent of U.S. deaths each year are associated with alcohol, drug, or tobacco use (Horgan, 1996); in 1988, the total cost to the United States for alcohol abuse was estimated to be $99 billion and for drug abuse, $67 billion (Rice, Kelman, & Miller, 1991). While substantial costs are attributable to chronic substance problems, a large share is related to episodic and short-term alcohol and drug use (Rice, Kelman, & Miller, 1991). Treatment is often directed toward the nonchronic population, which may indicate that chronic substance abusers are not well served in the treatment system.

The purpose of this chapter is to establish a conceptual framework for identifying indicators of community responsiveness to chronic alcohol and drug abuse. It addresses the following specific areas: *(a)* epidemiology and prevalence of chronic alcohol and drug abuse; *(b)* the selection of conditions representing chronicity; *(c)* the service needs of individuals with chronic drug problems; *(d)* the issues affecting service systems; and *(e)* data sources and indicators of chronic drug abuse and service monitoring.

In addressing these general topics, several issues require clarification. First, the concept of chronicity has not been adequately defined or operationalized in the alcohol and drug fields. Second, changes in the epidemiological description of alcohol and drug use, particularly a higher prevalence of polydrug abuse, have resulted in a more diagnostically complex substance abuse population. Third, chronic alcohol and drug abuse is often dealt with outside the medical care system, for example, in voluntary organizations such as Alcoholics Anonymous (AA) or in the criminal justice system.

EPIDEMIOLOGY AND PREVALENCE OF CHRONIC ALCOHOL AND DRUG ABUSE

While the alcohol and drug epidemiological and clinical literatures assume alcohol and drug abuse to be chronic conditions (Gerstein & Harwood, 1990; Institute of Medicine, 1990; Simpson, 1990; Taylor & Helzer, 1983; U.S. National Institute on Alcohol Abuse and Alcoholism, 1990; U.S. National Institute on Drug Abuse, 1991), neither field has fully operationalized the concept of chronicity or adequately addressed chronic patients as a special subpopulation. Statistics on clinical populations do not accurately reflect chronicity, since this population is not the only one targeted for treatment. The recent public health approach to alcohol-abuse treatment and prevention has emphasized episodic and transient alcohol "problems" rather than the more serious, long-term condition of "dependence" (IOM, 1990). While this is considered an important development, it has raised concern that chronic patients may not receive sufficient services. A recent Institute of Medicine (IOM) report on alcohol treatment officially advocated an emphasis on this problem-drinking population, characterizing those with "severe, chronic alcohol problems" as representing only about 5 percent of the problem-drinking population in need of some intervention (IOM, 1990). Regarding other drugs, little attention has been paid, in either studies or clinical practice, to distinguishing drug use from problematic or chronic use (Jones & Battjes, 1985).

Moreover, the broad condition of abuse and dependence cannot be defined accurately as chronic, in that a relatively large number of those who are dependent on alcohol or drugs at any given time will experience partial or complete remission (Jones & Battjes, 1985; Kandel & Yamaguchi, 1985; Roizen, Cahalan, & Shanks, 1978; Simpson, 1990). Numerous longitudinal surveys of the general population show individuals "maturing out" of alcohol problem status (Fillmore & Midanik, 1984; Roizen et al., 1978; Vaillant, 1983; Wilsnack et al., 1991). Similarly, the National Institute on Drug Abuse (NIDA) Report to Congress summarized the literature by stating that while many people experiment with drugs, few continue using them over time (U.S. NIDA, 1991). Thus, both the alcohol and drug literatures describe a chronic, relapsing condition with a great variety of trajectories in its "natural history," with improvement and recovery occurring in both treated and untreated segments of the population.

Measures of Chronicity

Given the lack of a clear delineation of chronicity, the following can serve as indirect measures to assess prevalence: alcohol and drug dependence, length of time in which alcohol and drug users remain in problem or dependence status, drug or alcohol use persisting from adolescence into adulthood, and chronic medical conditions stemming from alcohol and drug use. Indicators of these measures are not consistently available for both alcohol and drugs.

Alcohol and Drug Dependence

"Dependence" is typically used to assess the prevalence and severity of alcohol and drug problems. The diagnosis, however, does not refer to chronicity; it is made by counting three or more symptoms within a specified period, rather than emphasizing duration of symptoms over time. The Diagnostic and Statistical Manual of the American Psychiatric Association (DSM-III-R and the DSM-IV revision) (American Psychiatric Association, 1987) gives diagnoses of dependence by alcohol and drug type as well as for polysubstance use.[1]

As a diagnostic category, existing measures of dependence lack a temporal definition; variations caused by measuring different time frames and using diverse instruments have resulted in a range of prevalence estimates. Table 9.1 presents prevalence data from the Epidemiologic Catchment Area (ECA) studies, weighted to approximate a national estimate.

Table 9.1. Prevalence of Alcohol and Drug Dependence

Study	Criteria	Alcohol Dependence	Drug Dependence	Age
National Alcohol Survey	DSM-III-R dependence, 12-month rate	3.9%	NA	18+
	DSM-III-R dependence, 12-month rate	3.2%[1]	NA	
Epidemiologic Catchment Area	DSM-III-R dependence, 6-month rate	2.8%[2]	1.5%[2]	18+
		Any alcohol disorder	*Any drug disorder*	
		7.4%[2]	3.1%[2]	18+

Note: NA means that data were not available.
1. Caetano & Room, 1993 (data from 1990 general population survey).
2. Regier et al., 1990 (data from five ECA sites).

The studies are among the few to report both alcohol and drug dependence, with six-month rates of 2.8 percent for alcohol dependence and 1.5 percent for drug dependence using the Diagnostic Interview Survey (DIS) (Regier et al., 1990). Other studies include the Alcohol Research Group's (ARG) 1990 national survey, which used sets of measures based on DSM-III-R and DSM-IV criteria and found the prevalence of alcohol dependence to be 3.2 percent and 3.9 percent, respectively, for the general adult population in the United States. These rates differ because the latter study used a twelve-month time frame and different measurement instruments.

Within a dependence framework, individuals can be classified across a range of degrees of severity (Caetano, 1993; Gerstein & Harwood, 1990; Hasin & Glick, 1992; Woody, Cottler, & Cacciola, 1993). There is some indication that severity is associated with duration of symptoms and thus with chronicity, but this has not been thoroughly examined. The eight-year longitudinal follow-up of the ARG's national survey found that of those reporting five (out of nine) dependence symptoms in 1984, 56 percent still met dependence criteria in 1992; while of those reporting three to four symptoms, only 34 percent still met dependence criteria at the follow-up (unpublished data). Thus, for the purposes of assessing chronicity, the prevalence of severe cases can provide an approximate estimate.

Some extrapolations of need for treatment have been made using general population studies. NIDA's Household Survey data on frequency of consumption were used to estimate that 1.5 million individuals (or 0.7 percent) aged twelve or over were in "clear need" of drug treatment (Gerstein & Harwood, 1990). This figure comprises about 34 percent of those who reported using a drug in the previous month, but it is unclear what proportion of this number represents acute, as opposed to chronic, cases.

Differences exist in rates of problematic alcohol and drug use and dependence for men and women (Ferrence, 1980; U.S. NIDA, 1991; Weisner & Schmidt, 1992; Wilsnack et al., 1991). Table 9.2 shows general population rates of dependence according to DSM-IV criteria by sociodemographic characteristics. Men's rates are almost three times higher than women's. Data on dependence for drugs other than alcohol are not as readily available. One of the major gender differences in the drug field has to do with the type of drug used. NIDA's 1988 Household Survey found the population of lifetime intravenous drug users to be 27 percent women and 72 percent men; however, current nonmedical use of psycho-therapeutic drugs was higher for women than men (2 vs. 1.4 percent) (U.S. NIDA, 1991). Women's treatment needs often differ from men's, particularly because of higher rates of childhood sexual and physical abuse, and fewer economic resources and social supports (De Leon & Jainchill, 1981–82; Reed, 1987; Weisner, 1993). Dependence also differs by age. Individuals under age thirty have higher rates of dependence than older age groups (Table 9.2). This is the case for rates of drug use as well (U.S. NIDA, 1991). Prevalence rates of dependence among minority groups are higher than for whites (Table 9.2).

When ethnicity is examined, results are again confounded by age and gender (Anglin et al., 1988; Herd, 1988). Rates of abstention and prob-lems for African Americans vary by gender (with men reporting higher rates) and type of drug use (McNagny & Parker, 1992; U.S. NIAAA, 1990; U.S. NIDA, 1991). Studies of Hispanic populations have found similar important differences by gender and type of drug (De La Rosa, Khalsa, & Rouse, 1990). For example, use of illegal drugs and use of drug treatment facilities vary widely with the type of drug used, across and within Hispanic subgroups (De La Rosa et al., 1990). These rates by ethnicity are also affected by such factors as acculturation for Hispanics

Table 9.2. Percentage of Individuals
Meeting Criteria for DSM-IV Dependence

Characteristic	Alcohol Dependence
Gender	
Men	5.7
Women	2.2
Age (years)	
18–25	8.3
26–29	8.8
30–39	2.6
40–49	4.6
50–59	1.1
60+	0.8
Ethnicity	
African American	5.0
White	3.2
Hispanic	8.7
Other	2.7

Source: Alcohol Research Group, National Alcohol Sur-vey, 1990.

(Caetano, 1987; De La Rosa et al., 1990) and migration patterns and urban/rural location for African Americans (Herd, 1990).

Length of Time in Problem or Dependence Status

Natural history studies show that a substantial proportion of the drug-using population appears to end their addict careers over time (Nurco et al., 1975). Table 9.3 shows the proportion of adults reporting use of cocaine/crack and heroin at some point in their lifetime, as well as during the past year and the past month. Only a small number of each age group reported use during the past month, compared with those reporting lifetime and even twelve-month use; the proportion in each current time category decreased by age group. The large-scale Drug Abuse Reporting Program (DARP) study found the average length of addiction to be almost ten years (from first to last daily opioid use for the overall sample) (Joe, Chastain, & Simpson, 1990), an average similar to that found by Robins and others (Simpson, 1990, 243). The DARP study also found that about 25 percent of the treatment sample remained addicted at the twelve-year follow-up (Marsh, Joe, Simpson, & Lehman, 1990), a rate similar to that found in the three- to five-year follow-up in the Treatment Outcome Prospective Study (TOPS), which identified fewer than 20 percent as regular users (excluding marijuana). These findings were quite stable for heroin and cocaine across the methadone maintenance, outpatient drug free, and residential modalities.

The only large-scale alcohol study comparable to the drug treatment outcome studies (Polich, Armor, & Braiker, 1981) found a range of outcomes; while 18 percent were abstinent at two years and 9 percent at four years, only 54 percent of the sample were drinking with serious problems at four years. Studies of other populations have found higher rates (Vaillant, 1983), however, including a recent study in a private psy-

Table 9.3. Percentage of Individuals Reporting Cocaine and Heroin Use

Age (years)	Cocaine, Including Crack			Heroin		
	Lifetime	Past Year	Past Month	Lifetime	Past Year	Past Month
18–25	17.9	7.7	2.0	0.8	0.3	NA
26–34	25.8	5.1	1.8	1.8	0.3	NA
35+	7.0	1.6	0.5	1.6	0.4	NA

Source: Data from U.S. National Institute on Drug Abuse, 1991.
Note: NA means that data were not available.

chiatric hospital, which found that 29 percent were abstinent over four years and 55 percent had only occasional mild relapses (Nace, 1989). Results are clearly confounded by differences in type of primary problem. For example, a recent study found abstinence rates to be 71 percent at a twelve-month follow-up for the "alcohol only" dependent group, 66 percent for the alcohol and drug dependent group (other than cocaine dependence), and 62 percent for the cocaine dependent group (Miller, Millman, & Keskinen, 1990). Abstinence rates for drug use for the same groups were 96 percent, 90 percent, and 66 percent, respectively.

Natural history studies examining chronicity versus remission of alcohol problems in the general population have found sufficient instability over time and covariation by age cohort to caution against making generalizations (Fillmore & Midanik, 1984; Roizen et al., 1978). An eight-year follow-up of individuals in the 1984 National Alcohol Survey found that of those who reported three or more alcohol problems at time 1, 38 percent continued to report three or more at time 2 (Caetano & Kaskutas, 1993). Rates for women and men were similar, but varied by ethnicity.

Young men are at highest risk and report the greatest number of problems with alcohol and drugs. Many in this group, however, do not develop chronic problems (Caetano & Kaskutas, 1993; Fillmore & Midanik, 1984; Gerstein & Harwood, 1990). Longitudinal studies of men (Fillmore & Midanik, 1984) and women (Wilsnack et al., 1991) have found alcohol problem rates to vary according to age, with remission rates highest in younger age groups. In the specific case of problem-drinking women, about 27 percent of those aged twenty-one to thirty-four, 57 percent of those aged thirty-five to forty-nine, and 36 percent of those aged fifty or older reported two or more problems at a five-year follow-up (Wilsnack et al., 1991).

Thus, although young drug and alcohol users are at risk for chronic status, most "mature out" of their problematic use patterns. An estimate of chronicity cannot take prevalence for young people (i.e., as in the high school survey) as a proxy for chronic problem rates without adjusting for the proportion expected to "grow out" of drug use. Chronic cases would be targeted more accurately by focusing on the mid- to late twenties and older age groups.

In sum, while these samples have populations that vary from public to private clients and contain many epidemiological differences regarding combined alcohol and drug use and demographic characteristics, patterns and rates of relapse in the drug literature show that roughly 25 percent fall into the most extreme chronic group. A slightly larger proportion is found in the alcohol literature, although results are more mixed because of a lack of agreement about the definition of study populations and what is defined as relapse and success.

Alcohol or Drug Use in Adolescence Persisting into Adulthood

Research indicates that individuals who start drinking before age fifteen are more likely to continue to have problems than those who begin later. A substantial literature claims that most youth stop their problematic drinking in their twenties as they take on major life roles, such as marriage and joining the labor force (Fillmore & Midanik, 1984; Room, 1977). A large meta-analysis of thirty-four longitudinal data sets from fifteen countries found the greatest decrease in frequency of drinking to be among those aged twenty to twenty-four (Fillmore et al., 1991). Associations between age of initiation and progression and length of time addicted and between initiation and progression of drug use provide measures that can be used for synthetic estimates of chronicity (Anglin, Hser, & McGlothlin, 1987; Kandel & Yamaguchi, 1985). Findings indicate that initiation of illicit drug use generally decreases around age eighteen, drug use patterns become stabilized in the year after high school graduation, and the most intense use of alcohol and other drugs declines around age twenty-two (Johnston, O'Malley, & Bachman, 1991; Kandel & Yamaguchi, 1985). Although rates are greatly affected by gender, ethnicity, and type of substance (Kandel & Yamaguchi, 1985), roughly 30–40 percent of those who begin use early continue into adulthood and become chronic users.

Chronic Medical Conditions Stemming from Alcohol and Drug Use

The prevalence of chronic medical conditions resulting from alcohol and drug use provides another measure of chronicity. Table 9.4 shows that 4 percent of hospital discharges involve an alcohol-related diagnosis. Other medical problems accompanying chronic alcohol consumption include osteoporosis, ischemic heart disease, alcoholic pancreatitis, endocrine malfunctioning, reproductive incapacity, neurologic malfunctioning, and weakened immune system. Mortality rates from medical conditions related to chronic alcohol use also provide an estimate of chronicity. Table 9.5 shows data for four alcohol-related causes of death;

Table 9.4. Alcohol-Related Morbidity

	Discharges
Alcohol-related diagnosis (N = 1,100,000)[1]	27%
Alcohol-related disorder principal diagnosis (N = 600,000)	54%
Alcohol dependence syndrome	68%
Chronic liver disease and cirrhosis	16%
Alcohol psychosis	9%
Nondependent abuse	6%
Male/female rate of alcohol-related principal diagnosis	3:1
Alcohol-related disorder secondary diagnosis[2]	46%

Source: Age 14 and over data from 1985 National Hospital Discharge Survey, NCHS 1989 in U.S. NIAAA, 1990, *Alcohol & Health*, p. 20.
1. This represents 27,400,000 short-stay hospital discharges (excluding those that were pregnancy related).
2. Diseases and disorders of liver, pancreas, digestive tract, respiratory system, nervous system, and cardiovascular system, as well as drug abuse, mental disorders, injuries, accidental poisoning, infections, anemia, and malnutrition.

cirrhosis has the highest rates, 14.9 percent per 100,000 population.

Medical conditions related to drug use have not received the same research attention as those related to alcohol use; this may be in part a result of the political factors involved in studying medical complications of illicit substance use and a tendency to vacillate between defining drug abuse as a medical or a criminal problem. In addition, early research found that health problems associated with illicit drug use were related to contaminants in street drugs as well as to the drugs themselves (Cherubin et al., 1972). Interest is growing in this area, however, as a result of chronic drug use patterns, the increase in such diseases as tuberculosis, and the association between intravenous drug use and AIDS/HIV.[2] This latter association gives particular importance to chronic drug abuse and its effect on minority populations, who are overrepresented in the incidence and prevalence of AIDS/HIV (Chaisson et al., 1989; U.S. NIDA, 1991).[3]

Selection of Conditions Representing Chronic Alcohol and Drug Abuse and Rationale

Data sets and indicator systems measuring dependence, severity of dependence, long-term use of drugs, persistence of use past adolescence, and alcohol- and drug-related chronic medical conditions and mortality are the focus of this chapter. The discussion is limited to the population of chronic alcohol and drug abusers aged eighteen and older and ex-

Table 9.5. Average Mortality (per 100,000 Population) from Selected Alcohol-Related Causes, Ages 15–74 (1979, 1980, 1983–85)

	Cirrhosis	Alcohol Dependence Syndrome	Alcohol Psychosis	Alcohol Poisoning	Estimated Alcohol-Involved Mortality	
					Minimum	Maximum
Underlying cause of death[1]	14.9	2.7	0.5	0.2	28.5	43.8
Average age-adjusted mortality from selected alcohol-related causes underlying or contributing	10.8	2.0	0.2	0.2		
Average age-adjusted mortality from selected alcohol-related causes underlying or contributing according to multiple causes of death[2]	15.8	4.9	0.3	0.9	23.3	35.8

Note: U.S. rates; mortality counts averaged across the five years. Data also available by county (U.S. Department of Health and Human Services, *U.S. Alcohol Epidemiologic Data Reference Manual, Vol. 3, 2d Ed.: County Alcohol Problem Indicators, 1979–1985,* pp. 31, 204, 205).
1. Disease/injury leading to death (only one disease identified). Codes for causes of death are based on ICD-9 codes.
2. Underlying cause plus two sets of conditions listed as causes of death.

cludes problems of dual drug and mental health diagnoses and tobacco use, although the issue of indicator databases for these groups is addressed. Individual substances emphasized are alcohol, heroin, and cocaine. The chronic population may be identified at particular life stages, using the characteristics described above.

Adolescence

Although only 30–40 percent of adolescent users continue use past adolescence, those that do constitute a very high risk group. They are most likely to enter the specialized treatment system through the criminal justice or educational systems or emergency rooms, rather than through primary health care. Thus, a system monitoring chronicity might track high-risk adolescent users who come into contact with the above systems.

Young Adulthood

This group includes both those who began use in adolescence and continue to be dependent and those who began use as adults but meet criteria for severe dependence. They are most likely to enter the system through the workplace and employee assistance programs (EAPs), the criminal justice system (for alcohol- or drug-related arrests), the mental health system (for comorbid problems), or emergency rooms (for alcohol- or drug-related injuries). They can be identified by screening for length of use or severity of dependence and frequent polydrug use. Medical complications may or may not be present.

Middle-Aged or Older

Individuals with long drinking and/or drug use histories who meet criteria for severe dependence often have symptoms characterized by chronic medical conditions and by repeated alcohol- or drug-treatment admissions. This group may enter treatment through the criminal justice system because of alcohol- or drug-related arrests, including public intoxication; through workplace programs, although many may no longer be employed; or through emergency rooms and primary health care.

Comorbidity Issues

Combined alcohol and drug use is increasingly characteristic of substance abusers (Clayton, 1986; Hubbard, 1990). In addition, chronic substance abusers have high rates of multiple drug use and mental health comorbidities.[4] These individuals often enter the specialized alcohol and drug treatment system through the mental health system or emergency rooms, and sometimes through the criminal justice or welfare systems. While it is common to find individuals with alcohol problems also reporting concurrent psychiatric problems, research indicates that this group has different treatment requirements (Helzer & Pryzbeck, 1988; McLellan et al., 1994; McLellan et al., 1983. Women may have different patterns of emotional distress and psychiatric comorbidities (Blume, 1986; Vannicelli, 1984), and thus are an important group to consider in issues of comorbidity.

SERVICE NEEDS OF INDIVIDUALS WITH CHRONIC ALCOHOL AND DRUG PROBLEMS

Because outcome and evaluation studies have not focused specifically on the chronic population, data are not available to empirically assess core service needs. Nevertheless, a clear range of services from detoxification to long-term care is indicated, which would require mechanisms for identifying those at high risk for long-term problems from the pool of episodic, acute abusers. In view of the relapsing nature of chronic substance abuse, ongoing monitoring and provision of services are crucial, as are access to repeated detoxifications; low-cost, longer-term, non-hospital-based care, such as halfway houses and therapeutic communities; medical supervision; and methadone maintenance and other pharmacotherapies potentially developed for chronic alcohol dependence (Gerstein & Harwood, 1990; IOM, 1990). While the general treatment approach may not require a medical setting, the medical problems of the chronic population require attention. This population may often also require adjunct habilitative services, such as housing, welfare, and employment services, which are considered important for improvement (Gerstein & Harwood, 1990; IOM, 1990).

Ideal Service Course

Overall, research indicates that treatment for alcohol and drug abuse is effective in reducing substance use (Gerstein & Harwood, 1990; IOM, 1990; Tims, 1981) and that treatment in all modalities shows reductions in alcohol use, drug use, criminality, and other behavioral outcomes. A range of services needs to be available and may need to be repeated; longer treatment stays may be required. Ideally, individuals at high risk for chronicity or those who are chronic abusers would be identified at life stages as described above, and appropriate levels and modalities of services would be provided. For adolescents, this would require examination of severity and type of drug used and provision of treatment with ongoing monitoring. Substance abusers in their mid-twenties require screening for age of initiation, patterns of use, and severity of problems, and a range of services are called for, depending on the severity of dependence, comorbidities, and type of primary drug. These services would likely involve the specialized treatment system as well as the mental health and health care systems, employment, family counseling, and other services. Middle-aged and older individuals who remain alcohol-and/or drug-dependent most likely constitute a primarily chronic group who may require repeated monitoring in both the health care system and the specialized system, as well as such interventions as detoxifications, ongoing outpatient evaluation, alternative treatment methods such as AA, and methadone maintenance. They may also require treatment for alcohol- or drug-related medical conditions. AA and its related groups Narcotics Anonymous (NA) and Cocaine Anonymous (CA) potentially provide ongoing and chronic support, as well as supportive social networks.

Matching appropriate treatment to problems potentially improves outcome. Recent findings suggest that the "content" of treatment—addressing education and services to the areas that are problematic to the client (e.g., legal, family, medical, or job problems)—may be more important than the modality through which it is given (McLellan et al., 1994). Current research also emphasizes relapse management for chronic abusers as an important part of treatment (Leukefeld & Tims, 1990; Marlatt & Gordon, 1985; Tims & Leukefeld, 1986), as well as the matching of patient and program characteristics (IOM, 1990; McLellan et al., 1983).[5]

An ideal treatment system would address the issue of HIV at all stages of substance abuse problems, especially for individuals in high-risk groups. Rates of HIV infection are high enough in treatment populations to justify the inclusion of AIDS prevention in all alcohol and drug treatment efforts, particularly those directed toward minority populations (Chaffee, 1989).

Coordination among the specialized substance abuse treatment, medical, mental health, and social welfare systems is necessary for screening and identifying individuals whose use and problem patterns indicate high risk for chronic conditions, and for providing effective, integrated services. Efforts to increase client retention are important to further development of effective treatment for the chronic population (Leukefeld & Tims, 1990; Mammo & Weinbaum, 1993). On the whole, evidence suggests that strategies linking treatment programs with criminal justice and workplace constraints (e.g., attending treatment to remove legal or work sanctions) improve retention (Leukefeld & Tims, 1990). This has led to advocacy for long-term client aftercare and monitoring and the potential use of civil commitment for compulsory treatments, especially for intravenous drug users at risk for HIV transmission (Leukefeld & Tims, 1990).

An ideal service system would stress linkages between primary health care, substance abuse, and mental health treatment. While the prevalence of alcohol and drug abuse in primary care populations varies greatly by type of practice and funding sector, with public patients reporting much higher drinking rates and alcohol-related problems than private patients (Cherpitel, 1993), overall rates are sufficiently high to warrant screening and coordination of services. The current trend toward "carving out" substance abuse and mental health treatment from other health services in managed care organizations (MCOs) potentially presents difficulties in integrating these services with primary care (Freeman & Trabin, 1994).

Typical Service Patterns

Several typical service patterns exist. For the most part, treatment programs and modalities function independently rather than as a continuum of care, with the type of treatment determined by access to health insurance and other third-party funding and type of coverage. For example, nonmedical, outpatient, short-term services and methadone maintenance services are found in much higher proportions in public programs than in private programs (Gerstein & Harwood, 1990; IOM, 1990). Individuals with chronic problems are often members of population subgroups who lack third-party health coverage and access to the range of services and thus do not follow a continuum of care (Gerstein & Harwood, 1990; IOM, 1990). In some cases, the lifelong course of care may consist primarily of nothing more than repeated detoxifications.

Self-help or mutual aid groups are an important adjunct to alcohol and drug treatment. Although many such groups exist, foremost among them are AA, NA, and CA. More people attend AA and its related groups than approach specialized alcohol and drug programs (Weisner, Greenfield, & Room, 1995), and most individuals have attended such groups before going to treatment. The last survey conducted by AA (in 1992) (General Service Office, 1993) estimated 89,000 groups worldwide, with most in the United States. The age distribution of members was estimated at 19 percent under age thirty, 57 percent between ages thirty-one and fifty, and 24 percent over age fifty; 65 percent were men. The number of members was not reported, but the 1993 survey estimated 653,000 members in the United States and Canada, with the average member attending three meetings per week (General Service Office, 1993). Of those surveyed in 1992, 63 percent reported receiving other alcohol treatment services before coming to AA (General Service Office, 1993).

AA and NA have also become integrated with most public and private programs (IOM, 1990). AA takes an active role in promoting the development of supportive relationships, which are vital to maintaining recovery, and is thus seen as a valuable "aftercare modality" by some programs and as an inherent component of treatment by others (Gerstein & Harwood, 1990; IOM, 1990). Many agencies, such as California's social model programs and the nonmedical programs commonly found throughout the United States, are generally based on AA philosophy, which has become a major ideological influence in formal alcohol programs. Other more clinical programs integrate its philosophy with their professional diagnostic and clinical approaches. AA and NA provide long-term support to chronic drug and alcohol abusers, who are vulnerable to relapse. In many cases, freestanding self-help groups are the predominant or only available help to which individuals with chronic problems have access, having depleted both their insurance benefits and social margin with family and friends.

SERVICE SYSTEM ISSUES

The 1980s saw a shift in the public/private balance, with the private sector growing and the public sector shrinking. In 1990, ownership of the specialized treatment sector of alcohol and drug units and alcohol-only units was distributed as 18 percent public, 64 percent private nonprofit, and 18 percent private for-profit, compared with the 1982 distribution of 28 percent public, 65 percent private nonprofit, and 7 percent private for-profit sector (Gerstein & Harwood, 1990; Schmidt & Weisner, 1993). In many states and counties, most public monies are contracted to private nonprofit programs, thus accounting for the large private nonprofit sector.[6] To some degree, the sectors have mixed funding sources.[7] The major public source across sectors is state and local government, including the Alcohol, Drug Abuse and Mental Health block grant and state and local matching funds (Schmidt & Weisner, 1993). Managed care has become the predominant type of organization. The growing use of MCOs, designed to contain the costs of treatment by restricting unnecessary treatment and reducing the average length of care, represents the greatest change in the organization of substance abuse services in recent years. To date, this has primarily involved private treatments, but state and county systems and public insurance, particularly Medicaid, have increasingly adopted similar cost containment mechanisms, such as MCOs, preferred provider organizations, and utilization review and case monitoring strategies (Levin, Glasser, & Roberts, 1984; Rogowski, 1992). Little is known about the effectiveness of program organizations or the effectiveness of the integration of those services with primary care services within MCOs.

Until recently, alcohol and drug abusers were identified as separate groups, and separate sets of specialized treatment institutions with dramatically different features existed for their treatment. The primary modalities for alcohol treatment have been detoxification, recovery homes, halfway houses and other residential services (hospital based and non–hospital based), and outpatient programs. Ideologically, they range from medical, psychosocial, and behavioral to nonmedical. Many public treatment systems consist of programs that are intrinsically nonmedical, such as the social model programs in California and elsewhere. These modalities are described in the IOM study on alcohol treatment (1990). Recovering persons play a large role in treatment overall. The major pharmacotherapy is disulfiram. Recent research has resulted in the Federal Food and Drug Administration's approval of Naltrexone as a medication for individuals in treatment.

The primary modalities for drug treatment include methadone maintenance, therapeutic communities, outpatient drug-free programs, detoxification programs, and chemical dependency programs; these are described fully in the IOM Report (Gerstein & Harwood, 1990). Treatment often differs by the primary type of drug used. Methadone maintenance has become an accepted treatment approach for heroin users; it is sometimes combined with counseling, but often it is a "stand alone" service. The other dominant treatment approach for heroin use, and sometimes for cocaine abuse, is the therapeutic community, a nine- to eighteen-month, structured, residential program emphasizing resocialization and behavior modification, designed primarily for individuals who have been involved in criminal behavior. Outpatient drug-free programs include clientele who use cocaine and other drugs, but typically not opiates. Detoxification programs generally last five to seven days and focus on withdrawal and prevention of medical complications.

The chemical-dependency program model (sometimes located in a hospital setting) is the predominant one for both alcohol and drugs in the private sector. It traditionally lasts twenty-eight days, although cost containment through case-managed private health insurance and MCOs has shortened the average length of stay dramatically. It is also the most costly and least evaluated model (Gerstein & Harwood, 1990; Hubbard, 1990; IOM, 1990). This model is increasingly found adapted in outpatient programs, as inpatient treatment models have decreased.

Merging of Alcohol and Drug Programs

During the past ten years the organization of treatment has been reoriented, as alcohol and drug treatment systems in both the public and private sectors have merged. In 1990, 76 percent of the public and private programs defined themselves as combined alcohol and drug programs, 13 percent as alcohol only, and 11 percent as drug only (compared with 1982 figures of 26 percent alcohol and drug, 51 percent alcohol only, and 26 percent drug only) (Schmidt & Weisner, 1993). This was influenced to a large extent by clinical and epidemiological research that has revealed increasing rates of combined alcohol and drug use and problems (Clayton, 1986; Gottheil, 1986; Hubbard, 1990; Weisner, 1993). Multiple chronic dependence is not an unusual occurrence, indicating that chronic cases may be overrepresented in this group of polydrug abusers (Hubbard et al., 1989; Tims & Leukefeld, 1986).

A crucial issue for the field is that while programs have merged, a treatment model oriented to these combined problems has not been developed and evaluated. Thus, the typical model of care incorporates persons with both alcohol and drug problems into existing programs and assumes that both are being treated (Hubbard, 1990). The usual approach for such clients in alcohol programs is an inclusive one, which considers that all addictions have the same etiology and require the same treatment. The typical approach in the drug treatment sphere has been one of "staged care," in which one type of addiction is treated first; others, including alcohol, assumed to be secondary, are treated later (Hubbard, 1990). Evidence suggests that those with the most severe and long-standing problems are more frequently found in programs oriented toward maintenance rather than rehabilitation, such as alcohol and drug detoxification or methadone maintenance (IOM, 1990).

Entry Points to the Treatment System

The public alcohol and drug treatment system provides a wide range of services characterized by specialized programs (for the most part operated outside the medical care system), with some services also provided within the criminal justice, mental health, and educational systems. Except for medical treatment for alcohol-related health problems, individuals are referred from other institutions to a specialized treatment system and to specific programs. An ideal system would involve a continuum of services in which chronic patients would be identified and admitted at a level diagnostically appropriate for each course of care. Entry points, however, especially in the private sector, are largely determined by health insurance coverage or by the program with which the referring institution has established networks and referral procedures. It cannot be assumed that any particular program or funding sector provides a comprehensive continuum of services or that clients enter the system at any one place.

Factors Limiting Access and Use of Appropriate Care

In the alcohol and drug fields, chronicity is not the major target for treatment; chronic groups are sometimes "written off," handled outside the treatment system (in AA, for example), or provided medical care for advanced alcohol-related conditions in isolation of specialty treatment. The predominant focus of public and private treatment systems is on individuals whose problems are at "earlier stages" and who are considered to have the highest recovery potential. In the public system, variations in social policy, related to factors such as jail overcrowding and local policies for screening for alcohol and drug problems in public assistance caseloads, affect access to treatment and availability of care. Treatment practices by MCOs may also limit access and use of the range of services by cost-containment mechanisms such as utilization review, selective contracting, and case-monitoring strategies (Clark & Fox, 1993; Keeler, Manning, & Wells, 1988; Rogowski, 1992; Tischler 1990; Wells et al., 1991). Few formal controls are used to govern MCOs and to ensure that cost-containment efforts do not hamper accessibility or affect the quality of service (England & Vaccaro, 1991). As increasing numbers of states contract with MCOs, such restrictions may also affect the public sector.

Financing

The "two-tiered" public/private treatment system, described above, is the most pervasive structural factor affecting deviations from an ideal course of care. The sectors differ in client characteristics, services offered, and user capacity (Hubbard, 1990; Schmidt & Weisner, 1993; Yahr, 1988). The resulting effect on access for various population groups was a major concern of recent alcohol and drug studies by the IOM (Gerstein & Harwood, 1990; IOM, 1990). As noted above, the public sector, which has been the treatment system of last resort, targeting those who lack third-party funding or who have depleted their health care benefits, has declined in recent years. At the same time, cost containment in the private sector has led to a shift from inpatient to outpatient programs. On the whole, substance abuse programs located within MCOs have also been limited to outpatient programs.

Social Policy

The treatment system is often affected by strategies that target access to certain populations and de facto limit access to others. For example, the creation of diversion programs from criminal justice to alcohol treatment without the infusion of funds to develop additional treatment capacity has increased access for those arrested and decreased access for others. Some evidence suggests that the population with decreased access to treatment is the more chronic population (Weisner, 1986). Finally, the merging of alcohol and drug programs may affect access to treatment in that the balance of treatment capacity for primary alcohol versus drug problems may shift.

Geographic Issues

Urban versus rural status affects both the availability of treatment and the type of program (IOM, 1990). State of residence is also likely an important factor, since the public/private sector balance, need level, general availability, and program type vary greatly by state (IOM, 1990). Disparity is found in the service courses in the public and private systems and in the type of service provided across states, especially in allocation: per capita funding (state and federal government combined) ranges from $2.36 to $23.54. The extent of private services across states is not well correlated with the amount of public services, nor is there any relationship between need (e.g., measured by cirrhosis mortality or per capita consumption) and amount of service provided (IOM, 1990). Additional variation exists across states in program philosophy and type of public program funded (e.g., the use of twenty-eight-day programs by the public sector in Minnesota and the support of social model programs in the public sector of California).

Minorities and Women

Differential access is found for ethnic groups and for men and women. Compared with their general population problem rates, African Americans remain overrepresented in public programs, while Hispanics are underrepresented (De La Rosa et al., 1990). Women also have made strides, due to funding mandates and policies targeted at particular groups of women, most specifically the pregnant addict. Analysis of the Uniform Facility Data Survey (UFDS)—formerly the National Drug and Alcohol Treatment Utilization Survey (NDATUS)—found women in programs across the alcohol modalities at rates of 1:4, the same as the prevalence of problem drinking in the general population. However, for each of these population groups, rates differ between public and private programs (Schmidt & Weisner, 1993).

Thus, the financing of treatment, the uneven availability of the full range of services across funding streams, differences across states and communities both in overall treatment capacity and in the public/private balance of services, and larger social policy concerns outside the health care system all affect access to treatment in general and to appropriate treatment. This is especially true for the chronic population, in which individuals of low socioeconomic status, who often lack health insurance or have depleted their benefits, are overrepresented. Overall, the specialized treatment system, except for methadone maintenance programs, is often based on a "cure" concept rather than on maintenance or management of relapse and is not well oriented to the chronic substance abuser.

DATA SOURCES AND INDICATORS

Political considerations related to the management of illicit substances have played a large part in shaping multiple treatment goals and indicator systems for chronic substance abusers. The consideration of outcome measures directly confronts issues that have provoked deep ideological and political conflict and tremendous controversy in both fields (Marlatt, 1983; Roizen, 1987). These are characterized by controlled-drinking treatment strategies versus abstinence in the alcohol field and by harm reduction versus abstinence in the drug field. While the fundamental approach has been abstinence (Room, 1978), controversy remains regarding the role of harm reduction for some groups. Blackwell (1983) pointed to stable patterns of controlled use by formerly physiologically dependent heroin users, arguing that controlled use may produce greater stability over time than abstinence. Methadone maintenance, the most common harm-reduction strategy in drug treatment, has been found to result in reduced heroin use. Its use as a treatment, however, remains controversial (Gerstein & Harwood, 1990). There is no realistic estimate of goals for the chronic population; the lack of a focus on defining, identifying, and studying this population may have prevented such a dialogue.

The traditional measure of outcome in alcohol and drug treatment has been the amount of substance used (most typically measuring abstinence) following treatment, usually assessed at six or twelve months. The argument has been made that measures should respond more to the chronic relapsing pattern common among abusers and should include level of functioning, as well as abstinence levels, changes in drinking and drug use patterns, health status and problems, mortality, subsequent treatment use, legal status, work and family problems, time spent in employment or education, quality of life, and integration with other community services (IOM, 1990; McLellan et al., 1994).

Data Sources Relevant to Measuring Chronicity and Service Capacity

No data directly address the chronic population as a group, and only indirect measures are available for doing so. Existing data also vary in their application to community-level use. The pools of data available to establish the service needs of chronic populations include studies of individual clinical samples, epidemiological household surveys, epidemiological studies of populations in health and community institutions (e.g., welfare, criminal justice, and medical settings), and monitoring systems in place at the community and national level, such as in emergency rooms and jails. Though useful for assessing the broad scope of the problem, existing data sources are probably inadequate for estimating prevalence and service needs of the chronic population, because they do not use uniform definitions and, on the whole, are service rather than community based. Major data sources and the relevant information contained in each are listed at the end of this chapter. This section details the types of data that address the indicators most applicable for community use.

Persistence from Adolescent to Adult Use

Research suggests that measures of drinking and drug use in young populations can enable communities to make synthetic estimates by projecting the extent of chronicity in their adult populations. These projections, however, need to take into account the effect of treatment, which may change as more effective treatment strategies are developed and treatment access is increased, and the complexity of use patterns for different types or multiple types of drugs. These data are not expensive to collect and may be gathered by surveys of young populations, using methodologies similar to the NIDA high school survey.

Treatment History

Since the chronic nature of alcohol and drug abuse often requires repeated interventions, recurrent treatment clients are often referred to as a chronic population (Babor et al., 1992). For example, treatment history data from clients in the DARP sample (Marsh et al., 1990) showed that length of addiction was correlated with lifetime history. At the twelve-year follow-up, those who were no longer using opioids daily reported an average of five admissions, while those still using reported twelve. Over 80 percent of the DARP follow-up sample reported multiple treatment episodes (U.S. NIDA, 1991). Other treatment studies have also found most clients reporting prior treatment episodes (Hubbard et al., 1989; Polich et al., 1981), but they vary too much by type of drug use and treatment modality to warrant generalization. Further, they do not measure those not receiving treatment in the community or those for whom access is limited. Such an approach would also require coordinating data collection or identifying information across public and private programs.

Data sources at the community level for monitoring repeated treatment admissions would include carefully constructed management information systems to track the number of admissions, the setting, and the type of services received. The new Client Data System could be revised to provide these data in the public system, because it is designed to collect data on each client seen in programs receiving any public reimbursement (see List of Data Sources in this chapter).

Chronic Medical Conditions

Information on chronic medical conditions resulting from alcohol and drug use is mainly available from hospital discharge surveys and death certificates (Adams et al., 1990; U.S. NIAAA, 1990). A major strength of these measures is their availability at the county level. The deaths that NIAAA argues are clear measures of chronicity are cirrhosis (including chronic liver disease and cirrhosis deaths and portal hypertension), alcohol-dependence syndrome, and alcohol psychoses. The NIAAA "minimum estimated alcohol-involved mortality rate" (a crude measure of chronicity) provides ranges of 13.3 to 33.9 deaths per 100,000 population in counties in Wisconsin, with an overall state rate of 18.5.[8] County rates in California range from 15.4 to 47.9, with an overall average of 27.2. Data are available at the county level on mortality rates for four alcohol-related causes of death, some of which are relevant to measuring chronicity (Table 9.5). In using such measures, other indicators should include size of population; existing treatment capacity, including geographic dispersion; resources per modality; urbanization and sociodemographic characteristics of the population, such as ethnicity and age; and the existence of waiting lists in treatment programs. Population estimates of need can be projected by linking these types of data with data on current resources in multivariate models (U.S. NIAAA, 1991). The major usefulness of large data systems adapted to measure chronicity is their potential for providing prevalence data, adjusted for differences in population characteristics.

Other Community Indicators

Factors identified as affecting the need for services, which could be tracked over time in a community, include availability of alcohol and drugs (e.g., availability of alcohol in convenience stores and gas stations and availability and price of street drugs); rise in underage drinking, since age of initiation appears to be related to chronicity; introduction of new types of drugs into the community; overall availability of health care to at-risk populations; and changes in employment rates, rates of alcohol and drug-related arrests, and incidence and prevalence of HIV-positive cases. Current practices affecting the "management" of service selection and the intensity, duration, and quality of monitoring vary greatly between public and private payers and across communities and states. Variables that differ include case management, eligibility screening, and government or private sector operation.

Data systems that would measure prevalence, service needs, and treatment capacity for the chronic substance abuse and mental health dual diagnosis population are lacking. At the community level, some data are available in the national surveys discussed in the Annotated List of Data Sources at the end of this chapter. Some of these data sets have large samples that potentially provide some smaller area indicator information on prevalence and service needs. Service use statistics for populations with both problems are not uniformly available, because of the separate service systems typically existing.

As discussed above, voluntary services such as the mutual-help groups of AA, NA, and CA, while not part of the formal treatment system, provide services for many individuals, including those not choosing formal agency interventions, those who attend groups in addition to formal treatment, and those who fall through the cracks. City, county, or other regional listings of self-help meetings exist at the local level. These listings are updated approximately every six months and provide at least a loose estimate of trends in the size of this "informal" system at the local level. The General Services Office of AA conducts a national survey of AA membership every three years by sampling a number of groups roughly proportional to the registered number of groups in each area. NA plans to conduct its first national membership survey in 1996.

Recent changes in requirements for public block grant funding have begun to reverse the erosion that occurred during the 1980s in standardized data collection in treatment agencies and in the accountability required of state and local governments; however, these data collection efforts do not focus on measurement of chronic cases. In the private sector, insurance providers have begun to require eligibility screening before authorizing type and length of service. This screening arguably provides some identification of chronic cases, but this has not been examined.

Currently, research projects are collecting selected indicators to assess a range of substance abuse prevention efforts. Community-level intervention studies in California (Prevention Research Center) and Minnesota (University of Minnesota) are collecting data in selected communities on such varied areas as crime, health, schools, economy, demographics, and political participation. Indicators specific to alcohol and drug abuse are drunk driving arrests, narcotics arrests, liquor law violations, drunkenness arrests, fatal automobile crashes, nighttime crashes, alcohol availability, and mortality rates due to chronic alcohol and drug abuse. With the exception of the mortality indicators, however, these indicators do not focus on chronic alcohol and drug abuse. A Robert Wood Johnson project (Horgan, 1996) has examined the range of indicators, although it also focuses on alcohol and drug problems overall rather than on chronicity.

In sum, social indicators already available at the county level are limited predominantly to treatment admissions, arrest and welfare statistics, and chronic medical conditions. Each of these has limited usefulness to communities for measuring the incidence and prevalence of chronic substance abuse and service needs and experiences. Moreover, these indicators of chronic medical conditions are quite limited for drugs other than alcohol.

Recommended Indicators

Considering the availability and validity of indicators and the feasibility of new data systems or collection efforts, communities would benefit from collecting data on repeated treatment admissions, hospital discharge statistics by alcohol-related condition, and alcohol-related mortality. Suggested measures are shown in Table 9.6. In each case, modifications might be developed to improve the weaknesses of existing systems by working with relevant institutions. Surveys of high school students to assess the population at risk may be feasible for some communities. Screening in emergency rooms and the criminal justice system, especially for those over age twenty-five who began use in adolescence and/or are in the severity range of alcohol or drug dependence, would be a way to optimize access to high-risk populations for measurement. While costly, population-based epidemiological surveys conducted every few years to measure the prevalence of dependence, the duration of symptoms, and

Table 9.6. Potential Community-Level Indicators of Substance Abuse
Prevalence and Treatment Access

Indicator	Data Source
Prevalence	
Synthetic estimate (all rates per 1,000 population)	Derived from national studies, or extrapolated from high school or other local survey
• Age by gender	
• Age by gender by race	
Alcohol and drug use surveys	High school student surveys
	Population survey (sample of communities)
Alcohol/drug-related service encounters	
• Hospital admissions	Hospital discharge statistics
• Emergency room use	Emergency room statistics
• Criminal justice system (arrests/accidents)	Police reports
Access to care	
Synthetic estimates	
• Private treatment center cases	Treatment center–reported unduplicated caseloads
• Public treatment center cases	Treatment center–reported unduplicated caseloads
• All treatment center cases	Treatment center–reported unduplicated caseloads
• Treatment center service units	Treatment center–reported unduplicated caseloads
Unmet need	
Health status and coordination of care	Follow-back surveys with clients identified in general population surveys, treatment caseloads, and/or hospital admissions, emergency rooms, or the criminal justice system

the amount and type of treatment would provide an anchoring point
from which to develop such monitoring strategies. This might be done
on a sample of communities rather than universally, to reduce costs.

None of the efforts to collect epidemiological data on treatment populations, need, and treatment effectiveness has explicitly addressed chronicity. Most of these data sources, however, do provide information on
treatment history, severity of dependence, type of drug, and age of first
use and thus may be used as indirect indicators of chronic conditions.
They may also serve as pilot efforts, suggesting the kinds of data that

can be collected and addressing the difficulties in collecting particular indicators. The primary issue remains the lack of a definition of chronicity.

The most successful data are from national efforts, although these studies have limitations. Most of the epidemiological studies of general populations, for example, provide national prevalence estimates of use, problems, or dependence, but they have a variety of shortcomings in measuring chronicity. The lifetime measures of problems and treatment history collected cross-sectionally are limited by recall bias; longitudinal studies with protracted follow-up periods better assess chronicity. Although several national studies are large, they cannot be used for state or community-level rates because of the primary sampling unit–based sampling frames. Problems in data collection on clinical populations have highlighted the difficulties of obtaining prevalences of chronic alcohol and drug problems in so fragmented and decentralized a service delivery system as that in the United States.

The important differences between results drawn from data collection in the general population and those from treatment systems should be noted (Rounsaville & Kleber, 1985). While both data sources are crucial to estimating need and developing monitoring of care for chronic substance abusers, they cannot answer the same questions. Systems in place to track prevalence in the general population tend to respond to questions regarding prevalence and need for services in the population as a whole. Research and data systems in place within treatment agencies tend to provide data on trends and needs of the group receiving services.

Epidemiological surveys are clearly the preferred data to measure prevalence and monitor the effectiveness of community institutions to respond to chronic substance abuse problems. However, the limitations of such surveys as a community strategy have been detailed above.

The limitations of using repeated treatment admissions as a measure of chronicity include lack of clarity in determining how many treatments of what type and quality would characterize chronicity. In addition, treatment use is often determined by social, financial, and political factors rather than diagnostic ones (a large literature addresses the problem of unequal access). Finally, the bias with this indicator will be toward an older population, because they are more likely to have been to treatment.

Use of hospital discharge data and alcohol-related mortality statistics has limitations as well: lack of coverage for chronic conditions related to drug use other than alcohol; instability for smaller communities; the time lag between early manifestations of chronic use and the development of medical conditions, which prevents the timely setting of treatment policy; and representation of only the extreme segment of the chronic population. Some of the indicators making up the overall alcohol-related mortality rate stem from acute episodes rather than chronic use, which presents some bias in use of these statistics; the rarity of these types of deaths in the general population presents additional barriers to use. For small counties, data need to be averaged over five years to provide stable community estimates, which causes additional problems for planning treatment services. Finally, the uneven capacity of these statistics to measure chronic drug use as well as chronic alcohol use needs to be addressed.

CONCLUSION AND RECOMMENDATIONS

An examination of chronicity in the substance abuse field points to the importance of an indicator system that would provide communities with measures of need for services and the community response to that need. The current organization of the treatment system and the public health and prevention approach to treatment raise concern that the chronic population of substance abusers lacks access to the range of needed services. The lack of definition and operationalization of chronicity is an important issue in developing such an approach. The development of new health care policy, its mechanisms of supplying substance-abuse services, and the extent of those services will greatly affect the potential for tracking need and services in communities.

An approach that would monitor problems at different life stages provides the opportunity to use different sets of indicators, which may be appropriate for a particular stage of monitoring but not for others. Thus, while it may be logistically possible to conduct a school survey to interview adolescents, general population surveys are usually too costly for a county to conduct. On the other hand, measuring problems in individuals who have longer and more severe problems may be possible in the specialized treatment sector, health care agencies, and adjunct services, such as criminal justice and welfare. One feature of the treatment system for chronic substance abuse is its location primarily outside medical services institutions, which emphasizes the need not to focus solely on medical care. The recommended approach would include some reliance on synthetic estimates; however, some administrative systems could be developed or modified, such as improved management information systems in agencies and screening in emergency rooms.

Data collection should be focused at the local or county level, since that is where most services are organized. Additionally, public funds are most often channeled through this level of government, information on licensing of private programs may be available from the state, and social policy regarding institutional arrangements between different institutions, such as criminal justice, welfare, and substance abuse treatment, evolves here.

Finally, the heterogeneity of the chronic substance-abusing population is an important issue for communities making use of broad indicators from national data sources. Even rates examined by gender, age, and ethnicity show a wide range of variation. These dramatic differences in types and rates of problems and service needs across geographic and population groups argue strongly for indicators assessed and collected at the community level.

Attention to multiple drug abuse, including alcohol and other drug abuse and associated psychiatric problems, must be addressed in the study and development of social indicators. The alcohol and drug fields stem from separate research and treatment traditions and have not paid careful attention to interactions with each other. Today's chronic population may indeed be heavily represented by individuals who abuse more than one substance and who have psychiatric problems as well; therefore, data systems are required that provide meaningful measures of each and that can be collapsed for overall measures.

Finally, any progress in assessing the prevalence and needs of the chronic substance-abusing population and monitoring its care will require that the chronic population be actively defined, identified, and distinguished from the treatment populations with which it currently is enmeshed. Only then can the needs of each group be assessed and strategies be developed to monitor the availability and effectiveness of treatment in the community.

ANNOTATED LIST OF DATA SOURCES

Epidemiologic Surveys of the General Population

The *NIDA Household Survey on Drug Abuse (NHSDA)* is a large national survey conducted irregularly since 1971 and annually since

1990. Formerly under contract by NIDA, it is now funded by the Office of Applied Studies at the Substance Abuse and Mental Health Service Administration (SAMHSA). In the past it has included oversampling in large cities and a set of tangential studies aimed at sampling nonhousehold populations (DC*MADS) (Bray & Marsden, 1992). With regard to prevalence data, recent surveys include measures of age at onset of drinking one drink or more per month; frequency of being very high or drunk during the past twelve months; combined use of drug types and/or alcohol; age at onset of drug use for nonmedical reasons; frequency of use during lifetime; and problems experienced for each type of drug and alcohol in past year. It is a large survey and may provide some smaller-area information.

NIAAA-sponsored national alcohol surveys, carried out by the Alcohol Research Group (ARG), have been conducted as cross-sectional surveys roughly every five years since 1964, with longitudinal substudies included intermittently. Some surveys have included oversampling of African Americans and Hispanics (1968, 1984, and 1994). Survey data include twelve-month measures of frequency and a range of amounts of alcohol, and frequency of drunkenness. Lifetime measures include largest amount of alcohol; drinking five or more drinks at least once a week; twelve-month and lifetime measures of problems and alcohol dependence (DSM-III-R and DSM-IV); and treatment history. Information on drugs (by type) includes use in past year, whether medically prescribed, and use in combination with alcohol. Its sample size precludes the availability of small-area data.

The *National Longitudinal Alcohol Epidemiology Survey (NLAES)* is a large cross-sectional, rather than longitudinal, survey. It includes data on drinking and drug use quantity and frequency, combination use, age at first use, age at first problematic use, drug and alcohol dependence (DSM-III-R and DSM-IV), and drug and alcohol treatment history. Its large sample size may allow for some smaller area information on those measures.

The *Behavioral Risk Factor Surveillance System (BRFSS),* sponsored by the Centers for Disease Control (CDC), is a telephone survey in which forty states participate. It includes questions on alcohol use, drunk driving, and alcoholism risk, but no questions to represent chronicity. Average sample size is 1,500 per state per year.

The *National Health Interview Survey (NHIS),* a national in-person survey of the National Center for Health Statistics (NCHS), asks questions on drinking patterns for the previous twelve months, but not problems. Supplemental surveys focused on alcohol were conducted in 1983 and 1988. It is a very large survey with some applicability to smaller areas.

Epidemiologic Catchment Area (ECA) studies are surveys of the general population and some institutional samples (discussed below) in five major cities throughout the United States. They are one-time studies and include data on alcohol and drug dependence (DIS six-month and lifetime measures) and treatment history. National comorbidity studies by R. C. Kessler et al. can be considered successors.

Epidemiologic and Service-Related Data Systems in Alcohol and Drug Agencies

Client Data System (CDS), sponsored by the Office of Applied Studies at SAMHSA, has been in operation since 1990 and collects client-level data from all programs receiving state alcohol or drug funds, including federal block grant funds for alcohol or drug treatment. It includes a core of nineteen items. Those relevant to the issue of chronicity are number of prior treatment episodes in any drug or alcohol treatment program (5 + is the highest category); primary, secondary, and tertiary substance-abuse problems; frequency of use (but no data available on quantity); age at first use of drugs; and age at first alcohol intoxication). The CDS also includes an "Optional Data Set." Portions completed by states vary, but data include measures of drug and alcohol dependence based on DSM-III-R criteria, psychiatric comorbidities and combined alcohol or drug problems, health insurance coverage, and criminal justice referrals.

The *Uniform Facility Data Survey (UFDS),* formerly the *National Drug and Alcohol Treatment Utilization Survey (NDATUS),* conducted intermittently since 1974 and annually since 1989, is a point-prevalence mail census/survey of public and private alcohol and drug treatment and prevention units in the United States. A strength is that it includes both public and private agencies; a weakness is that it includes only agency-level data. Although the data have not been completely comparable from year to year, UFDS provides data on general sociodemographic characteristics of clients, types of services provided, primary problem, and funding information. Thus, while it is a potential database for communities to use to monitor client statistics and characteristics, it does not provide a definition of chronicity or request such data.

The *State Alcohol and Drug Abuse Profile (SADAP)* is an annual report of agency-level data collected by the State Alcohol and Drug Abuse agencies and submitted to the National Association of Alcohol and Drug Abuse Directors (NASADAD). Statistics are reported for agencies that receive any funds administered by each state's alcohol and drug agency. Relevant variables collected include primary drug of abuse; gender; age; ethnicity; type of service; number of alcohol, other drug, and methadone admissions; and source of funding and expenditures.

There are also *state data systems.* Each state's alcohol and drug agency has a system of gathering statistics on clients, which includes at least the information submitted to SADAP and in many cases more. California's Department of Alcohol and Drug Programs' client registration form ("Confidential Client Information"), for example, requires reporting of gender, age, race, ethnicity, and marital status; education; disability status; any previous admissions to drug detoxification, methadone maintenance, outpatient drug-free, drug residential, alcohol outpatient, or alcohol residential programs; primary, secondary, or tertiary drug or alcohol problems; DSM-III-R dependence; number of prior admissions; pregnancy status; usual route of drug administration; frequency of use; age at first use; number of arrests in last twenty-four months; and discharge status. States with these data systems can provide counties with chronicity data on their treatment populations, as measured by previous treatment, and can potentially redesign these forms to collect data more relevant to chronicity.

In addition to treatment statistics as discussed above, longitudinal *research studies* of treatment populations provide data useful for measuring chronicity in clinical populations. These studies typically consist of large national samples, and many are still in the design and data collection phase. They include the Drug Services Research Study (DSRS) and its alcohol component (ADDS), both conducted by Brandeis University; its retrospective evaluation component (SROS), conducted by National Opinion Research Corporation; the National Treatment Study (NTS), conducted by MayaTech Corporation; the Drug Abuse Treatment Outcome Study (DATOS), conducted by the Research Triangle Institute; and the National Treatment Evaluation Study (NTES), conducted by the Center on Addiction and Substance Abuse, Columbia University.

The *Drug Abuse Treatment System Survey (DATSS)* (Price & D'Aunno, 1992a; Price & D'Aunno, 1992b) is a longitudinal (1988 and 1990) national telephone survey of directors and clinical supervisors of drug treatment and drug/alcohol combined programs. The survey used a primary sampling unit method for sampling and examines the relationship of organizational characteristics of programs to outcome.

County-level alcohol indicators include some aggregate data on mortality rates for eight alcohol-related causes of death collected by counties and states, providing data relevant to measures of chronicity (e.g., mortality from liver cirrhosis, alcohol-dependence syndrome, nondependent abuse of alcohol, alcoholic psychoses, alcohol poisoning). NCHS collects these data using cause-of-death classification codes based on the International Classification of Diseases, Ninth Revision (ICD-9). Some counties collect data using a more extensive set of indicators.

Epidemiological Studies and Data Systems in General Health and Service Agencies

Research projects and data systems in place in health and social service institutions potentially provide data to estimate chronic alcohol and drug abuse in communities. However, as with the data sources discussed above, none is specifically designed to operationalize and measure chronicity.

The *National Short-Term Hospital Study* involved a probability sample of short-term general hospitals designed to measure the prevalence of alcohol and drug problems in such settings. It was funded by NIAAA and collected data on alcohol and drug dependence, severity, and treatment history, as well as in-person interview and service records data on health conditions relevant to issues of chronicity. Although this national sample of two hundred hospitals presents a national prevalence rate across hospitals, it cannot provide data on a smaller geographic area.

The *National Hospital Discharge Survey* is an ongoing study of discharge records conducted by the NCHS. Similar to mortality studies, it collects data from discharge records on alcohol psychosis, alcohol-dependence syndrome, alcohol gastritis, chronic liver disease and cirrhosis, and alcohol abuse, and has similar strengths and limitations for chronicity research (Sanchez, 1984).

The *Client Oriented Data Acquisition Process (CODAP)* collected data annually from 1975 to 1981. The NIMH required all agencies receiving federal grants or contracts for drug abuse treatment services to report to this system. Client-level data reported included demographic characteristics, prior treatment admissions, primary drug, year of first use, year of first continuous use and extent of present use, additional drug problems, employment, number of medical contacts, number of medical and psychiatric contacts. The CDS, although it collects less information, has the potential of replacing this instrument.

The *Drug Use Forecasting (DUF)* project, sponsored by NIDA, collects data on drug and alcohol use involvement in arrests in selected county jails throughout the United States. It is not a probability sample, but it collects data on drug use and treatment history.

The *Drug Abuse Warning Network (DAWN)* collects data on alcohol and drug "mentions" in emergency room admissions from medical records. It collects information on reported reasons for taking substances, reason for present contact (e.g., chronic effects, although not defined), form in which substance was taken, route of administration, and alcohol involvement. Since 1988, it has been able to produce national estimates as well as more specific estimates for twenty-one metropolitan areas, but it clearly cannot provide county-level data.

Notes

1. The diagnostic instruments typically used include the Diagnostic Interview Schedule (Robins, Helzer, Croughan, & Ratcliff, 1981; Robins, Helzer, Croughan, Williams, & Spitzer, 1981), the Composite International Diagnostic Interview (World Health Organization, 1990), the Structured Clinical Interview for DSM-III-R (SCID) (Spitzer et al., 1990), and the Alcohol Use Disorders and Associated Disabilities Interview Schedule (U.S. NIAAA, 1980).

2. Studies have found that intravenous drug users make up almost 34 percent of adult AIDS cases (Centers for Disease Control, 1987, 1989).

3. In 1988, AIDS associated with intravenous drug use accounted for over half of all AIDS cases among African Americans and Hispanics (Leukefeld et al., 1992); in 1990, over 29 percent of all intravenous drug users who had contracted AIDS were Hispanics (De La Rosa et al., 1990).

4. The ECA data found the proportion of individuals who met criteria for lifetime prevalence of alcohol dependence to be 24 percent of those meeting criteria for schizophrenia, 52 percent of those with antisocial personality, 12 percent for any anxiety disorder, 12 percent for phobia disorder, 22 percent for panic disorder, and 17 percent for obsessive-compulsive disorder (Regier et al., 1990).

5. Project Match, sponsored by NIAAA, is currently conducting outcome studies to systematically examine a variety of patient characteristics in relation to program characteristics.

6. The 1990 total market share of the public sector was $191,070,826; the private nonprofit sector, $522,970,642; and the private for-profit sector, $150,907,619.

7. In 1990, the private nonprofit sector received 42 percent from private

sources (28 percent from health insurance) and 55 percent from public sources; the private for-profit sector received 79 percent of its funds from private sources (63 percent from private third-party insurance); the public sector received almost all of its funding (89 percent) from public sources.

8. This rate is based on the following percentages: 100 percent of deaths from alcohol-dependence syndrome, nondependent abuse of alcohol, alcohol poisoning, and alcoholic psychoses; 41 percent of the cirrhosis mortality rate; 42 percent of the motor vehicle accident mortality rate; 47 percent of the homicide mortality rate; and 20 percent of the suicide mortality rate.

References

Adams, E. H., Blanken, A. J., Ferguson, L. D., & Kopstein, A. 1990. *Overview of Selected Drug Trends*. Berkeley, Calif.: Alcohol Research Group.

American Psychiatric Association. 1987. *DSM-III-R: Diagnostic and Statistical Manual of Mental Disorders*. Washington, D.C.: American Psychiatric Association.

Anglin, M. D., Booth, M. W., Ryan, T. M., & Hser, Y. 1988. Ethnic differences in narcotics addiction. II. Chicano and Anglo addiction career patterns. *International Journal of the Addictions 23*: 1011–27.

Anglin, M. D., Hser, Y.-I., & McGlothlin, W. H. 1987. Sex differences in addict careers. 2. Becoming addicted. *American Journal of Drug and Alcohol Abuse 13*: 59–72.

Babor, T. F., Dolinsky, Z. S., Meyer, R. E., Hesselbrock, M., Hofmann, M., & Tennen, H. 1992. Types of alcoholics: Concurrent and predictive validity of some common classification schemes. *British Journal of Addiction 87*: 1415–31.

Blackwell, J. S. 1983. Drifting, controlling and overcoming: Opiate users who avoid becoming chronically dependent. *Journal of Drug Issues*, 219–35.

Blume, S. B. 1986. Women and alcohol: A review. *Journal of the American Medical Association 256*: 1467–70.

Bray, R. M., & Marsden, M. E. 1992. Prevalence of use of illicit drugs, alcohol, and cigarettes among DC metropolitan area household residents in 1990. Presented at the 100th annual meeting of the American Psychological Association, Washington, D.C., August 14–18.

Caetano, R. 1987. Acculturation and drinking patterns among U.S. Hispanics. *British Journal of Addiction 82*: 789–99.

Caetano, R. 1993. The association between severity of DSM-III-R alcohol dependence and medical and social consequences. *Addictions 88*: 631–42.

Caetano, R., & Kaskutas, L. A. 1993. Longitudinal changes in drinking patterns among whites, blacks, and Hispanics: 1984–1992. Presented at the 1993 annual meeting of the Research Society on Alcoholism, San Antonio, Texas, June 20–24.

Centers for Disease Control. 1987. Human immunodeficiency virus infection in the United States: A review of current knowledge. *Morbidity and Mortality Weekly Report 37*: 133–37.

Centers for Disease Control. 1989. Years of potential life lost before age 65—
United States, 1987. *Morbidity and Mortality Weekly Report 38:* 27–29.

Chaffee, B. H. 1989. Prevention and chemical dependence treatment needs of
special target populations. *Journal of Psychoactive Drugs 21:* 371–79.

Chaisson, R. E., Bacchetti, P., Osmond, D., Brodie, B., Sande, M. A., & Moss,
A. R. 1989. Cocaine use and HIV infection in intravenous drug users in San
Francisco. *Journal of the American Medical Association 261:* 561–65.

Cherpitel, C. J. 1993. *Alcohol Use among Primary Care Patients: Comparing an
HMO with County Clinics and the General Population.* Berkeley, Calif.: Alcohol Research Group.

Cherubin, C., McCusker, J., Baden, M., Kavaler, F., & Amsel, Z. 1972. The
epidemiology of death in narcotic addicts. *American Journal of Epidemiology
96:* 11–20.

Clarke, R. E., & Fox, T. S. 1993. A framework for evaluating the economic
impact of case management. *Hospital and Community Psychiatry 44:* 469–
73.

Clayton, R. R. 1986. Multiple drug use: Epidemiology, correlates, and consequences. In M. Galanter (ed.), *Recent Developments in Alcoholism* (pp. 7–
38). New York: Plenum Press.

De La Rosa, M. R., Khalsa, J. H., & Rouse, B. A. 1990. Hispanics and illicit
drug use: A review of recent findings. *International Journal of the Addictions
25:* 665–91.

De Leon, G., & Jainchill, N. 1981–82. Male and female drug abusers: Social
and psychological status 2 years after treatment in a therapeutic community.
American Journal of Drug and Alcohol Abuse 8: 465–97.

England, M. J., & Vaccaro, V. A. 1991. New systems to manage mental health
care. *Health Affairs (Millwood) 10:* 129–37.

Ferrence, R. 1980. Sex differences in the prevalence of problem drinking. In O.
Kalant (ed.), *Research Advances in Alcohol and Drug Problems* (pp. 69–124).
New York: Plenum Press.

Fillmore, K. M., Hartka, E., Johnstone, B. M., Leino, E. V., Motoyoshi, M., &
Temple, M. T. 1991. The collaborative alcohol-related longitudinal project: A
meta-analysis of life course variation in drinking. *British Journal of Addiction
86:* 1221–68.

Fillmore, K. M., & Midanik, L. 1984. The chronicity of drinking problems
among men: A longitudinal study. *Journal of Studies on Alcohol 45:* 228–
36.

Freeman, M. A., & Trabin, T. *Managed Behavioral Healthcare: History, Models,
Key Issues, and Future Course.* Report submitted to the U.S. Department of
Health and Human Services, 1994.

General Service Office. 1984. *Alcoholics Anonymous 1983 Membership Survey.*
New York, Box 459 Grand Central Station, 10163.

General Service Office. 1991. *Alcoholics Anonymous 1989 Membership Survey.*
New York, Box 459 Grand Central Station, 10163.

General Service Office. 1993. *Alcoholics Anonymous 1992 Membership Survey.*
New York, Box 459 Grand Central Station, 10163.

Gerstein, D. R., & Harwood, H. J. (eds.). 1990. *Treating Drug Problems: Vol. 1. A Study of the Evolution, Effectiveness, and Financing of Public and Private Drug Treatment Systems.* Washington, D.C.: National Academy Press.

Gottheil, E. 1986. Overview. In M. Galanter (ed.), *Recent Developments in Alcoholism* (pp. 3–6). New York: Plenum Press.

Harrison, L. D. 1992. Trends in illicit drug use in the United States: Conflicting results from national surveys. *International Journal of the Addictions* 27: 817–47.

Hasin, D. S., & Glick, H. 1992. Severity of DSM-III-R alcohol dependence: United States, 1988. *British Journal of Addiction* 87: 1725–30.

Helzer, J. E., & Pryzbeck, T. R. 1988. The co-occurrence of alcoholism with other psychiatric disorders in the general population and its impact on treatment. *Journal of Studies on Alcohol* 49: 219–24.

Herd, D. 1988. Drinking by black and white women: Results from a national survey. *Social Problems* 35: 493–505.

Herd, D. 1990. Sub-group differences in drinking patterns among black and white men: Results from a national survey. *Journal of Studies on Alcohol* 51: 221–32.

Horgan, C. 1996. *Chartbook of Social Indicators for Substance Abuse.* Princeton, N.J.: Robert Wood Johnson Foundation.

Hubbard, R. L. 1990. Treating combined alcohol and drug abuse in community-based programs. In M. Galanter (ed.), *Recent Developments in Alcoholism* (pp. 273–84). New York: Plenum Press.

Hubbard, R. L., Marsden, M. E., Rachal, J. V., Harwood, H. J., Cavanaugh, E. R., & Ginzburg, H. M. 1989. *Drug Abuse Treatment: A National Study of Effectiveness.* Chapel Hill: University of North Carolina Press.

Institute of Medicine. 1990. *Broadening the Base of Treatment for Alcohol Problems.* Washington, D.C.: National Academy Press.

Joe, G. W., Chastain, R. L., & Simpson, D. D. 1990. Length of careers. In D. D. Simpson & S. B. Sells (eds.), *Opioid Addiction and Treatment: A 12-Year Follow-Up* (pp. 103–19). Malabar, Fla.: Robert E. Krieger Publishing Company.

Joe, G. W., & Simpson, D. D. 1990. Death rates and risk factors. In D. D. Simpson & S. B. Sells (eds.), *Opioid Addiction and Treatment: A 12-year Follow-up* (pp. 193–202). Malabar, Fla.: Robert E. Krieger Publishing Company.

Johnston, L. D., O'Malley, P. M., & Bachman, J. G. 1991. *Drug Use among American High School Seniors, College Students and Young Adults, 1975–1990: Volume 1. High School Seniors* (DHHS Publ. no. (ADM) 91–1813). U.S. Department of Health and Human Services.

Jones, C. L., & Battjes, R. J. (eds.). 1985. *Etiology of Drug Abuse: Implications for Prevention* (NIDA Research Monograph: A RAUS Review Report. DHHS Publ. no. (ADM) 85–1335). U.S. Department of Health and Human Services.

Kandel, D. B., & Yamaguchi, K. 1985. Developmental patterns of the use of legal, illegal, and medically prescribed psychotropic drugs from adolescence to young adulthood. In C. L. Jones & R. J. Battjes (eds.), *Etiology of Drug Abuse: Implications for Prevention* (pp. 193–236). (NIDA Research Monograph no. 56: A RAUS Review Report). U.S. Department of Health and Human Services.

Keeler, E. B., Manning, W. G., & Wells, K. B. 1988. The demand for episodes of mental health services. *Journal of Health Economics* 7: 369–92.

Leukefeld, C., Pickens, R. W., & Schuster, C. R. 1992. Recommendations for improving drug treatment. *International Journal of the Addictions* 27: 1223–39.

Leukefeld, C. G., & Tims, F. M. 1990. Compulsory treatment for drug abuse. *International Journal of the Addictions* 25: 621–40.

Levin, B. L., Glasser, J. H., & Roberts, R. E. 1984. Changing patterns in mental health service coverage within health maintenance organizations. *American Journal of Public Health* 74: 453–58.

Mammo, A., & Weinbaum, D. F. 1993. Some factors that influence dropping out from outpatient alcoholism treatment facilities. *Journal of Studies on Alcohol* 54: 92–101.

Marlatt, G. A. 1983. The controlled-drinking controversy: A commentary. *American Psychologist* 38: 1097–110.

Marlatt, G. A., & Gordon, J. R. (eds.). 1985. *Relapse Prevention: Maintenance Strategies in the Treatment of Addictive Behaviors*. New York: The Guilford Press.

Marsh, K. L., Joe, G. W., Simpson, D. D., & Lehman, W. E. K. 1990. Treatment history. In D. D. Simpson & S. B. Sells (eds.), *Opioid Addiction and Treatment: A 12-Year Follow-Up* (pp. 137–56). Malabar, Fla.: Robert E. Krieger Publishing Company.

McLellan, A. T., Alterman, A. I., Metzger, D. S., Grissom, G. R., Woody, G. E., Luborsky, L., & O'Brien, C. P. (1994). Similarity of outcome predictors across opiate, cocaine and alcohol treatments: Role of treatment services. *Journal of Consulting and Clinical Psychology* 62: 5–21.

McLellan, A. T., Woody, G. E., Luborsky, L., O'Brien, C. P., & Druley, K. A. 1983. Increased effectiveness of substance abuse treatment: A prospective study of patient-treatment "matching." *Journal of Nervous and Mental Disorders* 171: 597–605.

McNagny, S. E., & Parker, R. M. 1992. High prevalence of recent cocaine use and the unreliability of patient self-report in an inner-city walk-in clinic. *Journal of the American Medical Association* 267: 1106–8.

Midanik, L. T., & Clark, W. B. 1994. The demographic distribution of U.S. drinking patterns in 1990: Descriptions and trends from 1984. *American Journal of Public Health* 84: 1218–22.

Miller, N. S., Millman, R. B., & Keskinen, S. 1990. Outcome and six and twelve months post inpatient treatment for cocaine and alcohol dependence. *Advances in Alcohol and Substance Abuse* 9: 101–20.

Nace, E. P. 1989. The natural history of alcoholism versus treatment effectiveness: Methodological problems. *American Journal of Drug and Alcohol Abuse* 15: 55–60.

National Center for Health Statistics 1992. Advance report of final mortality statistics, 1989. *Monthly Vital Statistics Report 40* (suppl. 2), 1–52.

Nurco, D. N., Bonito, A. J., Lerner, M., & Balter, M. B. 1975. Studying addicts over time: Methodology and preliminary findings. *American Journal of Drug and Alcohol Abuse 2:* 183–96.

Polich, J. M., Armor, D. J., & Braiker, H. B. 1981. *The Course of Alcoholism: Four Years after Treatment.* New York: John Wiley and Sons.

Price, R. H., & D'Aunno, T. (1992a). *Drug Abuse Treatment System Survey: A National Survey of Outpatient Drug Abuse Treatment Services, 1988–1990* (NIDA, final report, grant no. 5RO1-DA03272). Institute for Social Research, Survey Research Center, University of Michigan.

Price, R. H., & D'Aunno, T. (1992b). The organization and impact of outpatient drug abuse treatment services. In R. R. Watson (ed.), *Drug and Alcohol Abuse Reviews, Vol. 3: Treatment of Drug and Alcohol Abuse.* Clifton, N.J.: The Humana Press.

Reed, B. G. 1987. Developing women-sensitive drug dependence treatment services: Why so difficult? *Journal of Psychoactive Drugs 19:* 151.

Regier, D. A., Farmer, M. E., Rae, D. S., Locke, B. Z., Keith, S. J., Judd, L. L., & Goodwin, F. K. 1990. Comorbidity of mental disorders with alcohol and other drug abuse: Results from the Epidemiologic Catchment Area (ECA) study. *Journal of the American Medical Association 264:* 2511–18.

Rice, D. P., Kelman, S., & Miller, L. S. 1991. Estimates of economic costs of alcohol and drug abuse and mental illness, 1985 and 1988. *Public Health Reports 106:* 280–91.

Robins, L. N., Helzer, J. E., Croughan, J., & Ratcliff, K. S. 1981. National Institute of Mental Health Diagnostic Interview Schedule: Its history, characteristics and validity. *Archives of General Psychiatry 41:* 949–58.

Robins, L., Helzer, J., Croughan, J., Williams, J., & Spitzer, R. 1981. *NIMH Diagnostic Interview Schedule III.* Rockville, Md.: National Institute of Mental Health.

Rogowski, J. A. 1992. Insurance coverage for drug abuse. *Health Affairs 11:* 137–48.

Roizen, R. 1987. *The Great Controlled Drinking Controversy.* New York: Plenum Press.

Roizen, R., Cahalan, D., & Shanks, P. 1978. "Spontaneous remission" among untreated problem drinkers. In D. B. Kandel (ed.), *Longitudinal Research on Drug Use: Empirical Findings and Methodological Issues* (pp. 197–221). New York: John Wiley and Sons.

Room, R. 1977. Measurement and distribution of drinking patterns and problems in general populations. In G. Edwards, M. M. Gross, M. Keller, J. Moser, & R. Room (eds.), *Alcohol-Related Disabilities* (pp. 61–87) (Offset publ. no. 32). World Health Organization.

Room, R. 1978. *Governing Images of Alcohol and Drug Problems: The Structure, Sources and Sequels of Conceptualizations of Intractable Problems.* Ph.D. diss. University of California, Berkeley.

Rounsaville, B. J., & Kleber, H. D. 1985. Untreated opiate addicts: How do they differ from those seeking treatment? *Archives of General Psychiatry 42:* 1072–77.

Sanchez, D. 1984. *NIAAA Quick Facts*. Rockville, Md.: National Institute on Alcohol Abuse and Alcoholism.

Schmidt, L., & Weisner, C. 1993. Developments in alcoholism treatment: A ten year review. In M. Galanter (ed.), *Recent Developments in Alcoholism* (pp. 369–96). New York: Plenum Press.

Simpson, D. D. 1990. Final comments. In D. D. Simpson & S. B. Sells (eds.), *Opioid Addiction and Treatment: A 12-Year Follow-Up* (pp. 239–52). Malabar, Fla.: Robert E. Krieger Publishing Company.

Spitzer, R. L., Williams, J. B. W., Gibbin, M., & First, M. B. 1990. *Structured Clinical Interview for DSM-III-R—Patient Edition (with Psychotic Screen)— SCID-P (W/PSYCHOTIC SCREEN)—Version 1.0*. Washington, D.C.: American Psychiatric Press.

Taylor, J. R., & Helzer, J. E. 1983. The natural history of alcoholism. In B. Kissin & H. Begeiter (eds.), *The Pathogenesis of Alcoholism: Psychosocial Factors* (pp. 17–67). New York: Plenum Press.

Tims, F. M. 1981. *Effectiveness of Drug Abuse Treatment Programs* (NIDA Treatment Report. DHHS Publ. no. (ADM) 84–1143). U.S. Department of Health and Human Services.

Tims, F. M., Fletcher, B. W., & Hubbard, R. L. 1991. Treatment outcomes for drug abuse clients. In R. W. Pickens, C. G. Leukefeld, & R. Schuster (eds.), *Improving Drug Abuse Treatment* (Research Monograph no. 106). U.S. Department of Health and Human Services.

Tims, F. M., & Leukefeld, C. G. (eds.). 1986. *Relapse and Recovery in Drug Abuse* (NIDA Research Monograph no. 72). U.S. Department of Health and Human Services.

Tischler, G. L. 1990. Utilization management of mental health services by private third parties. *American Journal of Psychiatry* 147: 967–73.

U.S. National Institute on Alcohol Abuse and Alcoholism. 1980. *Report to the President and the Congress on Health Hazards Associated with Alcohol and Methods to Inform the General Public of These Hazards*. Washington, D.C.: U.S. Government Printing Office.

U.S. National Institute on Alcohol Abuse and Alcoholism. 1990. *Alcohol and Health: Seventh Special Report to the U.S. Congress* (DHHS no. (ADM) 90–1656). U.S. Department of Health and Human Services.

U.S. National Institute on Alcohol Abuse and Alcoholism. 1991. *U.S. Alcohol Epidemiologic Data Reference Manual, Vol. 3, Third Edition: County Alcohol Problem Indicators, 1979–1985* (DHHS Publ. no. (ADM) 91–1740). U.S. Department of Health and Human Services.

U.S. National Institute on Drug Abuse 1991. *Drug Abuse and Drug Abuse Research: The Third Report to Congress from the Secretary, Department of Health and Human Services* (DHHS Publ. no. (ADM) 91–1704). Public Health Service; Alcohol, Drug Abuse and Mental Health Administration; National Institute on Drug Abuse.

Vaillant, G. 1983. *The Natural History of Alcoholism: Causes, Patterns and Paths to Recovery*. Cambridge: Harvard University Press.

Vannicelli, M. 1984. Treatment outcome of alcoholic women: The state of the art in relation to sex bias and expectancy effects. In S. C. Wilsnack & L. J. Beckman (eds.), *Alcohol Problems in Women: Antecedents, Consequences, and Intervention* (pp. 369–412). New York: The Guilford Press.

Weisner, C. 1986. The transformation of alcohol treatment: Access to care and the response to drinking-driving. *Journal of Public Health Policy 7:* 78–92.

Weisner, C. 1993. The epidemiology of combined alcohol and drug use within treatment agencies: A comparison by gender. *Journal of Studies on Alcohol 54:* 268–74.

Weisner, C., Greenfield, T., & Room, R. 1995. Trends in the treatment of alcohol problems in the U.S. general population, 1979 through 1990. *American Journal of Public Health 85:* 55–60.

Weisner, C., & Schmidt, L. 1992. Gender disparities in the treatment of alcohol problems. *Journal of the American Medical Association 268:* 1872–76.

Wells, K. B., Astrachan, B. M., Tischler, G. L., & Unutzer, J. 1995. Issues and approaches in evaluating managed mental health care. *Milbank Quarterly 73:* 57–75.

Wilsnack, S. C., Klassen, A. D., Schur, B. E., & Wilsnack, R. W. 1991. Predicting onset and chronicity of women's problem drinking: A five-year longitudinal analysis. *American Journal of Public Health 81:* 305–18.

Woody, G. E., Cottler, L. B., & Cacciola, J. 1993. Severity of dependence: Data from the DSM-IV field trials. *Addiction 88:* 1573–79.

World Health Organization. 1990. *Composite International Diagnostic Interview: Authorized Core Version 1.0.* Geneva: World Health Organization.

Yahr, H. T. 1988. A national comparison of public and private sector alcoholism treatment delivery system characteristics. *Journal of Studies on Alcohol 49:* 233–39.

10/ COMMUNITY-LEVEL INDICATORS FOR CHRONIC HEALTH CARE SERVICES

Robert J. Newcomer and A. E. Benjamin

The preceding chapters present a mosaic of ideas for describing chronic conditions, the service histories associated with these conditions, and potential measures for tracking their prevalence, treatment, and outcomes. One of the major values of this work is its perspective on conceptualization and measurement, cutting across groups that may not usually communicate with one another. Some chronic condition subsystems are more advanced in the resources available (e.g., aged with Medicare), but the experience gained from this group can be extended to others in Medicaid- or survey-based studies. Other groups may offer strengths in problem conceptualization, client empowerment, or delivery system coordination, which can be usefully extended to the others.

Our goals in concluding this book are to distill common themes and perspectives from these chapters and to propose a framework for organizing the discussion and development of community-level chronic-care monitoring systems. We emphasize conceptual dimensions that we think are appropriate for these conditions, offer suggestions as to the relative priority and salience of particular types of indicators, and propose a variety of options for their development, testing, and refinement. These integrative proposals are consistent with and supplemental to contemporary indicators efforts such as *Healthy People 2000* (U.S. Public Health Service, 1993) and the Institute of Medicine's (IOM) *Access to Health Care* (Millman, 1993), and the developing capacities for community-level data reflected in hospital discharge abstracts and claims data systems (e.g., Luft & Hunt, 1986; Roos, Roos, & Sharpe, 1987; Wennberg, 1987). We avoid the technical and political question of specifying normative indicator levels or the specific procedures that define standards of practice. The history of community data systems and indicators makes clear the incremental and political nature of this process. Years of blue-ribbon committee negotiations are usually required to reach agreement on minimum indicators. Additional time is required to obtain reasonably uniform data reporting among the participating states and communities.

UNDERLYING THEMES

Seven themes related to service systems for chronic-care populations, although developed with varying depth and urgency by each background paper, have emerged as universal among the preceding chapters. These are summarized here as an important basis for the service-system indicators and data collection priorities presented later.

Needs for Service Change over Time

A number of factors contribute to changing care needs among clients and their informal care systems, one of which is the changing experience with the problem or condition. With time, clients know their bodies better and know how to use the service system more effectively. Another factor is a potential change in the developmental needs and expectations of individuals as they age; this applies most obviously to children as they grow to adulthood. More subtly, but as emphasized with substance abusers and those with mental retardation or physical disability, there is a developmental cycle progressing from the age of onset of the problem to greater age. The developmental cycle in this context includes roles in society, the natural progression of degenerative conditions, and the emergence of comorbid conditions. Apparently, formal providers for people with mental or physical disability sometimes ignore the likelihood that these individuals will experience physiological changes with age and that they have risk factors affecting the functioning of their other body systems. Sometimes, too, as chapters 4 and 5 indicate, the needs go away.

A third dynamic involves the family and other elements in an individual's informal support system. For children and young adults (such as those with cognitive and mental disorders, substance abusers, and even those with physical disability), this usually refers to parents. For those with chronic degenerative medical conditions and physical impairment, often a spouse, siblings, or even one's children assume the role of informal support. In either set of circumstances, caregivers change in their ability to provide care over time, even holding client attributes constant. These changes can occur for physical and financial reasons or because of other responsibilities, such as other children, employment, or marital status. Because of these various factors contributing to changing service needs, we suggest that service plans be monitored and revised on a regular basis. All the background papers express a concern that the delivery system is not inherently set up to do this effectively but note that the process can be monitored effectively by service recipient studies.

Coordination between Primary and Specialty Care

Primary medical care is the touchstone for ongoing management of people with chronic conditions and for the early detection and treatment of those health conditions that may develop with age (e.g., cardiovascular, musculoskeletal, neurological, pulmonary) and produce their own risk for functional impairment. Specialty care includes surgical and medical specialties such as cardiology and oncology and ancillary services such as rehabilitative care and psychological counseling. People with chronic conditions are often under the care of specialists (e.g., pediatric neurosurgeons, cardiologists, psychologists) or specialty centers (e.g., spinal cord injury rehabilitation, geriatric assessment) at some stage of their service history for diagnosis and initial treatment. Under these circumstances, there is a tendency for the client to link more with specialist physicians than with primary care physicians. To whom does (or should) the client go for episodic problems, such as infections secondary to their condition, immunizations, and the monitoring of their general health status?

Coordination between medical and nonmedical service delivery systems may be even more problematic. How do clients deal with conflicting demands and recommendations from multiple providers? Do the providers even know of these conflicts? The fragmentation and categorical nature of much service funding further contributes to these problems. Delivery systems (with the possible exception of managed care under Medicaid) have few incentives to assume a comprehensive coordinative role.[1] Although these are common problems for clients and providers, it is typically left to the clients and their families to coordinate and negotiate multiple services. Families are seldom given training in how to negotiate needed delivery systems and may not have a good access point into care as needs change over time (e.g., those with physical disabilities trying to reenter the delivery system but without the contact point of the rehabilitation center). Self-help groups for some systems often fill the training role. This infrastructure is perhaps more developed for some childhood conditions, alcohol-abuse support, and some disability groups than for other age groups and conditions. Self-help groups are not uniformly available in all communities, nor are they equally accessible to all cultural and economic groups.

These concerns demonstrate that access to primary care and the various forms of specialty care and therapies is but one aspect of service delivery to be monitored. Often of more importance is how these providers exchange information and how well families and clients are trained to use and coordinate multiple providers. Claims systems can track the use of multiple providers, but surveys focused on the points of care coordination and the client's service coordination experience may also prove valuable.

Nonmedical Implications of Poorly Managed Conditions

The implications of impaired primary care (and poorly coordinated care more generally) extend beyond medical and health status risks to other care needs and care systems. For children, this includes school attendance and fatigue levels while in school, both of which affect educational attainment, self-esteem, and, in some cases, the ability to overcome developmental disabilities. For family members, this may result in such things as time lost from work, stress, depression, and marital and family conflicts. All these outcomes affect the quality of life for caregivers and their ability to continue in the caregiving role. Persons with chronic conditions are at risk for their psychological status, as indicated by depression, poor self-esteem, and a limited sense of self-determination. These may impair cognitive function and motivation, which in turn affect self-maintenance ability and academic and employment performance. The underlying causes of these consequences are varied and not always easily delineated. They include the use of medications that may affect cognitive function; poorly managed infections or other episodic problems that require absences from school or training programs; and the use of services outside the community, which removes clients from their home environment and friends and places extra time and expense burdens on families. Though potentially correctable, such secondary effects as these are too infrequently recognized by providers.

Within each of the populations examined here, the use of case managers or care coordinators is seen as one means of overcoming the departmental, organizational, professional, and even financial barriers to better integrated and coordinated services. Implementation takes many forms, ranging from information dissemination and referrals, assessment and care plan development, through benefit authorization and care monitoring. The breadth of service under the coordinator's role is also varied. Seldom does authority extend to medical care and the coordination that may be needed at that level, but this is an "evolving" program. We suggest that indicator systems include tracking of the authority and breadth of systems coordinated through such mechanisms, although true tests of effectiveness will have to come from focused experiments.

Barriers to Care from Other Services

The problems of, and barriers to, appropriate care are not solely a consequence of uncoordinated care. Among other factors, the regulations and funding levels in the community care system may inadvertently limit access or effective use by those with chronic conditions. For example, children who need to take medications in school to manage a chronic condition may be unable to do so because schools lack skilled care or have restrictions against medications. Architectural barriers may limit access to programs, buildings, and transportation systems to those with physical disability.

Another type of barrier is created by the categorical funding for special services. It is not unusual for benefit eligibility to require that the client be segregated into special programs or into an income- or means-tested program. Such requirements may reduce the willingness of families to accept such programs.

A third type of barrier is created by limitations on available community services. A good illustration of this is the restriction of in-home educational tutorial services to those homebound for two or more weeks only. Persons with frequent short-term illness, such as those under treatment for various chronic conditions, may be excluded from these programs and placed at risk of falling behind in their education. Barriers to care, whatever form they take, possibly contribute to community and state variation in service access and use. Community indicator data, focused community studies of policies and regulations, and client program experience may be useful means of explicating these effects.

Program Financing for Medical and Nonmedical Care

The source of payment for nonmedical care is recognized as a leading, but by no means the only, factor contributing to the poor coordination of regulations and benefits across these multitiered services. Health care is typically covered by private insurance or, for those meeting entitlement or other eligibility requirements, by Medicaid, Medicare, and the Veterans Administration (VA). Medicaid and the VA offer the most comprehensive benefits, covering medical, some institutional, and home-care services. Private insurance and Medicare do not usually cover nonmedical care. Community care, such as education, mental health, residential treatment, and sheltered workshops, is financed by a combination of federal, state, and local funds—but without a direct connection to health care delivery or incentive to coordinate with it. Efficiencies in one financial system that may produce saving in another are not typically rewarded, nor are processes that foster cost shifting typically sanctioned. More typically, each system eagerly pursues approaches that shift cost to other sources of payment. Access to much of the community care available is limited by income and other asset eligibility, Medicaid (or VA) payment levels, or third-party-payer rules. States and communities show great variation in eligibility and payment levels for these programs, which leads to much variation in the supply of these services. Also restricting supply are licensing requirements and restrictions (e.g., staff-to-client ratios) and requirements concerning the adequacy of training and experience in key delivery system elements. These affect the cost of operation and the cost of care.

Enrollment in managed care systems is one means by which payers and providers are seeking to control costs and create more vertical integration of economic incentives. This phenomenon is occurring at different rates across the country. One expressed concern for the chronically ill about these systems is their effect on access to care. One fear is that they will possibly reduce access to specialty care and the range of treatments available. Optimists expect that managed care will improve coordination between specialists and primary care providers and reduce the use of out-of-area providers. These scenarios are not mutually exclusive.

Effects arising from financing and regulatory policies and conditions are implicitly reflected in both program- and client-level data as a contributing factor (along with client conditions) in these trends. These kinds of variables need to be controlled when client treatment and outcome patterns are compared across communities or over time

Families and Other Informal Supports

Families and other informal social supports are seen as vital elements in the chronic-care system. Their roles vary depending on the age of the client and the age of the caregiver (e.g., parents are key factors for children and persons with developmental disabilities; spouses for the aged and those with chronic medical illness or physical disability; parents and siblings for substance abusers, those with mental illness, and unmarried people with disabilities). The appropriateness and accessibility of service or treatment options are often strongly affected by the informal resources available to the individual client. A community-care monitoring system should measure how the informal system is functioning and the effect of "chronic" condition management on this system's members. A number of substudies are suggested to empirically test assumptions about effective methods of strengthening informal care; among them, What effect do support groups have on the knowledge and use of formal and other informal care? Does the presence of nonmedical specialized services (e.g., home tutors, physical access to schools, home aides, personal attendants) affect the psychological status and social integration of clients and families?

When family members are not able to carry out a custodial role, other forms of supported or assisted living are often necessary (e.g., state hospitals, nursing homes, and less restrictive settings like foster care and group housing). This continuum of living arrangements, although often financed and regulated through different programs, is similar across disability and age groups. The willingness of advocates to endorse a given form of service (e.g., nursing home care) varies considerably across groups (e.g., older vs. younger people with physical disabilities). The distribution of people with chronic disability into various living arrangements may serve as a crude indicator of the informal care system, but data on the functioning of informal care (including its effect on caregivers) may have to be obtained through surveys of these caregivers.

Scope of the Indicator System

Each of the background papers came to its own conclusions and recommendations about appropriate indicators, but there was commonality in the conceptual dimensions emphasized. Among these were prevention, access to treatment, the nature of the treatment, treatment outcomes, client satisfaction, social or community adjustment and integration, and informal caregiver outcomes. For the most part, these dimensions derive from client- or case-level data, although they lend themselves to aggregation into community- or program-level measures. There was also commonality in the categories of service to be included in the care system. Medical care and health services formed a core, but social supports, education, and specialized therapies (e.g., psychological, occupational, physical) were also recognized as important. Also acknowledged were factors influencing program operations (e.g., regulations and reimbursement policies) and other environmental factors affecting supply, competition, or cooperation among elements in the various delivery systems. In terms of indicators, however, these dimensions were implicitly treated as constants in the short term or as an underlying basis for cross-community comparisons.

There is much more variation among the authors' recommendations about how the data for their suggested indicators can be compiled. Some rely heavily on survey-based measures, others on a balance between administrative records and surveys. These perspectives considered in the aggregate raise a number of provocative considerations as we contemplate the development of an indicator system for chronic conditions. How aggressive should monitoring be? Can sentinel indicators be used to trigger more in-depth analysis? Which elements of systems monitoring should be at the national level? What should be the frequency of monitoring? Can monitoring explicitly connect cause to effect? Is this necessary? Is longitudinal, panel-based measurement needed? Is the quality and reliability of existing measures sufficient to warrant their use as indicators? What is the role of population-based studies, and what is gained or lost by service recipient measures? Are cost-efficient means available for developing sample frames for population- or recipient-based surveys?

A FRAMEWORK FOR MONITORING COMMUNITY CARE

The extent and depth of information monitored are constrained by the data available, the resources required to generate it, and the political will to act on the information. Related to these issues is a fundamental question about the readiness of delivery systems (and their regulators) to focus on client-level outcomes versus the performance and cost savings within the "programs" themselves. Program performance is presently measured in terms such as user volume, units of service per recipient, frequency of use, cost per unit of care, and practice variations. In many situations, basic program operations data may produce more political responsiveness than information about who is served or what failings may be occurring.

In preparing a community indicator model, we have tried to balance these positions by identifying indicators reflecting both perspectives. The indicators are organized into a framework consisting of three levels. Each succeeding level becomes more precise in its measures. Level one, which we have termed "system and contextual," measures basic trends in service access, condition prevalence, expenditures, service supply, and health outcomes. Level two is more closely focused on "service access and process of care" for selected subgroups of recipients. These subgroups are defined by a diagnosed condition or the types of procedures used. Level three continues the focus on targeted subgroups and measures trends in health outcomes, social adjustment, and family "outcomes."

To be practical and responsive to the variations in state and community technical and financial capacity, most of the proposed level one and level two indicators can be built from readily available data. The outcome measures usually require primary data. Many refinements and operational details will be needed before proposals such as these can be implemented. Recognizing the preliminary nature of our proposal, we have tried to keep the presentation at a relatively conceptual level. This is done so that the discussion can address dimensions of interest, general depth of information desired, and the process for setting relative priorities, rather than operational details of measurement or the interpretation of specific indicator levels. We have expressly avoided making recommendations as to specific standards or norms, although we have suggested a process for doing this. Measures are discussed primarily from the point of view of data source priorities and how data might be aggregated. Certainly, the framework can be implemented with a variety of data sources as they become more widely available.

Although the initial selection of seven subgroups and multiple chronic conditions was intended to provide broad exposure to the problems and delivery systems, we recognize that the framework is built from the services required for a particular set of chronic conditions and the data available to monitor these services and their outcomes. Each condition uses a combination of medical care, both primary and specialty; nursing, educational, and social services; mental health or psychosocial counseling; specialized therapies, such as occupational, physical, respiratory, nutrition, speech, or hearing; and living arrangements. As other conditions are considered, the delivery system scope, as we have outlined it, may need to be reevaluated.

System- and Contextual-Level Indicators

System and contextual indicators have two principal interrelated purposes. The first is to provide an overview of selected conditions in a community. We propose the several dimensions shown in Table 10.1, but this list can be readily expanded or altered. These indicators provide an "alert" about potential problems in the subset of systems that are being monitored. The sentinel, or trigger, values that define a trend as problematic would be based on a comparison of community indicators over time, communities with each other, or communities against national or regional norms. System-level indicators are made somewhat more precise by stratifying the tabulations by demographic subgroups, such as age, gender, and race, and possibly combinations such as gender by race. The data used at this first level of monitoring are not generally intended to be specific to most chronic health conditions. That level of refinement is a feature of the two remaining levels in the proposed indicator framework. The determination of the causes of observed trends or of the pervasiveness of problems for particular health conditions within a community requires either second-level indicators or focused studies.

The second purpose of system-level indicators is to bring a consideration of state policy, community service supply, and other contextual effects into the interpretation of national and regional indicator trends. This is done by documenting and comparing community indicator trends as a basis for studying communities that have unexpected rates (after adjusting for population characteristics).

The proposed system-level indicators are generally derived from program-reported encounters and events or other relatively accessible administrative records. These data sources are largely in place, making it possible to quickly implement a national minimum and relatively uniform data set. Prevalence and incidence estimates are the area in which substantial capability may have to be developed. Synthetic estimation may be one means of reducing the cost and other logistical factors associated with generating these baseline values.

Table 10.1. System- and Contextual-Level Indicators

Indicator (Source)	Data Aggregation		
Access	Age	Gender	Race
• Community encounter counts of selected conditions (surveillance, encounter, or claims systems)			
• Prevalence/incidence estimates of selected conditions (derived from national or other surveys)			
• Unmet need (prevalence minus encounters)			
Prevention [1]	Age	Gender	Race
• Births to teenagers			
• Births to low-income women			
• Low-birthweight newborns			
• Births with physical deformity			
• Drug-dependent newborns			
• Work-related accidents			
• Vehicle accidents			
• Vehicle accidents, alcohol or drug related			
Health and other outcomes [1]			
• Mortality rate			
• Hospitalization per hospital rate			
• Nursing home placement rate			
• Other assisted living			
• Heart attack			
• Stroke			
• Spinal cord injuries			
Service supply	Service units	Units—estimated need	
• Physician			
• Hospital			
• Rehabilitation			
• Nursing home			
• Other therapeutic programs			
• Skilled/paraprofessional home care			
• Specialized living arrangements			
• Special education/employment training			
• Other social service			
Service expenditures	Expenditures per capita	Expenditures per recipient	
• Physician			
• Hospital			
• Rehabilitation			
• Nursing home			
• Other therapeutic programs			
• Skilled/paraprofessional home care			
• Specialized living arrangements			
• Special education/employment training			
• Other social service			

1. Estimated prevalence minus observed events or observed events.

The following discussion elaborates the rationale for the choice of the domains and measures in this level of our framework. This is a minimum indicator set. Many other readily available contextual measures could be added to this framework for routine tracking or comparative analyses. Among measures commonly seen in such analyses are per capita income, per capita public expenditures, and employment rates. Such data are available from existing data sources, such as the *Area Resource File* and *State and County Data Book*. We have not included such measures in our proposal simply because we consider the effect of these variables to be reflected in other measures in the model, namely, supply and expenditures. The refinement of the minimum domains and indicators will come only with experience in their use and interpretation.

Access

Access to care is a basic feature of system performance. Differential access is presumed to be a contributing factor in health status, service intensity, costs of care, and health and other treatment outcomes. Access indicators take varying forms. On the one hand are unadjusted rates, such as reported encounters and units of service used. Unadjusted rates can be tabulated for subgroups in the population, such as by age, gender, and race, to provide one basis for comparison of access or access barriers. The conversion from a simple rate to an adjusted rate is usually necessary if comparisons are to be made with other communities, national averages, or time periods, since adjustments have to be made for population size and the relative mix of age, gender, and racial groups. An important step in this standardization process is the selection of the denominator for these calculations. Is it the total population, a subset of people somehow defined as at risk, or the users of selected services? Such encounter data would be expressed respectively as rates per thousand population, rates per thousand persons at risk, or service units per recipient. Each derived rate serves as an indicator for different facets of community and delivery system operation.

The access measures proposed for level one indicators consist of two components, the first of which is reported delivery-system encounters (e.g., hospital discharges, emergency room visits, substance-abuse program participation). Such data are available from disease surveillance systems, claims data, hospital discharge abstract systems, or local use surveys. Encounter data may be biased, since they reflect those who actually received care rather than those needing, but not accessing, care. The second component is an estimate of the prevailing need within the population, differentiated by age, gender, and racial groups. Need can be expressed in alternative forms, such as by expected rates for particular health conditions or by service use.

The difference between prevailing need and observed encounters is one means of assessing bias in the encounter data. It is also a means of assessing the level of unmet need or problems in access within the population. Per capita measured encounters substantially above the prevalence estimate suggest that environmental or other local conditions may be contributing to a higher than expected prevalence/incidence. Substantially lower use or encounter rates may suggest problems of access to the care system. Either situation may require a community study to identify the underlying factors. In spite of the simple math involved, there are a number of potential pitfalls in this process, beginning with the availability of a population estimate of need and ending with completeness of the encounter data. Most communities (as well as programs or health plans) have access to information about the number of service or program recipients and even about persons eligible for these benefits on the basis of membership or other eligibility standards. Population-based estimates of the prevalence of conditions are less commonly available. Putting these two pieces of information together is helpful, first, for a comparison of the potential number of persons at risk for particular conditions (and their probabilities of requiring services within a given period), as we are suggesting for the measures of access and outcomes shown in Table 10.1; and second, for a comparison with the available service supply to assess its adequacy. These estimates can also be used in later stages of our framework to assess the proportion of persons with a condition (or at risk of a condition) who are actually using services or who are known to the relevant sectors of delivery system.

The usual method for compiling population-based estimates is through surveys, either area probability samples or catchment area samples. This is costly, complex, and not replicable in most communities. An alternative endorsed by the authors is a synthetic estimate of disease or condition prevalence (or incidence). Synthetic estimates use probabilities for a disease or condition derived from sources such as the National Health Interview Survey (NHIS) or community studies. These estimates can be per capita or more refined and specific to demographic and other characteristics (e.g., age, gender, sometimes racial, and living arrangement). These probabilities are applied to the demographic profile of the target geographic area, such as a substate region, community, or neighborhood. The major purpose of a synthetic estimate is to establish the expected number of persons affected by the particular condition(s). Separate estimates can be developed for the annual incidence of "new" cases or the prevailing number of persons in the population having the conditions.[2] Statisticians generally question the reliability of "small area" synthetic estimate applications, but the cost-saving simplicity of these estimates is compelling, at least as a starting estimate of prevalence/ incidence. The quality of, and bias in, the information obtainable from the encounter data systems is at least as problematic in many communities.

Prevention

Prevention, as outlined in the preceding chapters, takes multiple forms. Many years and multiple factors often contribute to the onset or severity of various types of physical disability, substance abuse, and mental illness. In these situations, national- or state-level surveys probably suffice to produce estimates of behavioral risk and health promotion trends within the general population. Data on risk factors and behaviors, such as diet, exercise, smoking, and alcohol consumption, are routinely collected in national surveys (e.g., the NHIS) and in state Behavioral Risk Factor Surveillance Surveys (BRFSS). Public policy (or health plan) responsiveness to the trends reported in such data are outside the scope of our proposed indicator framework.

Our attention is focused on those conditions in which the relationship between prevention and its benefit is short term and direct. Public health indicators related to this issue typically concentrate on health screening and immunizations as indicating access to primary care and the preventive care implied by these procedures. To this list, we add elements that emphasize children and accident-related injury. For conditions affecting children (some of whom will become adults with developmental disabilities), service intervention involves prenatal care to identify high-risk pregnancies, intervention to assure adequate nutrition, community health education efforts to reduce teenage pregnancy, and additional efforts to reduce drug or other environmental exposures for those who are pregnant. The adequacy of these interventions is in part reflected in birth rates among groups thought to be at high risk (e.g., teenagers, low income) or in the number of high-risk infants born (e.g., low birthweight, drug dependent). Another stage of prevention occurs once there is a high-risk birth (i.e., low birthweight, low income, drug exposed, or other developmental risk factors). Among the interventions appropriate to this population are an enrichment of the training for these children and adequate training of families in how to care for their child.

Basic incidence reporting on births is proposed for level one monitoring. Information about how much prenatal care was used and the nature of the counseling or other interventions intended to reduce risk behaviors can be obtained in a second-level analysis, such as a follow-up survey of birth mothers. Alternatively, Medicaid claims can be used to track physician use by those who gave birth to a high-risk infant. This type of tracking illustrates the level of refinement that might be incorporated into level two indicators. The rates of accident-related disability (e.g., spinal cord injuries, work-related accidents, vehicle accidents, alcohol- or drug-related vehicle accidents), another preventable condition, are also appropriate for community monitoring. Such rates may be a basis for assessing how well preventive policies and their enforcement, such as speed limits, helmet laws, and occupational safety, are being implemented.

Health and Other Outcomes

Among the more pervasively used outcome indicators of system performance at the client level are mortality, hospitalization rates, and rates of various conditions considered to reflect environmental factors (e.g., cancer), health screening adequacy (e.g., hypertension), or treatment complications or inadequate care (e.g., rehospitalization). These values come from a combination of data sources, including population surveys. We have supplemented this list of indicators with others suggested by our background paper authors as indicating additional underlying problems in primary care (e.g., stroke, heart attack as indicative of poorly managed diet, hypertension, or blood cholesterol) or of social risk factors (e.g., nursing home placement, other assisted-living arrangement placement rates).

The set of outcomes suggested for the initial level of tracking in Table 10.1 is limited to events reported in either hospital discharge abstracts, service claims, or surveillance systems. This decision was made because these sources are generally reliable and available and thus can become components in national or statewide systems without much delay. The relative importance of any one indicator is best determined by comparing the observed and the estimated rates.

This list can be easily altered with the addition of other available health or social conditions. We are not so much interested in being definitive about a minimum list of conditions as in trying to illustrate how they can be used at this general level of monitoring. For example, there are a variety of measures beyond health status that can indicate the effectiveness of other aspects of the delivery system, and some of them are especially appropriate as indicators of short-term or immediate effects from "treatment" intervention. These outcomes include educational status (i.e., attendance rates and attainment), social adjustment (as indicated by arrests and other problems with the criminal justice system), and violent acts (e.g., suicide threats/attempts, perpetrators or victims of violent acts). We suggest such measures as level three outcomes, which are tied to defined subpopulations and therefore track more readily into specific delivery systems. We have not included such measures in our level one minimum indicators because at this level of aggregation, they reflect multiple dimensions of community life and are not necessarily tied to chronic conditions.

Measures that reflect "failure" to enter the delivery system at the "ideal" entry point are another illustration of potential indicators. These cases can be indicated by the number of target clients identified by other delivery systems (e.g., in mental health, entry through the criminal justice system, hospital emergency room, or homeless centers, rather than mental health centers). We have elected to put such indicators in level two monitoring because we think they are more easily developed and interpreted if they are connected with defined populations; others may prefer such measures in level one.

A caveat in the use and interpretation of the sentinel health outcome and access indicators proposed for level one monitoring is that many aspects of appropriate and quality care are not encompassed in this level of measurement. For example, system adequacy in mental illness cannot be limited to mental health services per se; it should also address assistance with community living skills, managing relationships, or engaging in productive activity. The connection between who is receiving care in one system or program versus the others requires complex claims tracking or survey data, and as such is appropriate for special studies or targeted monitoring.

Service Supply

Using a service inventory in a comparison with prevalence or incidence estimates provides a context against which to evaluate observed service access and use rates over time or among communities.[3] Substantial differences between prevalence/incidence and the supply of service units available may suggest problems of under- or oversupply. These measures can also be useful for assessing changes in service supply after the implementation of policy changes and under varying local conditions (e.g., labor supply, operational costs, competition). For example: Is the supply of home care attendants affected by changes in reimbursement, service acuity levels, or other higher-paying employment opportunities in the community? Moving to this level of refinement requires several steps. First, the prevalence/incidence estimates discussed above have to be refashioned to yield estimates of expected use (i.e., the number of days or hours of treatment) among recipients of the service, or the average annual expected use among members of the target or at-risk population. Similarly, service supply units would need to be expressed in terms of days or hours or other appropriate units (e.g., beds) available during a defined period (e.g., week, month, annually). Aside from the heroic assumptions that facilitate these supply estimates, two complications remain: many services are not exclusive to particular diseases or conditions, and often, several services might be used as alternatives or substitutes for each other. One means around the problem of competing demand is to aggregate the prevalence estimates for all groups that use these services, creating an aggregate number of cases and units of use over a defined period. This produces an adjusted per capita use rate for the community population. Similarly, the units of service from all the substitutable services can be aggregated to yield an adjusted measure of service supply.

Much of the data on the supply of services is already widely available. The most comprehensive and inclusive national service supply inventory is the Area Resource File, a county-level database that includes county descriptors, the number of licensed health professionals (e.g., doctors, dentists, pharmacists, podiatrists, nurses), the number of hospitals and nursing homes (e.g., size, type, use, staffing, and services), and expenditure data (e.g., hospital expenditures, Medicare enrollments and reimbursements, Medicare prevailing charges). Not all data are updated annually, but many elements could be if the derivative key data sources were accessed directly.[4] One limitation of the Area Resource File for chronic-care delivery system applications is that it does not systematically include many of the social service (e.g., paraprofessional home care, transportation, meals programs, sheltered workshops, specialized housing), educational, recreational (e.g., exercise classes), support group, and criminal justice programs that define important parts of the chronic-care delivery system. A second limitation is that the service inventory is not specific to subpopulations or target groups. Either or both of these enhanced inventories may be present in many communities under the auspices of the United Way, the Chamber of Commerce, or other entities, but they are not universal. Aggregating the expanded service inventories across communities or states will be challenging but could be phased in as experience is gained using the available supply indicators.[5]

Another approach to service supply calculations is to create an inventory or listing of specific providers, which is useful as a sample frame for periodic surveys of providers. These surveys can monitor such things as the number of programs and their census, types of services provided, referral sources, source of payment for programs, staffing, and financial performance. This particular type of survey is discussed below as an example of a community survey. Because this approach is relatively expensive, we believe it should be reserved for targeted programs or special studies. Given the recognized importance of care coordination among those with chronic conditions, a high priority for a targeted program survey could be primary care physicians, selected specialists, hospital discharge planners, and case managers for the various chronically impaired populations.

Service Expenditures

Use and expenditure rates are widely used as basic indicators of system-level responsiveness and performance. Such measures reflect the absolute spending on public and other programs, and if standardized on the basis of total population or an identified target population, they reflect the community's relative generosity. Wide variation across communities can be observed using such measures. Spending levels per se can be misleading, because they are a function of the prevailing unit price for services and the efficiency with which patients receive treatment. These latter concerns can be monitored by using recipients as the rate calculation denominator, producing per recipient rates.

The generation of use and expenditure information is complicated by

fragmented funding for services. Public payments occur in multiple programs. Data on private payments may not be available at all, except
through self-reports from providers or recipients. Working within these
limitations, we have elected to focus monitoring on public programs such
as Medicare, Medicaid, special education, and mental health services.
Aggregated use and expenditures reports and statistics are usually available from the agencies responsible for administering these programs.
They are typically reported by categorical eligibility subgroup (e.g., elderly, children, persons with disabilities, low income, racial minority)
and by the general type of service (e.g., physician, hospital, employment
training). Within Medicare and Medicaid, spending can be further disaggregated by diagnostic group and other classifications, but this is rarely
possible in social service management information programs. This degree
of analysis is deferred to the second and third levels of our framework.

When possible, it is desirable to create two types of service aggregations. One measure is tied to each source of categorical funding considered separately; the second adds across the categorical funding to create
total spending and use values for each program area or service. The distinction between the two reflects community efforts to pool and substitute resources. For example, one can tabulate home care expenditures
from only the categorical funding available through Medicaid. This reflects the relative priority given to the service within Medicaid and the
consequence of this priority relative to the other services funded by Medicaid. These data can also be organized by subtotaling the expenditures
by categorical groups (e.g., elderly, Aid to Families with Dependent Children (AFDC), people with disabilities) eligible for Medicaid. Relative priorities for spending may vary by these groups. The alternative set of tabulations would total all sources of funding for home care (e.g., Medicaid,
Social Service Block Grant, state discretionary funds).

Refinements such as these vary in importance from community to
community or state to state, depending on the willingness of those jurisdictions to pool funding and to allocate state and other discretionary
funding to particular programs or services. Very different patterns of
spending are reflected when analyses are limited to specific categorical
funding sources. Home- and community-based care, supportive housing,
mental health services, and special education are among the services most
sensitive to state discretionary funding.

In Table 10.1, we have shown a suggested list of program or service
areas. We have organized this list to parallel the service supply inventory

to give a first approximation of the priorities and tradeoffs in service emphasis by community. This list of services can be further disaggregated if desired, but even in its truncated form, it yields indicators of the relative emphasis given to physicians, hospitals, and other institutional care versus therapeutic programs, education, and social services. The standard of the expected or desired rate of users (or expenditures) versus the observed use is elusive and may have to be community specific for many services. This is because of wide variations in historical practice patterns, available alternatives, and differences in demand across communities and regions of the country. Comparisons with the same community over time or with a normative treatment pattern currently seem to be the most viable approach.

Access and Process of Care

Level two of the proposed indicator framework is organized in terms of subgroups defined by particular diagnoses or health conditions. Alternatively, the subgroups could be recipients of particular procedures, if such information is more readily available. Two broad types of indicators are proposed: *(a)* access to care by the target group and *(b)* the intensity or process of care among recipients. Access and use rates are represented by group means for service units used. The process of care is reflected by the duration (or length of use) and service expenditures. These broad dimensions are organized by a variety of inpatient, outpatient, and other services. Observed rates can be standardized by comparison with the expected number of persons with a particular condition, with those at specified stages of the condition (disaggregated by age, income, racial, or other attributes), or with service users. All such standardizations are affected by the precision of the denominator estimate. In most situations, we anticipate that the denominator values for "risk" or condition prevalence will be synthetically estimated. Depending on the data source, a community delineation of conditions or risk groups may be more readily available by measuring recipients.[6]

The derived annual or annualized rates can be compared with a normative reference rate, with other communities, or with the same community (or another entity such as a health plan) over time. Providers (or communities) with outlier rates, either high or low, could have their specific practices reviewed in follow-up studies. Rates of use per capita or per the at-risk population below a norm would suggest problems with service access. Rates of use exceeding a norm would suggest such potential problems as an unbalanced case mix and inadequate utilization control. Use rates per recipient within a set of related services (up to a norm) would suggest the system's cost efficiency and areas where potential tradeoffs and substitutions may be occurring.

If justified by the number of cases and providers, use and expenditure rates can be tabulated by community, provider, health plan, or other subgroup, allowing the unit of analysis to be more precisely focused. In situations in which treatments or procedures occur infrequently, or when conditions have low incidence rates, it will be appropriate to aggregate cases over several years to calculate a statistically reliable average annual rate for use in comparisons. Table 10.2 provides a listing of commonly suggested dimensions of inpatient and outpatient care (e.g., Weiner et al., 1990), as well as items related to community care programs for those with chronic conditions, as suggested in the background chapters. For several practical reasons, this list illustrates rather than defines the processes of care that operationalize the framework. First, while a minimum national indicator set may eventually emerge, the initial test of utility and practicality is likely to be at the community level. Within any community or system of care, many factors influence tracking priorities, among them trends in level one and level three indicators or other processes thought to be problematic. Another factor involves the consumer for whom the analysis is conducted. A Peer Review Organization (PRO), for example, may have a set of concerns very different from those of the administrators of a health plan. Similarly, a health department may be more concerned with who is gaining access to care, while a health plan or public payer is trying to monitor efficiency.

All levels of decision making are affected by the issue of defining the standards of practice that form the basis for tests, procedures, and other treatments used to define the process of care. The development and refinement of practice standards is an ongoing process. It is our expectation that every delivery system will have its own process for negotiating standards for its providers. A final issue, related to this last point, is data quality and comparability across groups and jurisdictions. Reaching consensus about what can be reliably and appropriately reported across providers and payers takes time and cooperation. This is well illustrated by pilot efforts that tested the efficacy of the HEDIS health plan "report cards" and the Health Care Quality Improvement Program (HCQIP) within Medicare.[7] Such experience suggests that meaningful process and

Table 10.2. Access and Process of Care Indicators

Indicator	Data Aggregation		

Outpatient health care[1]
• Frequency of M.D. visits
• Emergency room visits
• Diagnostic tests and proce-
  dures
• Immunizations
• Therapeutic surgical proce-
  dures
• Tests/procedures for monitor-
  ing treatment/management
• Follow-up care/continuity after
  inpatient stay
• Specialty referral
• Rehabilitation
• Skilled home care
	Diagnosis/condition		Procedure group

Inpatient care[1] • Hospital • Nursing home • Rehabilitation • Other therapeutic setting	Diagnosis/condition		Procedure group

Social and educational services[1]
• Other therapeutic programs
• Paraprofessional home care
• Specialized living arrange-
  ments
• Education/employment train-
  ing
• Other social services
	Age	Gender	Categorical group

Service entry point[2] • Specialty center • Care management programs • Emergency room • Criminal justice system • Homeless shelters	Diagnosis/condition		Procedure group

1. Mean units per capita or per those at risk; expenditures by service recipients.
2. Observed cases as % known cases with condition.

outcome indicators can be identified. Gaining provider and payer assurance that appropriate and reliable data can be compiled for these indicators is much more difficult. It is also apparent that a universal indicator system based on service appropriateness or practice standards will require substantial lead time. Until this is in place, more basic treatment and procedure counts will have to suffice to trigger further study.

For purposes of a community indicator system, the reporting of care processes can be aggregated by each treatment or procedure, rather than grouped by an episode of care. Episode-based tracking is more appropriate for quality assurance tracking and will likely be the most common unit of analysis for individual providers or groups of providers. Developments along these lines are occurring at the micro scale in individual health plans and within Medicare quality assurance programs. One application of the level two indicators in these settings would be to help determine whether such in-depth analyses are needed.

Inpatient and Outpatient Care

Inpatient and outpatient care indicators can be organized and interpreted on several levels. One set of measures includes indicators for access to primary care (e.g., physician visits, emergency room visits, the pattern and amount of specialty care used) and the effectiveness of primary care (e.g., immunizations, diagnostic tests, procedures). Patterns of other service use (e.g., hospital, nursing home, inpatient rehabilitation, other therapeutic settings) could indicate problems in primary care effectiveness. A second set of measures is more directly tied to the processes defining the care received. These can be monitored in terms of tests and procedures for ongoing treatment and condition management, therapeutic surgical procedures, the use of rehabilitation, skilled home care, emergency room use, and hospitalization or other inpatient rates. Each of these various processes is expressed in rates of the service units used and by the expenditures associated with use. These indicators can be differentiated by diagnostic or condition-defined risk groups. Further refinement is possible by stratifying additional subgroups, such as persons receiving ongoing primary or specialty care from specific sources, individuals whose care follows an inpatient stay, and people in nursing homes or other specialized assisted-living situations.

Process-of-care indicators would be used to identify patterns of treatment that are outside the expected range of care. The expected range can be determined from historical patterns in a community or reference to other communities or to some synthetic estimate of use, given the population and condition mix of the population. A focused study into the possible causes of this variation, such as the proportion of these procedures that are inappropriate for a particular subgroup, would then be suggested by outlier rates. The monitoring of clinically determined inappropriate care adds substantially more complexity to the indicator model than we think is necessary. Among other things, analysis of the appropriateness of care has to control for severity or stage of condition and the status of any comorbid conditions. Probably, the unit of analysis must also shift to an episode of care. It is not intended that the proposed indicator system per se identify these relationships.

The tabulation of persons with a specific condition and their access and use of a defined set of services, unlike the system-level indicators, requires data that are directly linked to the individual. The principle sources for such data are service claims and payment systems (such as Medicare and Medicaid) and survey data. Claims data can be structured around beneficiaries, enrollees, or other identifiable target groups (e.g., age, gender, racial groups, payers, health plans, health condition, geographic area). Available clinical information on encounter and payment records sometimes includes the patient's presenting symptoms, diagnoses, type and number of ambulatory encounters, diagnostic tests, surgical and other therapeutic procedures, prescriptions filled, and duration and level of hospitalization or other care.

Population- or user-adjusted rates derived from claims data have been used in a number of analyses of treatment and practice patterns within communities, medical groups, health plans, individual providers, and special groups, such as employees. Beyond concerns about consistency of definition and recording quality, the major criticism of these data systems is that they measure only those who have received care. The use of these measures with a synthetic prevalence or incidence estimate reduces this concern by tying observed access rates to an expected rate.

PROs[8] and others have developed and used a vast number of area-level files (e.g., *Hospital Data by Geographic Area for Aged Medicare Beneficiaries: Selected Procedures and Diagnoses*), which illustrate the many possible tabulations from Medicare claims files. Hospital-based procedures and outcomes of treatment have been measured in terms of hospital stays, readmission, length of stay, and mortality. Processes have been measured in terms of the number of expenditures, per recipient expenditures, length of stay for a variety of common procedures (e.g., coronary bypass, hip and knee replacement, prostatectomy), and the outcomes or complications (e.g., rehospitalization, deaths) presumed to be related to a procedure. Procedure rates and outcomes may also be tabulated by diagnostic categories (e.g., heart disease, cancer, stroke).[9]

These data can be compiled by provider, zip code, county, Metropolitan Statistical Area, and state; and they can be for limited time frames.[10] The main point is that Medicare claims system data can be used for a number of selected and focused analyses, not all of which have to be under way on an ongoing basis. Medicare, as noted earlier, is limited to eligible persons over the age of sixty-five or those with a qualifying disability.[11]

Similar tabulations and analyses are technically possible with Medicaid claims. Although less readily available (and subject to more variation in recipient eligibility and state administrative tenacity), Medicaid provides a potentially useful claims system for that proportion of persons with developmental disabilities, children with chronic illness, and adults with chronic mental illness who are recipients under this program. The substance-abuse population, another chronic-care target group, is more difficult to track through these two claims systems, because their service use may occur in either of these systems, in private insurance, or under indigent care. Working-age adults with chronic (but not disabling) medical conditions will most commonly be identifiable only in private insurance claims.

Monitoring systems limited to Medicare, Medicaid, or both these reimbursement sources are most appropriate for analyses of public-payer program users. These results can be extended to the utilization experiences of a broader public, if the experience of public-program beneficiaries can be accepted as a marker for how well the larger delivery system is working. This is what we propose for the "public health" application of the indicator framework. Health plans, employers, and similar groups using this framework would not have this restriction, because they would be able to direct their monitoring to the data available on their plan members.[12] Claims data, regardless of the population or database, reflect traditional patterns of exclusions and coverage; this limitation can produce a variety of problems in using or interpreting these data. One illustration of the subtlety of these problems is the Current Procedural Terminology (CPT) coding system used in health care. This reasonably standard system is used on bill forms to characterize most services delivered by physicians, laboratories, and other noninstitutional providers. The CPT contains thousands of codes for surgical procedures and diagnostic tests, but only a few codes for nonsurgical and nondiagnostic services (e.g., medical encounters or counseling).[13] This absence of detail for nonsurgical procedures to some extent reflects reimbursement criteria and may affect reporting precision. A second problem is that CPT detail is absent on many encounters. In spite of these problems, CPT codes have been used for some time to assess appropriateness of care (e.g., Brook, Williams & Rolph, 1978; Lohr & Schroeder, 1990).

Another limitation of claims data is that some services, such as preventive services, are minimally covered by insurers, which may produce incentives for care to be documented inaccurately. For example, physicians may document a disease-related diagnosis (even if one does not exist), so that the patient can obtain third-party reimbursement for what would otherwise be an uncovered service (such as a Pap smear). Additional record-system error can occur because administrative records may not contain data on claims and procedures if there is no reimbursement, such as in the case when a deductible has not yet been met or the benefit cap has been exceeded (e.g., Weiner et al., 1990).

Problems such as these suggest that trend lines estimated from claims data may contain systematic error. It may be possible to adjust the "observed" rate estimates to correct for this; however, the rigor needed to test and validate practice and treatment indicators is open to debate about the question of the indicator's purpose. Wide variations in treatment data quality across time or place compromise comparisons, as do variations in the ability to identify patients at risk of the same occurrence. Less rigor may be needed when the indicator is used primarily to trigger a focused in-depth follow-up of potential problem outliers. More rigor would be needed when these measures are used as guides for monitoring and evaluating such outcomes as the quality of care.

Social and Educational Services

Claims systems comparable to those in health care do not exist in education, criminal justice, and the various home and institutional programs so vital to those with chronic conditions and disability. Reimbursement for these latter programs is typically directed to the administrative unit or provider, which then enrolls a caseload. Reimbursement is not usually tied to specific client-based service encounters; consequently, there may not be a client-specific billing claim. To generate client-based data in most communities, it will be necessary to first compile client or recipient lists and then generate encounter data from the provider's case records. Such an effort is technically feasible, but tracking individual clients comprehensively within a single delivery system will require substantial cooperation. Tracking across service systems is even more complex, because of confidentiality considerations and differences in benefit eligibility. The expense associated with this kind of data collection suggests that these efforts be time limited and used only for focused problem monitoring. Surveys of service recipients will in many circumstances be a more efficient and effective means of obtaining use patterns and any service substitution between systems.

Client and caregiver surveys and provider surveys offer the possibility of further refinement, by adding the dimensions of preference and service satisfaction among clients and their support system members (including their ability to make choices and decisions in the course of care) and a consumer's perspective on treatment accessibility and the quality of its coordination. As worthwhile as these data are, their collection is costly and complicated. We suggest that these surveys generally be limited to in-depth studies of selected service systems components, such as case management or other service coordination and intake systems, or to situations that appear to be problematic on the basis of secondary data measures.

Aggregated use and expenditures reports and statistics are usually available from providers. These data are rarely reported specific to conditions, although many providers can potentially compile them in this form. More typical is reporting by categorical eligibility subgroup (e.g., elderly, children, persons with disability; low income; racial minority). Data limitations such as these suggest that the derived access and use indicators function principally as sentinel or trigger criteria.

Distinct sets of social and educational services would be needed to reflect the service access and use rates for each subgroup of chronic conditions. Nonmedical therapeutic programs and paraprofessional home care are illustrative of the nonmedical care available and being used. Additionally, specialized living arrangements may be used as an alternative to home- and community-based informal care or higher care institutions. All segments of the chronic-care population have a subset of members potentially served by alternative living settings. Education, employment training, and other social services illustrate the services that might be directed at specific subgroups to help them become more self-sufficient and achieve other similar self-actualization goals.

Service Entry Point

The determination of benefit eligibility, the development of care plans, the coordination of multidisciplinary care, the authorization of payment for services, and even the recruitment of those needing care are among the functions included in case management. Case, or care, management takes many forms in its staffing, range of cases seen, and intensity and duration of involvement. In some systems (e.g., Medicaid community-based care), for example, a social worker case manager may provide entry into all covered benefits. In many HMOs, the primary care physician (PCP) plays this central intake and coordination role. Whatever the ambiguity of role and scope, this approach to managed care is commonplace in virtually all the chronic care areas that have been examined in this book.

The endorsement and pervasiveness of service coordination has arisen in part to assist families and clients in effectively using and coordinating the range of services being received and in helping reassess care plans as needs change. Another stimulus for this coordination mechanism is the attempt to control cost and direct people into less expensive levels of care if feasible and appropriate.

Tracking care coordination and program entry processes is desirable, and we suggest that it be done indirectly in two ways. The first approach is to identify the entity(ies) responsible for this role in each community. Separate programs or agencies will usually be responsible for the various categorical subgroups within the chronic care population. Counts of the number of clients served by these programs can then be compiled and compared with the estimated number of users to yield an indicator of a program's penetration into its target population. This approach is subject to data comparability problems related to how active cases are defined, how long they are maintained as "active" cases, and the program's ability to differentiate encounters from an unduplicated count of ongoing clients (within and across subgroup systems). It is expected that active cases in a given period will be well below the number of persons defined as "at risk" and hence eligible for this service, should their needs require it.

Although these problems cannot be easily resolved, the use of a complementary approach offers a frame of reference for judging how well the process is doing in reaching those at high risk or in crisis. The second approach monitors the case volume showing up outside "ideal" entry points. For all groups, use of the emergency room is a prime example of a breakdown in care coordination and of crisis avoidance. For chronic substance abusers and people with mental illness, intake into the criminal justice system and into homeless shelters suggests gatekeeper program malfunction. The measures that are already in the framework (e.g., hospitalization, nursing home and institutional placements) may also be possible indicators of problems in care coordination.

Entry into health care settings can generally be tracked and reported with condition- and categorical-level population aggregations. The same level of condition specification will likely be absent in homeless shelters and the criminal justice system, although rough classifications into mental illness or substance abuse may be possible. At this level of monitoring, incidence reporting in the service entry system would not be at a client level. Consequently, the number of persons who appear in both case management caseloads and these other entry points cannot be easily determined. That level of detail could be sought in a more in-depth analysis.

Client and Family Outcomes

Chronic conditions, by definition, are not "cured." Instead, the therapeutic goals are appropriate management, avoidance of complications, and avoidance of secondary conditions. A wide variety of potential operational, use, and performance measures have been suggested or appear in the many systems used to track service use within Medicare and other delivery systems. These measures of clinical health status are often referred to as "outcomes." For purposes of this discussion, we distinguish between clinical outcomes (e.g., functional status, secondary complications), which are included here as level three indicators; processes (e.g., the use of specific services or procedures), included as level two indicators; and appropriateness of care (e.g., compliance with recognized standards of care), which we have generally excluded from the framework. Also included as outcomes are patient- or client-centered goals, including those related to social adjustment and maintenance of family and other support systems. In combination, the clinical and goal outcomes reflect the expert consensus of our contributing authors regarding their appropriateness and salience.

Outcomes and their presumed connection to treatment should not be confused with the "cause and effect" outcomes characterized by a clinical trial or quasi experiment. As with the system-level indicators, our intention is to recommend measures that reflect potential problems with the delivery system. These indicators would then be a basis to trigger more in-depth treatment process monitoring or other special studies.

This limited emphasis on outcomes is influenced by the consensus that is growing among health plans and others trying to develop treatment standards and performance criteria. These groups argue that monitoring systems should be built largely around process and appropriateness measures, which present more actionable information. These measures are preferable to clinical outcomes, many of which have a long lead time and multiple contributing factors. All these factors are particularly true for most chronic conditions. In-depth process analysis can be complex and costly and should be limited to highly targeted issues. The joint consideration of level two process indicators and level three outcomes can help in this targeting.

Our discussion assumes that the community is the level of analysis, but much of it can extend to specific health plans, enrolled populations (e.g., employee groups, individuals under treatment), or other target populations (e.g., groups with a specific diagnosis). Indicator standardization can similarly have several denominators yielding rates tied to the per capita population, the population at risk, and actual users or recipients of care. The interpretation of outcome rates is a work in progress. It is evolving with the development of clinical pathways and other consensual standards of care within the health and human services fields.

This level in our framework, summarized in Table 10.3, extends beyond the aggregate outcomes in level one and organizes data by condition-specific measures of the frequency of acute episodes and rates of secondary complications. Physiological status (e.g., pulmonary function, blood pressure, blood sugar) and functional status (e.g., the ability to perform activities of daily living and instrumental activities of daily living) are used to reflect how well a condition or risk group is being medically managed. Psychological status (including cognitive function, depression, anxiety), social adjustment, and caregiver outcomes indicate treatment outcomes as well as the level of assistance that may be necessary.

Systems-Level Outcomes

We have differentiated health outcomes into two groupings. The first is compiled from claims records, hospital abstracts, and similar secondary sources. Such data, when organized in terms of diagnostic, condition,

Table 10.3. Client and Family Outcomes

Indicator	Data Aggregation	
Systems-level outcomes • Mortality rate • Rates of health conditions or complications secondary to primary problem (e.g., stroke, renal failure) • Average total costs for selected episodes of care	Diagnosis/condition	Procedure group
Health outcomes and satisfaction • Condition-specific physiological measures (e.g., frequency of attacks, pulmonary function) • Functional status (e.g., disability, developmental capacity) • Psychological status • Satisfaction with care • Expressed unmet need for care	Diagnosis/condition	Procedure group
Educational status (by age, gender, race) • Graduation rates • Attendance rates	Diagnosis/condition	Procedure group
Social adjustment (by age, gender, race) • Suicide threats/attempts rate • Violent crime arrest/acts rate • Marriage/divorce rate • Employment • Income • Independent living • Community participation • Homelessness rate	Diagnosis/condition	Procedure group
Family and caregiver outcomes • Parental mental health • Parental physical health • Parental work force participation • Sibling mental health • Familial support • Satisfaction with care • Expressed unmet need for care	Diagnosis/condition	Procedure group

or procedure groups, permit a ready overview of the overall performance of the delivery systems represented in these databases. We refer to these as system outcomes. The second set of outcomes generally requires either chart reviews or self-reported data. These measures are discussed later as health outcomes.

Three basic indicators are proposed, each cross-tabulated by diagnosis/condition and/or procedures. The most general is mortality rate, which is commonly used as an indicator of treatment complications. This measure is refined by the second type of indicator, the annual incidence rate of specific conditions or outcomes within the various target groups. The listing of conditions to be monitored is again illustrative rather than definitive, and it could vary depending on the age group being considered. Using the elderly as one group, rates of stroke or congestive heart failure might be useful markers for how well chronic cardiovascular problems are being managed within the delivery system. Similarly, renal failure might be useful as a marker for the management of diabetes. The types of conditions or complications monitored is ultimately a decision that ties back to practice standards or other criteria. Following the model of the BRFSS, we can imagine a tracking system that includes a nationally determined minimum set of secondary conditions or outcomes that is monitored uniformly and a variable set that is selected by the community.

The third system-level measure is cost. This measure is distinguished from the level two process-level indicators in that it specifies all procedures received during an episode of care, rather than a simple aggregation of costs by procedure. A number of decision rules are necessary to define "episode" and the services or treatments related to this episode. Surgical procedures (e.g., bypass or angioplasty) are usually relatively discrete events, which illustrate one form of episode. The hospital stay and all services received over a specified period (e.g., 1, 3, 6, or 12 months) could, in such cases, define the episode of care. Limiting episodes of care to a defined set of possible complications (e.g., treatment for infections, rehospitalizations, and additional surgery) may refine this process.

Establishing a consensus on episodes-of-care criteria may be time consuming, especially for the more ambiguous episodes associated with ongoing management of chronic conditions. Because of this and data management considerations, we recommend that episodes-of-care monitoring be done only on a highly targeted basis. Monitoring could be triggered by level two indicators showing high rates of service or procedure use or high per recipient expenditures for selected treatments or by level three indicators showing high rates of complications. The feasibility and political willingness to do this may be higher within health plans or with specific providers than across whole programs such as Medicaid or Medicare. The system-level rates can be compared with statewide, regional, or national rates as one basis for determining and interpreting the "normal" levels of performance.

An emphasis on claims-based indicators biases the monitoring toward the richer data sources of Medicare and Medicaid, with the limitations to generalizability discussed previously.[14] In spite of this, we suggest that the initial emphasis on, or basic tracking of, health outcomes be limited to indicators derived from these secondary sources. This recommendation is in part pragmatic, because these are the most accessible data sources; but the conditions tracked here are responsive to the concerns of those with chronic conditions: namely, avoiding complications or conditions secondary to the initial condition.

Health Outcomes and Satisfaction

The background chapters were unanimous in their endorsement of refined measures of outcomes of care. This took several clinical forms, including *(a)* physiological measures that track how well particular conditions are being managed, *(b)* functional status as indicative of the prevention of disability and the maintenance of the ability for self-care, and *(c)* psychological status to ensure that this dimension of well-being was not ignored. Two other client outcomes deemed very important were client satisfaction with care and client expression of unmet needs. These latter two dimensions are thought to represent client impressions of the quality, appropriateness, and accessibility of the care system.

All of these measures require data that are most readily obtained from surveys, either of service recipients or of known program-eligible persons.[15] Clinical outcomes, like the other indicators, would be normalized by use of practice standards or other comparative bases. Normalizing satisfaction data or unmet-need data is more problematic. Satisfaction levels, such as among HMO members or among participants in community program demonstrations, tend to be high. This might be expected, since the dissatisfied may have left the plan or program. Recognizing this, we propose a two-level approach to satisfaction measurement. The first level involves tracking rates of disenrollment (or attendance, in the case of a training program) and the proportion of eligible persons who participate in the program (this often comes from synthetic estimates). Comparatively high rates of disenrollment and low rates of participation could stimulate a survey of participants, disenrollees, or eligible nonparticipants. These surveys could obtain information about client and family treatment and service outcomes; perceptions of the factors affecting service access, use, and satisfaction; and rates of complications and service substitutions.

As in our discussion of surveys, we believe that outcome surveys should be kept to a minimum within any community. Moreover, they should generally be limited to areas identified as potentially problematic by combinations of indicators. Aside from cost savings, this targeting acknowledges that the basic elements in the delivery system are common across the country, even if they are not necessarily delivered with the same intensity or eligibility standards. Periodic national studies of particular program recipients (or those considered to be at risk of becoming program participants) may be a reasonable basis for monitoring the general problems that individuals with particular conditions may be experiencing. Community outcomes surveys would be most appropriate when indicators of access, rates of complications, or per recipient expenditures suggest that particular services and subpopulations are experiencing problems.

In making this recommendation, we recognize at least two assumptions about the data sources and the derived indicators we are relying on to help stage or prioritize these special studies: *(a)* a large enough portion of the "at risk population" is represented in available data to provide a reasonable picture of the experience of these groups and *(b)* the experience of those not receiving Medicare or Medicaid services is comparable to that of those who are. Either or both of these assumptions can be generally tested with national surveys. A third assumption is that public-payer programs should receive first priority in a monitoring system, because it is unlikely that providers are functioning better under public payment than under private insurance. None of these assumptions necessarily applies to monitoring systems set up within health plans or other managed entities.

Once a decision is made to conduct a survey, the additional decision of whom to survey must be resolved. Should it be the recipient population, the larger population at risk, or a sample of providers who report on their clientele? While this decision rests on the "question" being investigated, there are also practical considerations. When the target or "at risk" population can be readily identified, surveys can be conducted directly with the client or caregiver. Some samples are more readily constructed than others. For example, pregnant teenagers, children in special education programs, the elderly or people with disabilities receiving SSI/

SSP or Social Security payments, and those recently discharged from the hospital can be relatively easily identified. Within specific health plans or practices, it may also be possible to identify people with specific diagnoses, such as arthritis. Groups such as chronic substance abusers or persons with chronic mental illness may be more difficult to identify unless they are selected from among service recipients.

We believe that in most circumstances the priority should go to recipient samples, because communities will usually be more likely to reform and refine current programs than to expand them greatly or create wholly new programs. The larger question of who is reached or not reached by current programs and services will usually be addressed more appropriately by national or other multisite studies. Provider surveys (such as a community version of the National Ambulatory Medical Care Survey) or data systems that report many client attributes (such as the nursing home minimum data set) can be useful resources for some client outcome data. Surveys conducted directly with clients have the additional advantage that information can be obtained about the experience of using the service system which is not available through any other means.

Educational Status and Social Adjustment

The background chapters identified a variety of dimensions that define delivery system effectiveness in realms other than health care. Some of these dimensions were introduced in level one as basic system indicators. We refine these indicators by making them specific to chronic conditions and adding other dimensions of the care system. These outcomes include educational status (i.e., attendance rates and attainment), social adjustment (as indicated by arrests and other problems with the criminal justice system, employment, income, independent living, homelessness, marriage rates, and other aspects of community participation), and violent acts (e.g., suicide threats/attempts, commission of violent acts, victim of violent acts). While all these measures can be compiled for the target chronic conditions, they are not necessarily of equal significance for all groups. For example, employment and educational attainment are particularly important indicators for children with disabilities and the population with mental retardation/developmental disabilities (MR/DD). Social adjustment and violence measures are especially meaningful for monitoring treatment effectiveness in such populations as people with chronic mental illness and chronic substance abusers.

These outcomes can be compared with synthetic estimates of use and outcome as one means of evaluating system performance. As with the other indicators, there is no consensus standard to use in determining when rates define something as problematic; at present, this is best done by comparing rates with those in other communities or over time.

A fundamental issue affecting the use of these indicators is that survey data will be required for condition-specific profiles. Outside health care, few secondary systems are organized to generate such cross-tabulations. To the extent that this is true, decision rules must be formulated defining when such in-depth data collection is needed and the appropriate sample frame for the survey. Regarding the first issue, level one indicators of social adjustment may serve as the appropriate trigger for level three measurement, although as we suggested earlier, such studies should usually follow national-level surveys. Similarly, the emphasis of most community surveys should be on recipient samples. Reforming the operation of local programs is generally more manageable than changing the other factors affecting program use or performance.

Family and Caregiver Outcomes

Family and informal caregiver outcomes are commonly measured in clinical practice and in evaluations of programs serving persons with chronic functional and cognitive limitations. This is generally done to ascertain what factors affect the maintenance of informal care and identify any adverse effects on those providing this assistance. Three types of measures are typically compiled: parental or spousal mental health (measured in terms of depression, stress, or burden), parental or spousal physical health (measured by functional capability and health service use), and parental or spousal work force participation (measured in hours of employment). Another type of data is caregiver-reported satisfaction with care or expressed unmet need for care. All these measures are usually obtained from self-reported survey data, perhaps linked to service claims and encounter systems for direct measures of diagnoses and use.

Monitored less commonly, but often of considerable interest, is the effect that caregiving may have on the mental health (e.g., self-esteem, depression) of siblings and other family members and on the stability of the family (e.g., divorce rates). These issues are generally more salient among families caring for persons with MR/DD and children with physical disability, but problems may be experienced by members of any extended informal care system. Outcomes such as these would be monitored most readily through cross-sectional or retrospective survey data. Sample frames for these caregiver and family surveys are generally limited to parents, spouses, or other identified primary caregivers. These sample frames may have to be modified to include all family members, if it is shown that reliable family histories cannot be obtained from a family representative.

For all the reasons discussed earlier in this section, surveys into caregiver issues should be conducted on a targeted basis and usually with similar recipient-based sample frames. In this instance, the primary triggers would be adverse outcomes among clients: high rates of institutionalization, lower than expected access to care, or higher than expected rates of secondary complications. Caregiver surveys are also indicated when a survey of clients is necessary and the caregiver will be reporting on behalf of the client or participating in some manner in the interview.

CONCLUSIONS

Community-level indicator systems have an established role in public health and human services planning. These systems are best represented by vital statistics, surveillance systems, the U.S. Census, and a variety of inventories of service supply and use. Some of these data are compiled and reported annually, others at intervals ranging up to ten years. These data serve to measure changes over time and to provide an empirical basis for planning. In-depth information on the factors contributing to trends has generally required focused studies. National databases are much more pervasive and developed for health care than for conditions related to social and educational needs and are more capable of monitoring use and expenditures for health care than for other human services. Population surveys, which generate much of the information on health status and service use, produce national rather than statewide (much less community-level) estimates. Neither the surveys nor other data sources fully span the variety of health care interventions (e.g., disease and disability prevention, screening, diagnosis, treatment, custodial management, and rehabilitation) or other elements (e.g., education, criminal justice, and social service) that define the complex systems of care for populations affected by chronic conditions.

Our task has been to explore the components of a community-level indicator system that might be useful in filling important gaps in current data systems. Other efforts to build national systems from community-level data systems have shown this to be a multidecade undertaking and one with a high likelihood of eventual collapse or dismemberment. Most successful systems produce information that is useful to state and local governments.

To enhance practicality and reduce cost, we have proposed a staged progression of measurement and data complexity. The first level uses a uniform minimum set of indicators. These indicators could perhaps be used as the basis for a state or national aggregation, but their more immediate uses are to help reveal community variation from national trends and to trigger more in-depth evaluation of community trends. The second and third levels of indicators are focused respectively on the process and outcomes of care among targeted subpopulations, such as those defined by diagnosis or health condition. The trends identified in either level could provide the basis for focused, time-limited studies of program sectors and their interrelationships with other sectors and of the experiences of the target clientele. In combination, such information would be used to determine whether the underlying trends are problematic for the intended clientele or their families and, perhaps, to yield insights into ways to improve operations.

Specific measures have been used to illustrate what we think is an operationally feasible and meaningful community indicator model. Indicators in this framework are chosen because they potentially relate to specific delivery system components or other contextual factors. They are not intended to establish causal relationships. The assumptions underlying any measure or set of measures require careful consideration by those who will use it and or be affected by its output, and very likely, they will not be without controversy. Substantially more debate will undoubtedly arise over how to interpret indicators, once they produce trend data.

Our proposal reflects the consideration of several basic issues discussed previously. We call attention to four of the most important to highlight the assumptions affecting our framework's structure. First, we believe that outcome measures should have some conceptual linkage to appropriate care, but in an indicator system, the ability to actually link the process of care with particular outcomes is unattainable and even unnecessary. Any efforts to make these linkages empirically are left more appropriately to quality assurance systems or experiments. These efforts, moreover, could likely be a focus of a national study or another targeted study rather than be conducted on a community-by-community basis. Second, we have tended to ignore the utility of longitudinal data collected on particular clients, relying instead on trends aggregated by subpopulation and time period. Case-level longitudinal data and studies have been viewed as a consideration only in focused studies.

A third issue is the relative merit of user-based surveys versus claims and other secondary data as the basis for the indicator measurement. While we recognize many problems with secondary data, we have recommended that they receive priority. This in part reflects the widespread availability of these data and the likelihood that some of these systems have other incentives influencing their continuing refinement. It also reflects concern about the cost, quality control, and periodicity of community surveys. Most of the background chapter authors favored consumer surveys as the only likely source of information on satisfaction, fit between preferences and needs, and degree of autonomy that clients and families have in the selection of treatment. From our perspective, these consumer surveys should be conducted on a very targeted basis within a community and only after the secondary indicators reveal substantial potential problems. The basic information on consumer satisfaction and perceptions should generally be gained from national or regional surveys.

The fourth consideration is that public policies and other community attributes form an important context affecting the supply of services, access, and demand. Within a single community, especially when monitored for only a few years, these attributes are largely constant in terms of their demonstrable effect on the community indicators. State and local attributes (e.g., economic base, per capita income, benefit eligibility criteria) take on more importance in extended-time series or in cross-community or cross-state comparisons. Counterbalanced against these effects is the tremendous burden of tracking policy and regulatory changes and the analytic challenge of linking multiple and time-lagged policy effects to particular outcomes. Recognizing this, we have omitted policy domains and regulations from the indicator set. Such measures are most feasibly tracked and used in the context of an analysis that is tied to particular patterns of service access or use rates, rather than in routine monitoring. While the preceding considerations were among the parameters influencing the scope of the indicator framework, another set of considerations arises as we consider implementation. Paramount among these is that justification of a community-level indicator system includes the reasonable expectation that something can be done with the information. This, of course, is not always true.

This book has been written from the perspective that public health departments or a combination of governmental agencies would be expected to oversee the indicator models and act on the trends that emerge. This perspective does not preclude the application of these models by managed care systems, HMOs, employer groups, and provider groups, or the use of such entities as the unit of analysis. Within such systems, access to data may improve, and a more direct incentive exists for the organization to respond to the information generated. We encourage experimentation with multiple auspices and perhaps complementary responsibility between public and private entities.

Regardless of the administrative auspices, how much information can be developed and acted on at any time must be assessed pragmatically. The framework suggested here is organized into an information hierarchy that triggers studies to identify root causes and actionable problems. Studies that are limited in time and scope seem to be the most appropriate for tracking how changes in local conditions, state policy, or other factors may be effecting access, effectiveness, and efficiency in the delivery system.

If focused studies lead to action, is there a way of triggering these focused studies that is less complicated than every community having its own indicator system? Under many circumstances, it may be easier and less costly to have a sample, rather than the universe, of communities within a state. Sample data could be a basis for assessing the direction of change, given trends in the age structure or economic base, shifts in benefits and eligibility for public and private programs, and changes in service technology. Sample communities could be selected to be representative in probability or in predefined contexts (as in service mix, economic resources, cultural mix). All large communities or metropolitan areas could perhaps be included in the sample, with some other stratification used to select the smaller sites.

The use of sample communities has a number of particular advantages, among them that development and maintenance of the information infrastructure can receive support from the whole system (i.e., other communities in the state or nation). The training and staff development related to these systems can be of manageable size. Further, the cost of the data systems and the time needed to get them operational can be minimized. The focused, or target-issue, studies might also be conducted within a subset of sample communities, rather than in each community identified as being problematic. Such an approach is consistent with surveillance systems used for disease and condition reporting in public health and with epidemiologic catchment area studies. A further advantage is that population-based and time-series (such as panel designs) studies are more feasible with a delimited set of communities than with the more general or universal geographic coverage designs.

Community-level program data are currently being compiled by claims systems, by administrative agencies charged with program oversight, and by providers for use in managing their operations. Such data can be a valuable local and national resource, if it is systematically organized. We have proposed a framework for doing this. However, implementation of this (or any) framework, resolution of the basic questions of administrative auspices, negotiation and interpretation of the measures, and the choice of universal versus target-community monitoring are complex technical and political activities. These are best taken on by blue-ribbon committees within organizations such as the Centers for Disease Control and Prevention, the National Center for Health Statistics, or a consortium of entities, including representatives of state and local government. Perhaps too, this process could be folded into the structure, planning, and implementation of the Healthy People 2000 program.

Notes

1. Within managed care systems as they are being implemented today within health maintenance organizations (HMOs) and other health plans, a primary care provider (usually a physician but sometimes a nurse practitioner) is the access point to many services, including those of specialty care. A similar point of coordination does not exist in fee for service. In managed care, the incentives may be to underuse specialty and ancillary services.

2. Prevalence estimates that differentiate the number of persons with particular stages or impairment levels associated with a particular disease or condition (rather than simply estimate the number having the condition) produce a potentially useful refinement in systems monitoring. These estimated rates are a proxy for a population estimate of need and can be compared with measures of service-system encounters to assess how well that system is doing in reaching its target population. This application would be appropriate for a level two indicator and is exemplified by diagnostic screening as a marker for the functioning of the primary system. The stage of a condition during which diagnosis is first made is one indicator for how well primary care is screening for these conditions. Diagnoses in which early detection is associated with a higher cure or control rate (e.g.,

cancer, diabetes, hypertension, cardiovascular problems) are frequently suggested for this purpose. Having an estimate of the expected number of cases at stage one or two, as in this example, provides a reasonable basis for assessing the appropriateness of the number and proportion of cases diagnosed during a given period. Another reason for differentiation within conditions is that the sectors of the delivery system (or the intensity of its use) may vary by stage or severity, such as in the case of arthritis and dementia. Estimated prevalence or incidence with this level of refinement can be compared with the rates of conditions known to particular sectors of the delivery system as a measure of both access to needed care and the adequacy of available supply.

3. An inventory or listing of specific providers, not just a tabulation of providers, can also be useful as a sample frame for periodic surveys of providers. These surveys can monitor such things as the number of programs and their census, types of services provided, referral sources, source of payment for programs, staffing, and financial performance. Among the possibilities would be using samples that supplement national data systems, such as those conducted among physicians and hospitals nationally, or paralleling their design among other community care providers. This particular type of survey is discussed later as an example of a community survey. It is relatively expensive and should be reserved for special studies.

4. For example, hospital bed and services information (including health promotion and rehabilitation programs) can be obtained on a regular basis from the American Hospital Association; listings of Medicare- and Medicaid-certified providers (both institutional and noninstitutional) can be obtained from the Health Care Financing Administration; physician listings are available from the American Medical Association.

5. One difficulty is the negotiation and maintenance of uniform service definitions across time and space. A second problem is variation in the state or local infrastructure for doing this. Populations such as the aged, through the network of area agencies on aging, may be able to do this more readily than any other subpopulations we have considered. In most circumstances, the use of service supply as a measure of the adequacy of the service system will have to be limited to aggregated population rates rather than be refined into subpopulations.

6. Standardized rates could be calculated by dividing the observed values by the population and perhaps multiplying by 1000 to produce a rate measured in use or expenditures per 1000 persons.

7. A variety of useful, yet seemingly simple, indicators were tested under these programs. Within HEDIS, for example, rates of prenatal care and very low birthweight deliveries are being used as indicators of access and outcome, respectively. Rates of cholesterol screening and ambulatory visits among those defined as having cardiovascular risk provide an example of tracking more applicable to the adult population. Outcome measures for this group include procedure rates for cardiac catheterization and cardiac bypass surgery, and hospital admission rates for angina.

8. PROs, operating under contracts from the Health Care Financing Administration's Health Standards and Quality Bureau (HSQB), have the potential

to become major providers of information affecting the aged and people with disabilities (Institute of Medicine, 1990). This is accomplished by collecting information on the outcomes of care for Medicare patients and linking it to data on the patient's clinical care abstracted from medical records. To facilitate this, HSQB commissioned a new abstracting system, the Uniform Clinical Data System, and began its pilot use by PROs. This project serves as a prototype for subsequent PRO activities, but it could eventually produce nationally representative data.

9. Also available on an ongoing basis are Medicare Inpatient Claims and Summary Inpatient Claims by Current DRG and by hospital from the AHA.

10. Among other data sources for such information are the Medicare Hospital Mortality Rate File (HCFA), National Mortality Statistics (National Center for Health Statistics, NCHS), Rehospitalization by Geographic Area for Medicare Beneficiaries: Selected Procedures (HCFA), and the Linked Medicare Use and NCHS Mortality Statistics File (HCFA).

11. Enrollment in managed care, especially in capitated systems (e.g., beneficiaries enrolled in Medicare risk-contract HMOs or under the Medicare Hospice Program), adversely affects the breadth of claims data available in current data systems. Individual Practice Association (IPA) or network-based health plans have much more experience in routinely compiling individual (i.e., case-level) encounter information than HMOs, which operate with a staff model. The IPAs commonly process reimbursement claims for their service encounters, while staff model plans historically have had no reimbursement incentives for such systems.

12. For those covered only by private insurance or health plan membership, it will be necessary to negotiate with the appropriate fiscal intermediary for access to data. Such arrangements have been infrequent historically, but the advent of market-area-based reimbursement formulas makes this more likely. Most health plans are shifting to management information systems that track encounters for total quality improvement purposes (if not billing), but it may be years before these systems are operational and capable of producing reliable encounter information across a full range of conditions.

13. The National Drug Code (NDC), managed by the Food and Drug Administration, is another source of information available on all pharmacy claims. This information can be used to identify the formulation and strength of any drug covered by insurance. No information will be available when coverage does not include drugs (such as in outpatient services).

14. Medicare reflects the experience of a large portion of the aged, except in areas with a high Medicare HMO enrollment, and that portion of the population with disabilities who are qualified for Medicare. Medicaid reflects varying portions of children with disabilities; adults with physical, developmental, or mental disabilities; and medically indigent chronic substance abusers. The proportion of these risk groups served by the Medicaid program is affected in part by the income eligibility standards used within each state. Working-age adults with chronic medical conditions will likely be substantially underrepresented in both data systems. Hospital discharge abstracts can compensate for some of these limitations, but that narrows the outcomes to those associated with hospital use.

15. Chart or case record reviews could be used to obtain some of the clinical data. This may be practical within a health plan or individual program, but for most situations a survey would be more practical.

References

Brook, R. H., Williams, K. N., & Rolph, J. E. 1978. Controlling the use and cost of medical services: The New Mexico Experimental Medical Care Review Organization—A four year study. *Medical Care 16* (suppl.): 1–76.

Institute of Medicine. 1990. *Medicare: A Strategy for Quality Assurance.* Washington, D.C.: National Academy Press.

Lohr, K. N., & Schroeder, S. A. 1990. A strategy for quality assurance in Medicare. *New England Journal of Medicine 332:* 707–12.

Luft, H. S., & Hunt, S. S. 1986. Evaluating individual hospital quality through outcomes statistics. *Journal of the American Medical Association 225:* 2780–84.

Millman, M. (ed.). 1993. *Access to Health Care in America.* Washington, D.C.: National Academy Press.

Roos, L. L., Roos, N. P., & Sharp, S. M. 1987. Monitoring adverse outcomes of surgery using administrative data. *Health Care Financing Review* (annual suppl.): 5–16.

U.S. Public Health Service; U.S. Department of Health and Human Services. 1993. *A Public Health Service Progress Report on Healthy People 2000: Surveillance and Data Systems.* Washington, D.C.: Government Printing Office.

Weiner, J. P., Powe, N. R., Steinwachs, D. M., & Dent, G. 1990. Applying insurance claims data to assess quality of care: A compilation of potential indicators. *Quality Review Bulletin 16:* 424–38.

Wennberg, J. 1987. Use of claims data systems to evaluate health care outcomes. *Journal of the American Medical Association 257:* 933–36.

APPENDIX A / *National Center for Health Statistics (NCHS) Data Sets*

Data Set (Acronym)	Sample	Smallest Geographic Area	Periodicity
1994 Access to Care Survey (ACS)	National follow-up survey drawn from respondents to NHIS; survey to characterize the experience of obtaining medical care and to provide detailed information on the nature of access problems (survey)	Region	1994, first data collection; completed once
Hispanic Health & Nutrition Examination Survey (HHANES)	Cross-sectional study of noninstitutionalized, selected Hispanic subgroups, aged 6 months–74 years; data include prevalence of selected diseases, substance use, body weight, and other health indicators (survey)	County/borough	1982–84, data collection; study completed once
National Ambulatory Medical Care Survey (NAMCS)	Annual survey, data on use of nonfederal, office-based physicians who provide ambulatory medical care services (survey)	Four geographic regions	1973, first data collection; 1992, most recent data available; annual from 1973–81, 1985, & 1989–present
National Health & Nutrition Examination Survey I (NHANES I)	Probability sample of 32,000 U.S. civilian noninstitutionalized population, aged 1–74; established baseline data for NHANES I Epidemiologic Follow-Up Study (survey)	Region	1971–75, data collection; study completed once

Continued

Data Set (Acronym)	Sample	Smallest Geographic Area	Periodicity
National Health & Nutrition Examination Survey II (NHANES II)	Nationwide probability sample of 27,801 civilian noninstitutionalized U.S. population aged 6 months–74 years (survey)	Region	1976–80, data collection; study completed once
National Health & Nutrition Examination Survey III (NHANES III)	Random sample of personally interviewed persons living in households in eighty-one selected counties (survey)	Region	1988–91 (phase I), 1991–94 (phase II); data collected once
NHANES I Epidemiologic Follow-up Study, 1982–84 (NHEFS)	Identify chronic disease risk factors associated with morbidity and mortality; sample drawn from NHANES I respondents aged 25–74 (survey)	Region	1982–84, data collection; study completed once
National Health Interview Survey (NHIS)	Nationwide household interview survey of noninstitutionalized civilians; incidence of acute conditions, hospitalizations, disability days, prevalence of selected chronic conditions, and self-reported health status (survey)	Census region	1969, first data; completed annually
National Hospital Discharge Survey (NHDS)	Nationally representative sample data on patients discharged from nonfederal short-stay (<30 days) and general hospitals (survey)	Census region	1965, first data collection; 1992, most recent data available; completed annually

National Medical Care Utilization & Expenditure Survey (NMCUES)	Data on health, access to and use of medical services, associated charges, payment sources and health insurance coverage for civilian noninstitutionalized population (survey)	National	1980, data collection; study completed once
National Mortality Followback Survey (1986 NMFS)	Representative sample of death certificates (for persons aged 25 and older), next-of-kin informant questionnaires, and facility abstract records (survey)	State	1986, only data collection; completed once
National Mortality Followback Survey (1993 NMFS)	Representative sample of death certificates (for U.S. residents aged 15 and older), next-of-kin informant questionnaires, facility abstract records, and medical examiner reports (survey)	State	1993, first data collection; ongoing data collection
National Nursing Home Survey (NNHS)*	Nationally representative data on characteristics of nursing homes, their services, residents, and staff (survey)	SMSA	1973–74, first data collection; 1985, most recent data available; completed irregularly (1973–74, 1977, 1985, 1995); 1996, nursing home data gathered in NMES/IPC
National Nursing Home Survey Follow-up (NNHSF)	Longitudinal study that follows a cohort of residents and discharged residents from the 1985 NNHS (survey)	Region	1987–90 data collection; study completed once

Continued

Data Set (Acronym)	Sample	Smallest Geographic Area	Periodicity
Vital Statistics Number of Deaths	Data collected from death certificates including residence, age, race, sex, and underlying and multiple causes of death (vital statistics)	State (cities ≥10,000)	1933, first data collection; 1991, most recent data available; annual collection
Supplements to the National Health Interview Survey			
Cancer Risk Factors Supplement	National samples of approximately 49,000 (1987) and 24,500 (1992) households; data include information about diet, screening practices, tobacco use, occupational exposure, cancer survivorship, medical care, and attitudes/knowledge about cancer and diet (survey)	Region	1987, first data collection; 1992, most recent data available; irregular collection
Child Health Supplement	Approximately 17,000 children randomly selected from NHIS respondents; data set includes household composition, child care, behavioral problems, use of health services, chronic disease presence/impact, accidents, injuries, and poisoning (survey)	Region	1981 and 1988, data collection; survey completed twice

Disability Supplement	Three-part survey that screens for disability and includes income and assets; sensory, mobility, and communication impairments; functional limitations by ADLs and IADLs; caregivers; mental health; services and benefits; children; and perception of disability (survey)	Region (some data by SMSA)	1994–95, first data collection; first phase could be available in 11/95; planned for one time including three phases
Health Insurance Supplement	Nationwide household interview survey of noninstitutionalized civilians; includes detailed HMO/health insurance data, job lock, employment information, out-of-pocket expenses, denial of application; 1995 will include managed care programs (survey)	Region	1963, first data available; 1992, most recent data available; biennial data collection as part of the NHIS, and additional surveys irregularly
Health Promotion, Disease Prevention**	One of nine special topics studied in the NHIS (current estimates) in 1991 (survey)	Census region	1991, first data collection
Supplement on Aging	Established baseline data to study changes in functional status and relationship between social and health factors and death (survey)	Region	1984, data collection; study completed once
Longitudinal Study of Aging I (LSOAI)	Longitudinal study to follow up cohort from Supplement on Aging; follow-up interviews done in 1986, 1988, and 1990 (survey)	Region	1986–1990, data collection; study completed once, including four contacts

Continued

Data Set (Acronym)	Sample	Smallest Geographic Area	Periodicity
Longitudinal Study of Aging II (LSOAII)	Baseline data to be established in supplement to NHIS '94; nationally representative sample of approximately 10,000 civilian, noninstitutionalized persons aged 70 and older (survey)	Region	1994, data collection; three follow-up contacts, two years apart, to begin in 1996

Note: The information about these data sets was compiled in 1995 and reflects the availability as known at that time.

* In 1991; National Health Provider Inventory Nursing Homes and Board & Care Homes; looked only at facility information (no individual resident data). Survey will be compiled irregularly.

** Although data are collected annually, not all the same information is collected each year. As of 1994, this study is called "Year 2000 Objectives." The data collection from 1991 serves as baseline data for the Year 2000 Objectives. Other topics included hearing; unintentional injuries; pregnancy and smoking; child health; environmental health; AIDS knowledge and attitudes; income; and drug and alcohol use.

Data Set (Acronym)	Sample	Smallest Geographic Area	Periodicity
Analysis of State Medicaid Program Characteristics	Database contains information on eligibility and provider reimbursement policies, service coverage, administration and finance/demographics, economic, and medical sector characteristics (admin)	State	1982, first data available; collected annually except for 1985
Continuous Medicare History Sample File (CMHS)	5% sample of beneficiaries regardless of use	National	1974, first data available; 1985, most recent data available; collected 1974–85
Medicaid Statistical File*	Data summarized from Form HCFA-2082 including all expenditures; reported by state Medicaid agencies; included are data on the recipients, payments, type of eligibility and service, coinsurance, long-term care, etc. (admin)	State	1987, first data collection; 1993, most recent data available; completed annually
Medicaid Statistical Information System (MSIS)	Data set contains fewer data elements than the Medicaid Tape-to-Tape; however, includes 25–29 states (varies from year to year); data currently in process of being validated for research (admin)	Zip code	1986, first data collection; 1992, most recent data available; collected quarterly

Continued

353

Appendix B/ *(continued)*

Data Set (Acronym)	Sample	Smallest Geographic Area	Periodicity
Medicaid Tape-to-Tape	Pilot project geared toward providing uniform data for research; sample includes data from four to five states (varies by year) (admin)	Zip code	1980, first data collection; 1992, last data collection (project ended)
Medicare Annual: Person Summary File	5% sample of aged and 25% sample of disabled Medicare population (admin)	State	1978, first data collection; 1995, most recent data available; annual data collection
Medicare Automated Data Retrieval System (MADRS)	All Medicare Parts A and B Bill and Payment records (admin)	County	1984, first data collection; 1991, most recent data available; monthly collection
Medicare Beneficiary File System	All Medicare claims (bills and payment records); samples used vary from file to file (admin)	Zip code	1984, first data collection; 1991, most recent data available; monthly collection
Medicare History Sample	5% sample of all Medicare use records; longitudinal study by person including hospital and ECF stays, billing amounts, and utilization data (admin)	County	1974, first data collection; 1995, most recent data available; annual data collection

Data set	Description	Geographic area	Dates
Medicare Hospital Mortality Rate File	Medicare patient mortality by diagnostic categories and hospital/state (admin)	Hospital service area	1986, first data collection; 1991, most recent data available; discontinued
Medicare Provider Analysis & Review (MEDPAR)	100% of Medicare short-stay hospital inpatient billing and medical data classified by DRGs (admin)	County	1983, first data collection; 1995, most recent data available; quarterly collection
National Ambulatory Medical Care Survey (NAMCS)	Annual survey, data on use of nonfederal, office-based physicians who provide ambulatory medical care services (survey)	Four geographic regions	1973, first data collection; 1992, most recent data available; annual from 1973–81, 1985, and 1989–present
Skilled Nursing Facility Medicare Cost Report Minimum Data Set	Costs, statistical, financial, and other information from the Medicare Skilled Nursing Facility cost reports (admin)	Facility	1988, first data collection; 1995, most recent data available; annual collection
Uniform Clinical Data Set (UCDS)	A proposed national database for Medicare's quality review program; data set will include clinical data (1,800 variables per patient), generic quality reviews (random 5% sample of Medicare admissions for problems that are independent of diagnosis), and *disease-specific* reviews of care focused on defined clinical conditions (e.g., management of patients with acute myocardial infarction)	Hospital service area	Scheduled nationwide implementation in 1996

Note: The information about these data sets was compiled in 1995 and reflects the availability as known at that time.

*In some cases, data from selected state Medicaid statistical files are available from the early 1980s; within the state files, the geographic area may be as small as an individual respondent.

APPENDIX C / *Data Sets from Sources Other Than NCHS and HCFA*

Data Set (Acronym) [Sponsor]	Sample	Smallest Geographic Area	Periodicity
Annual Census of Patient Characteristics for State & County Mental Hospital Inpatient Services [NIMH]	Inpatients in all state and county mental health hospitals at end of year (admin)	State	1949, first data collection; 1992, most recent data available; completed annually
Area Resource File (ARF) [Health Resources & Services Administration]	A comprehensive file of all facilities in the U.S. with three or more beds that provide medical, nursing, personal, or custodial care, including health professions, revenues, health status, mortality and natality, health training programs, and socioeconomic and environmental characteristics (admin)	County	1963, first data available; 1992, most recent data available; ongoing collection
Behavioral Risk Factor Surveillance System (BRFSS) [CDC]	State, population-based telephone survey to assess health-related behavioral risk factors associated with the leading causes of premature death and disability; core questions standardized; states can add questions as needed; majority of states have ongoing surveillance effort (survey)	State (county in 1994)	1982, first 24 states collected data (by 1994 all states participating); data availability varies by state

Name	Description	Geographic level	Data collection
Client Data System (CDS) [Office of Applied Studies, SAMHSA]	State-reported data on clients or codependents in drug and/or alcohol programs for which the provider receives government funding (admin)	City	1990, first data collection (some states); 1993, most recent data available; ongoing collection
Client Oriented Data Acquisition Process (CODAP) [NIDA]	Required reporting from facility admission and discharge records including data on legal/nonlegal drugs (admin)	State	1975–81, data collected annually
Community Epidemiology Laboratory (CEL) [Alcohol Research Group]	An area probability sample of a county in Northern California ($N = 3069$) to measure prevalence and epidemiology of alcohol and drug problems in the general population (survey)	County	1989, first data collection; one-time data collection, will be available in 1999
Continuous History Disability Sample (CHDS) [SSA]	20% annual sample of persons filing for SSA benefits	County	1975, first data available; annual collection
Current Population Survey (CPS) [Bureau of the Census]	Multistage clustered sample of civilian noninstitutionalized population; data set includes demographic characteristics and labor force status, including occupation, industry, hours worked, duration of unemployment (survey)	SMSA of 250,000 population and larger	1968, first data collection; 1993, most recent data available; completed monthly
Drug Abuse Treatment Outcome Study (DATOS) [NIDA]	Nationwide, purposeful sample of methadone maintenance, residential treatment, and outpatient drug-free programs; data include client characteristics, drug use patterns, type of and time in treatment and aftercare services; will include a twelve-month follow-up interview (survey)	National (possibly regional)	1991, data collected (baseline); completed once

Continued

Data Set (Acronym) [Sponsor]	Sample	Smallest Geographic Area	Periodicity
Drug Abuse Treatment System Survey (DATSS) [Institute for Social Research, University of Michigan]	National telephone survey (split panel design) of directors and clinical supervisors of drug and drug/alcohol combined treatment programs to examine the relationship of organizational characteristics of programs on treatment practices (survey)	Representative sample of SMSAs	1984, 1988, 1990, 1995 data collection; no data yet available; collected irregularly
Drug Abuse Warning Network (DAWN) [Office of Applied Studies, SAMHSA]	Nonrandom sample of ER and medical examiners to identify drug abuse morbidity and mortality and monitor drug use trends (survey)	SMSAs 1988+; (national before 1988)	1975, first data collection; 1993, most recent data available; ongoing collection
Drug Use Forecasting (DUF) [National Institute of Justice]	Data on drug and alcohol use involvement among arrestees in selected booking facilities throughout the U.S.; study incorporates urine analysis to verify self-reporting (survey)	County	1987, first data collection; 1993, most recent data available; quarterly collection
Epidemiologic Catchment Area (ECA) Program Community Surveys [NIMH]	Complex, multistage, stratified household sample in St. Louis, Mo.; Baltimore, Md.; New Haven, Conn.; Durham, N.C.; and Los Angeles, Calif.; also included respondents from nursing homes, prisons, and mental hospitals (survey)	Census tract	1980, first data collection; 1985, most recent data available; two waves at four of the five sites

Healthcare Cost & Utilization Project (HCUP) [AHCPR]	Approximately 10% sample (phase I and II) and 20% (phase III) of acute care, nonfederal hospitals, including data on hospital characteristics, discharge records, physician characteristics, and population (admin)	Zip code	1970–77 (I), first data collection; 1980–87 (II), most recent data available; 1988–94 (III), next planned data collection
Hispanic Health & Aging Studies–1993 (HHAS) [NIA, NIH]	Longitudinal, epidemiological study of noninstitutionalized Hispanic men and women aged 65 years and older; the study will look at rates of specific diseases/disabilities, factors affecting health status, health care services utilization, and traditional vs. nontraditional support systems; five separate studies in Texas, New Mexico, Colorado, Arizona, and California (survey)	Census tract	Data collection began in 1993; data not yet available; two waves planned, 4–5 years longitudinal
Hospital Owned & Operated Long-Term Care Beds Survey [AHA]	Sample derived from approximately 900 U.S. hospitals that stated on the most recent annual survey that they had long-term care beds (survey)	County	1989, first data available; 1991, most recent data available; irregular collection
Inventory of General Hospital Mental Health Services [AHA]	Survey of approximately 2,000 organizations offering psychiatric services (survey)	County	1969, first data available; 1992, most recent data available; biennial collection
Length of Stay by Diagnosis, Geriatric [Commission on Professional Census Regions & Hospital Activities]	Approximately 25% sample drawn from medical record abstracts sent to CPHA by participating short-term hospitals	National	1967, first data available; 1992, most recent data available; annual collection

Continued

Data Set (Acronym) [Sponsor]	Sample	Smallest Geographic Area	Periodicity
Longitudinal Client Sample Survey of Outpatient Mental Health Programs [NIMH]	Nationwide survey of outpatient services in state, county, private, and nonfederal general hospitals, multiservice mental health centers, and residential treatment centers for disturbed children (survey)	National	1990, data collection; one-time study; data available in 1995
Monitoring the Future [NIDA]	National sample of high school students (grades 8, 10, and 12) on drugs, alcohol, and cigarettes, including prevalence, use, age at start of use, attitudes on drugs and alcohol (survey)	Region	1975, first data collection (1976, follow-up started); 1993, most recent data available; annual collection
National Data Base on Aging [National Association of Area Agencies on Aging]	Voluntary annual survey that collects data on network of state and area agency on aging programs (survey)	Area agency	1981, first data collection; 1984, most recent data available; annual collection
National Disease & Therapeutic Index (NDTI) [IMS America]	Survey sent to panel of approximately 3,000 physicians covering 24 major specialty groups (survey)	Census region	1958, first data available; 1987, most recent data available; monthly collection, rolling six years of data
National Electronic Injury Surveillance System for Occupational Related & Other Injuries [U.S. National Institute for Occupational Safety & Health]	Data from ninety-one hospital ERs nationwide; after 1992, data are on persons younger than 17 years and older than 55; data from 1982 to 1986 include data on all ages from sixty-six hospitals (surveillance)	National	1981, first data available; 1987, most recent data available; ongoing collection

National High School Senior Survey [NIDA]	See "Monitoring the Future"		
National Household Survey on Drug Abuse (NHSDA) [Office of Applied Studies, SAMHSA]	Multistage probability sample surveyed for nonmedical use and abuse of drugs (survey)	Census region	1971, first data collection; 1995, most recent data available; annual collection since 1990
National Longitudinal Alcohol Epidemiologic Survey (NLAES) [NIH]	Representative sample of adults in the U.S.; designed to be a longitudinal public health reporting system to examine epidemiology of alcohol and drug abuse (survey)	State	1992 data first available in 1995; waves II and III dependent on funding
National Longitudinal Survey of Labor Market Experience of Youth (NLSY) [U.S. Department of Labor]	Study of youth cohort (aged 14–21 as of 1/1/79); data include education/training, geographic region of residence, labor market, parental influence, marital/family status, financial characteristics, health problems, and job description; blacks, Hispanics, and lower SES whites are over-sampled (survey)	SMSA	1979, first data collection; 1992, most recent data available; completed annually
National Master Facility Inventory	See Area Resource File		
National Medical Expenditure Survey (NMES) [AHCPR]	National probability sample survey; includes data on health status, use of health care services, sources of payment, employment, income, and demographics (survey)	Region	1977, first data collection (NMCES); 1987, most recent data available; completed irregularly; 1996, next planned data collection

Continued

Data Set (Acronym) [Sponsor]	Sample	Smallest Geographic Area	Periodicity
NMES/Institutional Population Component (IPC) [AHCPR]	National probability sample survey of mental retardation facilities and residents and nursing homes and residents; includes data as above (survey)	Region	1977, first data collection (NMCES); 1987, most recent data available; completed irregularly; 1996, next planned data collection (household and nursing homes only)
National Short Term Hospital Study [National Institute on Alcohol Abuse & Alcoholism, NIAAA]	National sample of ninety-six general hospitals designed to measure the prevalence of alcohol and drug problems among inpatients, health conditions relevant to issues of chronicity, and the impact of abuse/dependence on utilization of hospital resources (survey)	Region	1994, data collection; one-time study
National Electronic Telecommunications Systems for Surveillance (NETSS) [CDC]	Database designed to collect, transmit, analyze, and disseminate weekly and annual reports on notifiable diseases, injuries, and some nonnotifiable diseases (surveillance)	County	Connects all state health departments; allows individual case records to be sent to CDC on ongoing basis
National Treatment Survey	See "Uniform Facility Data Survey"		

Survey [Agency]	Description	Geographic level	Data availability
New Beneficiary Survey (NBS) [SSA]	Interviews with three types of beneficiaries who began receiving SS benefits in 1980–81: retired workers, persons with disabilities, and wife/widow beneficiaries; data include demographics, marital/childbearing history, employment, income/assets, and health (survey)	First wave by SMSA; second wave national	1982, first wave of data collection; 1991, second wave of collection
State Alcohol & Drug Abuse Profile (SADAP) [Office of Applied Studies, SAMHSA]	Survey of state alcohol and drug abuse agencies; includes data on treatment and prevention, funding, and number and characteristics of clients in treatment (survey)	State	1982, first data available; 1992, most recent data available; collection annually
Surveillance, Epidemiology, & End Results (SEER) Program [National Cancer Institute, NIH]	Sample of cancer cases from selected states and metropolitan areas obtained from hospital and lab records, tumor registries, and death certificates; represents approximately 12% of the population (survey)	Census region	1973, first data collection; 1991, most data available; completed annually
Survey of Income & Program Participation (SIPP) [Bureau of the Census]	Census-based, nationally representative sample of noninstitutionalized persons; study designed to measure the economic situation of persons aged 15 and older; survey looks at types of income received, disability, assets, taxes, and labor force status (survey)	County	1983, first data collection; 1991, most recent data available; data collection is ongoing

Continued

Data Set (Acronym) [Sponsor]	Sample	Smallest Geographic Area	Periodicity
Survey of Rehabilitation Hospitals & Programs (SRHP) [AHA]	Monitors the number of inpatient and outpatient programs, their census, types of services, source of payment, staffing, and financial performance (survey)	City	1979, first data collection; 1991, most recent data available; collected irregularly
Uniform Facility Data Survey (UFDS), formerly the National Drug & Alcoholism Treatment Utilization Survey (NDATUS) [Office of Applied Studies, SAMHSA]	Annual survey to assess the extent of all public and private sector treatment providers; data include type of services, client capacity/census, funding and sources, and client demographics (survey)	State	1974, first data on drugs available (added alcohol in 1979); 1992, most recent data available; irregular before 1989, annual since 1989

Note: The information about these data sets was compiled in 1995 and reflects the availability as known at that time.

Name Index

SUBJECT INDEX

Access to Care Survey (ACS), 62n15, 347
access to health care, 6, 13n1, 27, 40–41,
145–46, 313–15, 321–30, 323; chronic
disease and, 169; for elderly, 225; limits
on, 156–57; mental health services, 152;
mental illness and, 249–52; and substance abuse, 286
Accreditation Council on Services for People with Disabilities, 123
Act for the Relief of Sick and Disabled Sea-
men, 17
activities of daily living (ADL), 137, 139,
173–74, 176, 188–89
activity limitations, 1, 139–41
administrative databases, 4, 46–48, 140,
227
Adoption Assistance and Child Welfare Act
(1980), 113
Agency for Health Care Policy and Research (AHCPR), 40, 47, 52, 248
AIDS, 269, 273, 294nn2&3
Albert Einstein College of Medicine, Pediat-
ric Home Care Team, 83
Alcoholics Anonymous, 273, 275, 284
Alcohol Research Group (ARG), 264, 290
Alzheimer's disease, 209–11
American Cancer Society, 62n9
American Congress of Rehabilitation Medi-
cine (ACRM), 145–46
American Diabetes Association, 208
American Hospital Association (AHA), 24,
222, 230n8, 359
American Medical Association (AMA),
22–24, 62n9, 231n9
American Psychiatric Association, Diagnos-
tic and Statistical Manual (DSM), 238,
262–65
American Public Health Association
(APHA), 24, 34, 63n19
American Public Welfare Association, 24

American Statistical Association, 16
Americans with Disabilities Act, 2, 113,
155
Annual Census of Patient Characteristics,
252, 356
area agencies on aging (AAA), 221
Area Resource File, 51–52, 220, 313, 356
arthritis, 69, 170–76, 182–92. *See also*
rheumatoid arthritis
Arthritis Impact Measurement Scales
(AIMS), 185
Assessment Protocol for Excellence in Public Health (APEXPH), 34
Association of State and Territorial Health
Officials, 19–20, 63n19
asthma, 69, 71, 78–80, 87
autism, 99

Baltimore, Maryland, 25
bed-disability rates, 27, 62n14
behavioral dysfunction, 20, 88, 114
Behavioral Risk Factor Surveillance System
(BRFSS), 18, 37–38, 59, 63n22, 128,
290, 315, 333, 356
birth and death registrations, 16–17, 59,
93
blood glucose levels, 207–8
bone fractures, 186–87
Bureau of Economic Research, 62n13
Bureau of Health Professions, 45
Bureau of the Census, 16, 27, 139, 206,
338

Canadian Diabetes Advisory Board, Expert
Committee, 208
cancer, 6–7, 27, 36–37, 79, 141
cardiovascular diseases, 141, 203–4, 222–
23, 268, 333
case management, 3, 119, 121, 242, 245–
46, 306

Supplemental Security Income/State Supplemental Payment (SSI/SSP), 121

Surveillance, Epidemiology, and End Results Program (SEER), 18, 36–37, 363

surveillance and data systems, 31, 32, 316, 338

survey and certification program for quality monitoring, 49

Survey of Income and Program Participation (SIPP), 139–40, 363

Survey of Rehabilitation Hospitals and Programs (SRHP), 221, 364

Task Force on State and Community Data (1993), 37, 48

Technology Assistance Act, 163

Technology-Related Assistance for Individuals with Disabilities Act (1988), 155

total quality management (TQM), 4, 53–55

Toward a Social Report, 18, 27

Traumatic Brain Injury Centers System program, 162

Treatment Outcome Prospective Study (TOPS), 266

Uniform Clinical Data Set (UCDS), 48, 52, 231n11, 355

Uniform Facility Data Survey (UFDS), 280, 291, 364

U.S. Conference of Local Health Officers, 63n19

U.S. Congress: on access to health care, 41; drug abuse report to, 262; on health insurance, 40, 50–51; on mental retardation, 120; quality assurance efforts of, 9; social reporting to, 27

U.S. Marine Service, 17

Utilization and Quality Control Peer Review Organization, 50–52

visual impairment, 7, 141–42

"The Vitality of the American People" (Sydenstricker), 21–22

vital registration system, 18, 20, 59

vital statistics, 338; administration of, 17; death certificate data, 350; and health information, 16–18, 44–45, 193

WHO-WHL Hypertension Management Audit Project, 205

Women, Infants and Children (WIC), Supplemental Food Program, 106–7

World Health Organization (WHO), 17, 23, 29–30, 56, 60